Axel Loewe

Modeling Human Atrial Patho-Electrophysiology from Ion Channels to ECG

Substrates, Pharmacology, Vulnerability, and P-Waves

Vol. 23
Karlsruhe Transactions on Biomedical Engineering

Editor:
Karlsruhe Institute of Technology (KIT)
Institute of Biomedical Engineering

Eine Übersicht aller bisher in dieser Schriftenreihe erschienenen Bände finden Sie am Ende des Buchs.

Modeling Human Atrial Patho-Electrophysiology from Ion Channels to ECG

Substrates, Pharmacology, Vulnerability, and P-Waves

by
Axel Loewe

KIT Scientific Publishing

Dissertation, Karlsruher Institut für Technologie (KIT)
Fakultät für Elektrotechnik und Informationstechnik, 2016
Referenten: Prof. Dr. rer. nat. Olaf Dössel
Prof. Dr. med. Eberhard Scholz

Part of this work was supported by Deutsche Forschungsgemeinschaft (DFG) (grant DFG SE 1758/3-1).
This work was supported by Karlsruhe House of Young Scientists (KHYS).

Impressum

KIT Scientific Publishing

Karlsruher Institut für Technologie (KIT)
KIT Scientific Publishing
Straße am Forum 2
D-76131 Karlsruhe

KIT Scientific Publishing is a registered trademark of Karlsruhe Institute of Technology. Reprint using the book cover is not allowed.

www.ksp.kit.edu

Print on Demand 2016

ISSN 1864-5933
ISBN 978-3-7315-0528-0
DOI 10.5445/KSP/1000054615

Acknowledgments

First, I would like to express my sincere gratitude to Prof. Olaf Dössel for the opportunity to work under his guidance towards this thesis in the stimulating environment at the Institute of Biomedical Engineering at Karlsruhe Institute of Technology (KIT) since June 2013. I am thankful for his unparalleled motivation, confidence, encouragement, and interest in this work, as well as for the generous opportunities regarding professional and educational training. I would also like to thank Prof. Eberhard Scholz for the scientific collaboration, as well as for serving as a thesis committee member and his referee on my thesis.
A particularly big share of my gratitude goes to Gunnar Seemann for valuable scientific discussion, critical feedback on various manuscripts and in particular this thesis, as well as invaluable mentoring in all conceivable ways.
A lot of the studies presented in this thesis were conducted in collaboration with other scientists. In particular, I would like to thank Pyotr Platonov (his enormous responsiveness is remarkable) and Fredrik Holmqvist from Lund in Sweden, Georg Schmidt, Petra Barthel, and Daniel Sinnecker from Munich, Kristin Tøndel from Oslo in Norway, Fathima Fischer and Dierk Thomas from Heidelberg, as well as Armin Luik and Mathias Krause from Karlsruhe. Moreover, I would like to thank Meir Bar-Tal and Biosense Webster for support and discussions regarding the atrial flutter vulnerability project.
I would also like to thank a number of current and former colleagues: Mathias Wilhelms for introducing me to the world of computational cardiac modeling and for contributing to continuity in atrial modeling at IBT, Walther Schulze for familiarizing me with the scientist's life, Yuan Jiang for supporting our work on myocardial ischemia while being on duty all around the world, and Martin Krüger for supplying the cohort of anatomical models and leaving

them in an exceptionally good shape, for promoting the cardiac modeling at IBT in the scientific community, and for his countless contributions despite being out of the field for several years. Furthermore, I would like to thank Tobias Oesterlein for bringing the clinical focus into numerous discussions, Gustavo Lenis for his unparalleled enthusiasm and readiness when it comes to signal processing challenges, Danila Potyagaylo for keeping up the Zen spirit, Thomas Fritz for ensuring an atmosphere of productive chaos and creativity as well as for his services in matters of quality assurance regarding pieces of humorous art, and Manfred Schroll for fighting the everyday hassle of an administrator and providing a supreme IT infrastructure.

Furthermore, I would like to thank all students who contributed to the work described in this thesis through their own theses and research projects, in particular Robin Andlauer, Yannick Lutz, Emanuel Poremba, and Andreas Wachter.

Finally, I want to express my deepest gratitude to my family for their invaluable support along my way and to my future wife Katharina – for just everything.

Contents

Abbreviations

AF	atrial fibrillation
AFlut	atrial flutter
AP	action potential
APD	action potential duration
BB	Bachmann's bundle
BCL	basic cycle length
bpm	beats per minute
BSPM	body surface potential map
cAF	chronic atrial fibrillation
CFAE	complex fractionated atrial electrogram
CS	coronary sinus
CT	crista terminalis
CV	conduction velocity
DF	dominant frequency
DI	diastolic interval
EAS	earliest activated site
ECG	electrocardiogram
ECGI	electrocardiographic imaging
ERP	effective refractory period
GPU	graphics processing unit
HC-PLSR	hierarchical cluster-based partial least squares regression
hERG	human ether-à-go-go-related gene
IAC	interatrial connection

ICB	intercaval bundle
IVC	inferior vena cava
LA	left atrium
LAA	left atrial appendage
LAAb	left atrial abnormality
LAE	left atrial enlargement
LHS	latin hypercube sampling
LIPV	left inferior pulmonary vein
LPC	lower posterior connection
LSPV	left superior pulmonary vein
MDP	maximum diastolic potential
MPC	middle posterior connection
MRI	magnetic resonance imaging
MV	mitral valve
MVR	mitral valve ring
ODE	ordinary differential equation
PCA	principal component analysis
PDE	partial differential equation
PLSR	partial least squares regression
PLT	AP plateau
PM	pectinate muscle
PSO	particle swarm optimization
PTF	P-wave terminal force
PTF-V_1	P-wave terminal force in lead V_1
PV	pulmonary vein
PWD	P-wave duration
RA	right atrium
RAA	right atrial appendage
RIPV	right inferior pulmonary vein
RMSD	root mean square difference
RSPV	right superior pulmonary vein
RTT	round trip time

RVI	reentry vulnerability index
SN	sinus node
SNR	signal to noise ratio
SVC	superior vena cava
TI	triangulation index
TRR	trust-region-reflective
TV	tricuspid valve
TVR	tricuspid valve ring
VCG	vectorcardiogram
VW	vulnerable window
WL	wavelength
WT	wild-type

CHAPTER 1

Introduction

1.1 Motivation

Atrial fibrillation (AF) is the most common sustained arrhythmia in humans [1]. Although not being lethal itself, AF is associated with severe complications, such as cerebral stroke and increased mortality. 25% percent of all strokes are accounted to AF [2]. With more than 8 million people affected in the European Union alone, AF represents a huge socio-economic burden. Besides the higher mortality and impaired quality of life, AF causes estimated costs of $\approx$26 billion € in the European Union [3, 4]. As an age-related arrhythmia, the number of patients is estimated to double within the next decades [4, 5]. Therefore, good therapeutic and preventive strategies are of paramount importance.

Despite considerable research efforts and progress regarding the understanding of mechanisms driving AF, state-of-the-art therapy comprising pharmacological treatment and catheter ablation is not effective in up to 50% of patients in the long run [6, 7]. The development of post-ablational atrial flutter (AFlut) poses a particular problem [8]. Besides further clinical and wet-lab research, computational models of atrial electrophysiology are a promising complement and might serve as a remedy for the AF burden [9, 10].

Mathematical representations of the cardio-vascular system spanning multiple spatio-temporal scales and levels of integration provide means to gain mechanistic insight [9, 11, 12]. Therefore, computational modeling is an emerging and aspiring complementary approach to animal experiments and clinical trials [13]. *In silico* methods have the advantage of yielding quantitative results, of providing a controlled environment allowing to study how changes of certain parameters affect the system, of causing no harm to patients or animals, and of being capable of bridging gaps across levels of integration [14]. The latter is of particular importance considering that a lot of the fundamental changes happen on very low levels of integration: e.g. mutations of genes altering the properties of cardiac ion channels or drug therapies targeting specific binding sites of ion channels. The phenomena of interest, e.g. AF, often happen on the organ level on the other hand. Multi-scale simulations of such effects are often insightful and imperative for a comprehensive assessment because the altered fundamental biophysical properties enter the system in a complex and mostly non-linear way, often resulting in non-intuitive changes on higher levels of integration. Moreover, experimental data are available on very low levels of integration (e.g., ion currents) and very high levels of integration (e.g., the ECG) with missing links on intermediate levels in many cases. Model-based approaches can bridge this gap arising from a lack of data, thus foster our understanding and facilitate the development of tailored therapeutic approaches.

Within the scope of this thesis, computational models of human atrial patho-electrophysiology ranging from the ion channel level up to the electrocardiogram (ECG) on the body surface are developed, advanced, and employed aiming at tailored therapies at different levels of individualization:

- **Mechanism-specific**: Elucidate basic mechanisms, such that the physicians can apply them to a patient's individual situation.
- **Group-specific**: Develop therapeutic approaches that are optimal for a specific sub-population of patients (e.g. specific atrial substrates defined by comorbidities, genetic variations, or disease induced remodeling).
- **Patient-specific**: Optimize a therapy based on a personalized model of the patient.

By employing the models and applying the insight derived from them, both the patients' and the socio-economical burden of AF can hopefully be reduced eventually.

1.2 Aims of the Thesis

The following major challenges are addressed in this thesis:

- Development of a method to integrate measured ion current data into models of cardiac electrophysiology robustly by means of parameter estimation.
- Multi-scale characterization of atrial substrates regarding their arrhythmic potential. Substrates comprise effects of remodeling due to chronic AF and familial AF substrates represented by two mutations of the human ether-à-go-go-related gene (hERG).
- Investigation of the dynamic mode of action of antiarrhythmic agents on pathologic substrates.
  - Comparison of amiodarone and dronedarone under consideration of the atrial substrate, as well as the circadian variation of heart rate and drug concentration.
  - Evaluation of the experimental data base regarding the mode of action of vernakalant.
- Optimization of pharmacotherapy considering the genetic profile of the patient aiming at the prevention and therapy of familial AF.
- Implementation of a mesh-type-agnostic pipeline to augment anatomical models with a priori knowledge regarding myocyte orientation, interatrial connections, and ablation lesions.
- Development of a comprehensive methodology to determine the vulnerability to AFlut considering individual anatomical and electrophysiological properties aiming at an *in silico* evaluation of planned AF ablation patterns to overcome the *learning by burning* paradigm and reduce the incidence of post-ablational AFlut.
- Evaluation of factors influencing P-wave morphology in the body surface ECG.
  - Contribution of the left and the right atrium.
  - Effect of the location of the earliest activated site in the right atrium and the conductive properties of the posterior interatrial connections.
  - Influence of left atrial hypertrophy.

1.3 Structure of the Thesis

Part I outlines the medical fundamentals and the basic principles of computational cardiac electrophysiology.

- **Chapter 2** gives a brief introduction to cardiac anatomy and electrophysiology. The atrial arrhythmias flutter and fibrillation are introduced and state-of-the-art pharmacological and interventional therapeutical approaches are presented.
- **Chapter 3** provides an overview of state-of-the-art techniques regarding computational models of cardiac electrophysiology. The models cover various scales ranging from single ion channels via integrated cell models and excitation propagation in tissue up to the body surface potential level.

Part II presents studies regarding the effect of alterations of cellular electrophysiological properties using *in silico* methods.

- **Chapter 4** presents and evaluates methods to integrate experimental data in mathematical models by reparametrizing the mathematical formulations. In this way, models reflecting gene mutations, the effect of pharmacological agents, or the distinct properties of sub-populations can be obtained.
- **Chapter 5** characterizes different atrial substrates leveraging computational models. Besides two gain-of-function mutations of the human ether-à-go-go-related gene (hERG), a model representing chronic atrial fibrillation induced remodeling is formulated and characterized.
- **Chapter 6** introduces methods to investigate the mode of action of pharmacological agents *in silico*. The compounds amiodarone and dronedarone are characterized regarding their dynamic effects on pathological substrates. Regarding vernakalant, relevant gaps in the experimental data are identified. Finally, hypothetic and existing multi-channel blockers are designed and optimized paving the way for tailored pharmacotherapy of familial atrial fibrillation.

Part III describes a novel method to quantify the vulnerability to atrial flutter in personalized models.

- **Chapter 7** presents methods to augment anatomical models with a priori knowledge regardless of the underlying type of mesh. In this way, information regarding myocyte orientation and interatrial connections can be included in the models. Moreover, methods to introduce standard ablation patterns, as well as user-defined lesions are presented.
- **Chapter 8** presents a pipeline of methods to identify vulnerable paths in the atria along which atrial flutter can be sustained. The novel approach considers the individual anatomy of the patient as well as heterogeneous, anisotropic, and heart rate dependent tissue properties.

Part IV presents three studies elucidating the genesis of the P-wave and determinants of morphology.

- **Chapter 9** quantifies the contribution of the two atria to the P-wave in different leads in a temporally resolved manner.
- **Chapter 10** shows how the location of the earliest activated site and the conductive properties of the posterior interatrial connections affect the P-wave. In particular, the effect of these two contributors on P-wave terminal force in ECG lead V_1 is evaluated.
- **Chapter 11** presents methods to dissect the effects of left atrial hypertrophy and dilation on the P-wave.

Chapter 12 summarizes the findings presented in this thesis.

During the almost three years of research leading to this thesis, I published four journal papers and 13 conference contributions as first author and an additional journal publication is under review. As a co-author, one journal paper and eight conference contributions were published and two papers are under review. Five conference contributions are currently under review. Moreover, I supervised eight student theses that partly form the basis of the work presented here (cf. *List of Publications and Supervised Theses* at the end of this thesis).

PART I

FUNDAMENTALS

CHAPTER 2

Medical Fundamentals

In this chapter, the basic medical fundamentals are presented that are essential to understand the studies presented in Parts II to IV and put them into context. After a brief discussion of atrial anatomy and physiology, cardiac electrophysiology is summarized. Then, the atrial arrhythmias flutter and fibrillation are introduced and state-of-the-art pharmacological and interventional treatments are presented. The interested reader is referred to the cited references for a more in-depth introduction to the different topics.

2.1 Atrial Anatomy and Physiology

The heart is a cone-shaped, hollow muscle and located in the pericardial sac within the thorax. The four-chambered system is anatomically and functionally divided in two halves by the septum. Each half consists of an atrium and a ventricle that are separated by the atrioventricular plane and connected via valves controlling the blood flow (Figure 2.1). While the ventricles fulfill the pumping function of the heart by ejecting blood from the left ventricle into the aorta and from the right ventricle into the pulmonary arteries, the atria are in the focus of this thesis. The atria collect the blood continuously flowing from the veins and entering the heart. In this way, they allow uninterrupted venous blood flow to the heart and prevent circulatory inertia [16]. The right atrium (RA) collects blood from the systemic circuit via the superior vena cava (SVC), the inferior vena cava (IVC), and also the blood perfusing the heart itself from the coronary sinus (CS). The RA ejects and passes blood to the right ventricle via the tricuspid valve (TV). The right ventricle ejects into the pulmonary circuit which leads back to the left atrium (LA) via the lungs where the blood is oxygenated. Blood enters the LA through (normally) four pulmonary veins (PVs) and leaves it via the mitral valve (MV) into the left ventricle. The left ventricle pumps blood out of the heart into the systemic circuit via the aorta. As the systemic circuit leads back to the RA, the circulatory loop is closed.

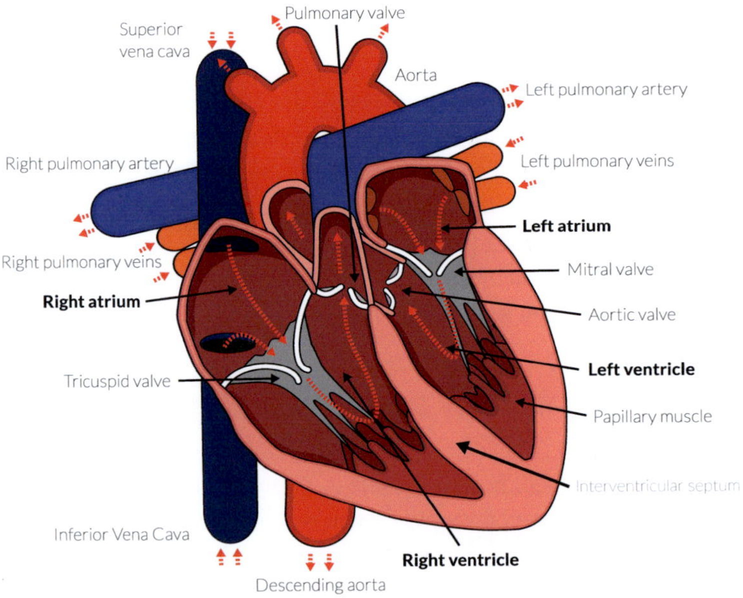

Figure 2.1: The human heart and the great vessels. Blood flow is indicated by dashed red arrows. Reproduced from [15] with permission.

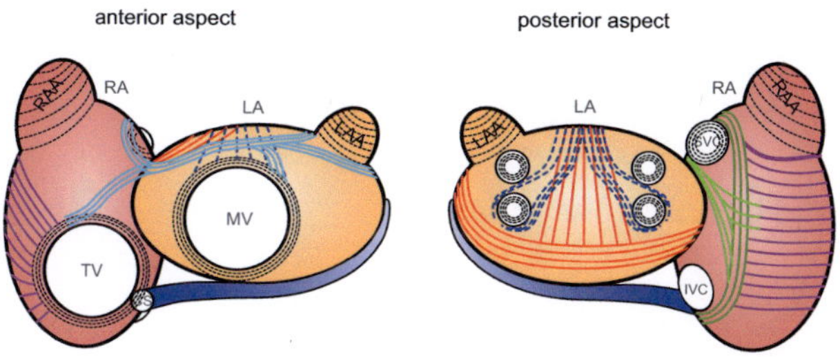

Figure 2.2: Schematic representation of the major muscular bundles in the atria. Blue: septo-atrial bundle in the subendocardium, red: septo-pulmonary bundle in the subepicardium, light blue: BB, green: CT, pink: PMs, black: circular myocyte orientation around the appendages, as well as vessel and valve orifices, blue CS. Reproduced from [23] with permission.

2.1.1 Atrial Anatomy

The atrial anatomy is characterized by prominent muscular bundles, particularly in the RA, and regions with distinct properties (Figure 2.2). The LA is located posteriorly in the thorax with its posterior wall being adjacent to the oesophagus. As the endocardial surface of the LA is smooth [17], it exhibits a simpler structure than the RA. The ear-shaped left atrial appendage (LAA) being located supero-anterior of the left superior pulmonary vein (LSPV) is an exception with its rough endocardial surface [18].
The RA can be divided in four regions: the smooth and the rough parts of the posterior wall, the septum, and the right atrial appendage (RAA). The most important bundles in the RA are the crista terminalis (CT) [19, 20], 15 to 20 pectinate muscles (PMs) [21], the intercaval bundle [22], Bachmann's bundle (BB) [19], and the tricuspid valve ring (TVR). The CT separates the rough free wall from the smooth part and runs on the posterior wall from the right side of the SVC orifice via the right side of the IVC orifice towards the CS region where it smooths out. The width of the CT reduces from the SVC to the IVC [20]. The vestibule supports the leaflets of the TV. The PMs run from the CT along the lateral and anterior wall to the vestibulum. The tent-shaped RAA overlaps the root of the aorta [20].
The atrial wall exhibits a spatially varying thickness ranging from 1 mm to 3 mm. In the RA, the prominent muscular bundles dominate the wall thickness

distribution. In the LA, the wall is thicker on the posterior and the inferior side compared to the roof (2.9±1.3 mm vs. 2.3±1.0 mm) [24, 25]. The existing literature on atrial wall thickness is reviewed in [23].

2.1.1.1 Interatrial Connections

The atria are electrically isolated from the ventricles by a valve plane and isolated from each other by the atrial septum. While both sides of the septum are covered with myocardium, an isolating layer separates the RA from the LA [26, 27]. Interatrial conduction is thus only possible via distinct interatrial connections (IACs). BB is the most prominent IAC with a width of 4.6 mm [28] and is located supero-anteriorly. It extends between the atrial appendages and even encircles them partly after splitting in two branches [19]. The inferior part of BB in the RA connects with the TVR. BB serves as an IAC by bridging the interatrial groove [29, 30]. As the outer surface of the CS is covered with myocardium, it forms an IAC as well [31].
While the IACs formed by BB and the CS are present and conductive in most humans, additional IACs on the anterior and posterior side show significant interindividual variability in terms of presence, location, and conductive properties [26, 32–34]. Particularly the middle and lower IACs on the posterior side that are present in 67% and 87% of the population [23] are vulnerable to conduction block due to their thin and fragile nature and are thus often non-conductive in elderly or diseased subjects [35].

2.1.1.2 Atrial Myocyte Orientation

Atrial myocardial tissue is composed of discrete myocytes. The myocardium forms a functional syncytium because myocytes are electrically coupled to, on average, eleven neighbors via gap junctions [36]. Single myocytes are not spherical but have a shape which roughly corresponds to a prolate spheroid and tend to align along their longest semi-principal axis. As the gap junctions are concentrated at the poles of the cells and because the number of membrane crossing per unit length is lower, the conductivity is higher along the principal axis than perpendicular to it [36].

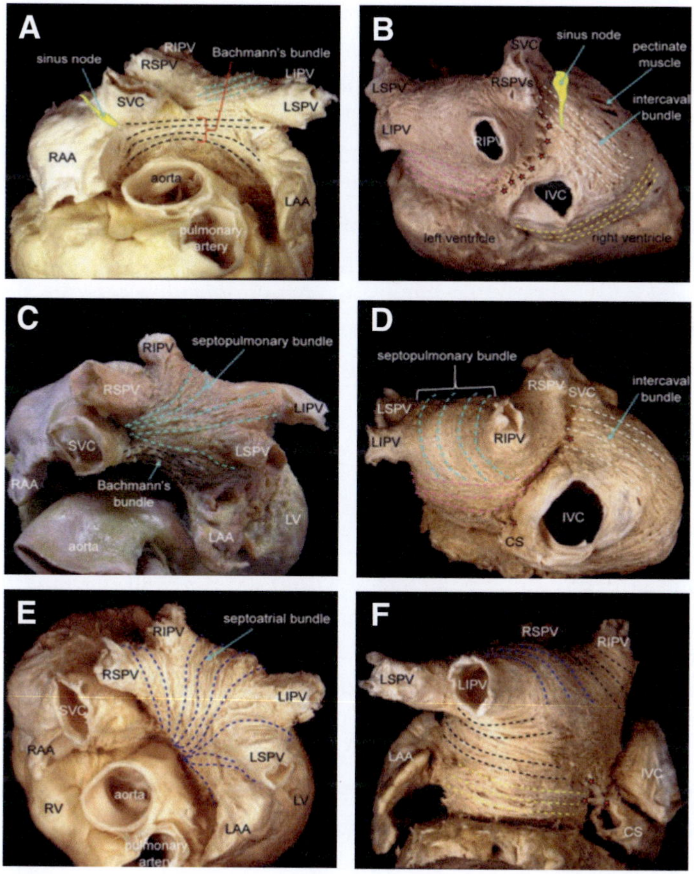

Figure 2.3: Major muscular bundles in the atria indicated by dashed lines overlaid on photographs of hum atrial dissections. Stars indicate bundles bridging the interatrial groove. Reproduced from [23] with permission.

The orientation of myocytes within atrial tissue is not distributed uniformly. The cells are rather aligned along major bundles determining the preferential orientation. These bundles are visible on a macroscopic scale (Figure 2.3) and follow distinct patterns [19, 22, 37, 38].

The most prominent bundles can be found in the RA with myocytes aligned along the CT, PMs, and BB (Figure 2.3A). At the junction of the PMs with

the CT and the TVR, perpendicular orientation can be observed (Figure 2.3B). The tissue between the discrete PMs is aligned similarly. Myocytes are aligned tangentially around the TVR and the SVC [38]. The intercaval bundle is located in the RA between the CT and the septum. The superior part encircles the SVC while the inferior part extends towards the IVC orifice and connects with the CT on the posterior wall [22] (Figure 2.3E). Around the IVC, no preferential orientation can be identified [37].
The LA wall is composed of two layers: the subepicardial and the subendocardial layer with discontinuous myocyte orientation between the layers. The most prominent structures are the septo-pulmonary bundle in the subepicardium (Figure 2.3C+D) and the septo-atrial bundle in the subendocardium (Figure 2.3E+F).

2.1.1.3 Sinus Node

The sinus node (SN) driving the heart under physiological conditions is a complex structure in crescent shape within the RA wall reaching from the SVC orifice downward in the projection of the terminal groove [39]. Its size has been reported to be 29.5 mm in length, 1.8 mm in height, and 6.4 mm in width measure using immunohistochemical methods [40]. Earlier electron microscopy measurements reported 13.5$\pm$2.5 mm in length, 1.2$\pm$0.3 mm in height, and 5.6$\pm$1.4 mm in width [41]. Functional studies indicated significantly bigger surface areas as large as 75 mm $\times$ 15 mm [42]. The location where the excitation of the SN is captured by the RA myocardium is defined as the earliest activated site (EAS) and has been shown to express tremendous interindividual variability. The EAS ranged from the mid-septal region to the junction with the RAA during epicardial mapping studies [42, 43]. Moreover, interindividual variability has been described and is accounted to vagal stimulation, different exit pathways in the SN, and switching between different distinct groups of pacemaker cells [44, 45].

2.1.2 Atrial Electrophysiology

This section introduces the basic concepts governing cardiac electrical activity from the single ion channel via integrated cardiac myocytes, and excitation propagation in tissue up to the body surface electrocardiogram (ECG).
The plasma membrane confines the intracellular space of each myocyte. The membrane itself is built of a phospholipid bilayer and impermeable for ions and most water-soluble molecules. However, dedicated, selectively permeable ion channels, pumps, and transporters are integrated in the membrane allowing for exchange between the intracellular and the extracellular space. The plasma membrane allows to maintain different ion concentrations inside and outside the cell causing a non-zero transmembrane voltage V_m according to the Goldman-Hodgkin-Katz equation [46]:

$$V_m = -\frac{R \cdot T}{F} \ln\left(\frac{P_{K^+} \cdot [K^+]_i + P_{Na^+} \cdot [Na^+]_i + P_{Cl^-} \cdot [Cl^-]_o}{P_{K^+} \cdot [K^+]_o + P_{Na^+} \cdot [Na^+]_o + P_{Cl^-} \cdot [Cl^-]_i}\right), \quad (2.1)$$

with R being the gas constant, T being the absolute temperature, F being Faraday's constant, and P_x being the membrane permeabilites for sodium, potassium, and chloride ions. $[X]_i$ and $[X]_o$ are the respective intracellular and extracellular concentrations. Under resting conditions, V_m accounts to approximately –80 mV in human atrial myocytes.

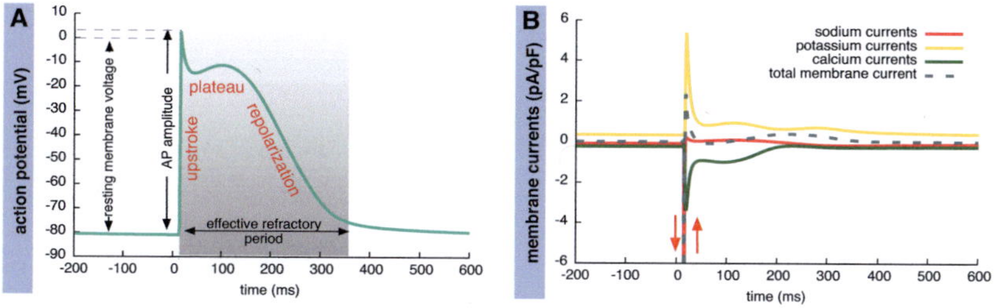

Figure 2.4: The course of the transmembrane voltage V_m during a cardiac action potential with its different phases (A) and the membrane currents carried by the different ions (B). The sodium current reaches an amplitude of ≈–70 pA/pF. The calcium exchange with the sarcoplasmic reticulum is not considered. Courses were computed using the Courtemanche et al. model [47]. Figure inspired by [48].

Ions can flow passively through the membrane along their electro-chemical gradient if ion channels that are permeable for the specific type of ion are open. Ion channels are composed of several subunits with the α-subunit forming the pore, while β, γ, and potential further subunits serve auxiliary functions [49]. Passage through the pore is goverened by gates that open and close depending on V_m, the presence of ligands, temperature, or mechanical force. Voltage-sensitive channels change their conformation depending on V_m. The interested reader is referred to [50] for a detailed review of ion channels in the heart.

V_m can not only be influenced by changes of parameters in Equation (2.1) but also by applying external stimuli. If a stimulus raises V_m above a certain threshold ranging between –50 mV and –60 mV, fast sodium channels open and initiate an action potential (AP) (Figure 2.4A). After this depolarization phase carried by outward I_{Na}, sodium channels inactivate and the AP plateau is entered due to the balance of repolarizing currents carrying K^+ out of the cell and depolarizing currents carrying Ca^{2+} from the sarcoplasmic reticulum into the cytosol (Figure 2.4A+B). After an AP was elicited, the cell is in a refractory state for a certain time. The time before a new AP can be elicited is called the effective refractory period (ERP) and is mainly determined by the state of the inactivation sodium gates. The initial state is restored due to active ion transport by the sodium calcium exchanger (I_{NaCa}), the sodium potassium ATPase (I_{NaK}), and the sarcoplasmic endoplasmic reticulum calcium ATPase ($SERCA$) [51].

As introduced in Section 2.1.1.2, adjacent myocytes are connected via gap junctions and form a functional syncytium. The gap junctions are non-selective connections formed by one connexon in each plasma membrane. In this way, excitation propagates within cardiac tissue once one cell is activated and the current sink formed by the adjacent cells is not too large to be driven by the active cells. The gap junction density and their distribution in combination with the AP upstroke velocity dV_m/dt determines the conduction velocity (CV) in the tissue and its anisotropy.

2.1.2.1 Sinus Rhythm

The cells of the cardiac conduction system do not exhibit a stable resting membrane voltage but depolarize spontaneously. The cells of the SN are the ones that depolarize the fastest and thus drive the cardiac rhythm as the primary pacemaker. In rest, the autorhythmicity rate of the SN is about 60 to 100 beats per minute (bpm).
From the EAS where the RA myocardium captures the excitation originating from the SN, the wave propagates fastest along the CT, BB, and the PMs due to the higher conductivity and pronounced anisotropy within these anatomical structures [42, 52–54]. Earliest LA breakthrough is normally conducted via BB, thus the LA is activated from the supero-anterior side [55]. Physiological CV values are reported to be between 500 mm/s and 1200 mm/s (see [23] for a review of available literature) and tend to exhibit larger variance under pathologic conditions [9]. Anisotropy is commonly assumed as 2:1 to 3:1 for the common myocardium [56–58] and between 4:1 and 12:1 for fast conducting bundles [23, 54, 59].

2.1.2.2 The Electrocardiogram

The spread of the depolarization wave is carried by electrical currents. Sodium influx at the back of the wavefront in combination with capacitive outflow at the front depolarizing adjacent cells causes a positive current in the intracellular domain in direction of wave propagation. The broader repolarization front gives rise to currents from regions that are still active to already repolarized regions in combination with potassium outflow at the waveback leading to a negative current in direction of wave propagation. These currents act as sources for an electrical field reaching to the body surface. Thus, the electrical activity in the heart can be measured on a macroscopic scale by evaluating the potential differences on the body surface in the ECG. The depolarization of the atria is reflected in the P-wave of the ECG. The interested reader is referred to [60] for a detailed description of the genesis of the body surface potentials. Routinely, a 12 lead ECG is recorded using nine electrodes. The three Einthoven leads I, II, and III are defined as the bipolar signals between the extremities. For the unipolar Goldberger leads aVR, aVL, and aVF, the mean

of the two other limb leads is used as a reference signal. The Wilson leads on the chest are measured with respect to Wilson's central terminal defined as the mean of the three limb leads I, II, and III.
The vectorcardiogram (VCG) is the projection of the field integral vector on the frontal, sagittal and transversal plane. The VCG can be estimated from a subset $\mathbf{S_{ECG}}$ of the 12 lead ECG (V_1-V_6, I, II) using the inverse Dower matrix **D** [61]:

$$\hat{\mathbf{S}}_{\mathbf{VCG}} = \mathbf{D}\,\mathbf{S_{ECG}}\,, \tag{2.2}$$

with

$$\mathbf{D} = \begin{pmatrix} -0.172 & -0.074 & 0.122 & 0.231 & 0.239 & 0.194 & 0.156 & -0.010 \\ 0.057 & -0.019 & -0.106 & -0.022 & 0.041 & 0.048 & -0.227 & 0.887 \\ -0.229 & -0.310 & -0.246 & -0.063 & 0.055 & 0.108 & 0.022 & 0.102 \end{pmatrix}. \tag{2.3}$$

2.2 Atrial Flutter

Atrial Flutter (AFlut) is a supraventricular tachycardia with a consistent excitation pattern. It is perpetuated around a large central obstacle, which can be an anatomical structure, unexcitable scar tissue, or a functional line of block [62]. The cycle length is between 250 ms and 135 ms [63]. As this fast rhythm can not be sustained by the ventricles, 2:1 or 3:1 conduction block at the AV node is frequently observed. AFlut is categorized in two major types: *typical AFlut* (also termed *type I*) and *atypical AFlut* (*type II*).
Typical AFlut is maintained in the RA by mostly counterclockwise reentry around the TV annulus (Figure 2.5A). The CT acts as a conduction barrier due to the slow transversal conduction. The floor of the RA between the inferior TV annulus and the IVC forms the critical isthmus for this type of reentry (*cavotricuspid isthmus*) [64]. In $\approx$15% of the cases, the excitation rotates in a clockwise direction [62].

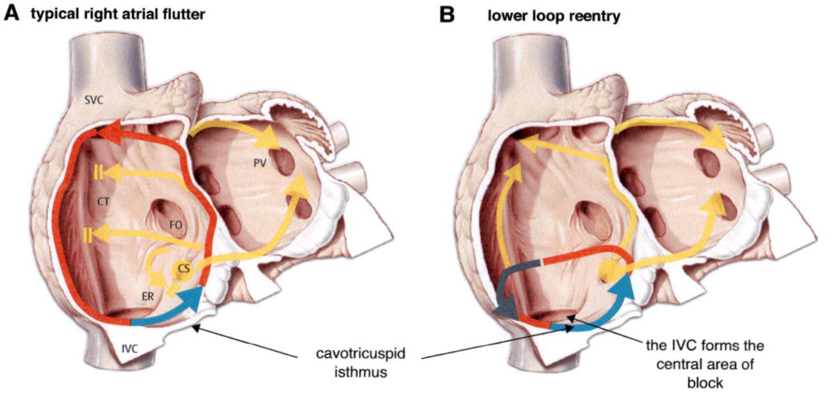

Figure 2.5: Paths maintaining AFlut in the RA (red arrows). Flutter is sustained along the TV annulus in typical flutter (A). Both atrioventricular annuli have been removed for clearer visualization. The blue arrow indicates the cavotricuspid isthmus representing the crucial narrowest part in typical AFlut (A) and lower loop reentry (B). Yellow arrows indicate pathways activating the atrial myocardium but not driving the flutter. The dark gray arrow in (B) indicates a zone of slow conduction allowing to sustain the flutter along the shorter circuit compared to (A) where the CT forms a line of functional block in transverse direction. Reproduced from [62] with permission from the publisher.

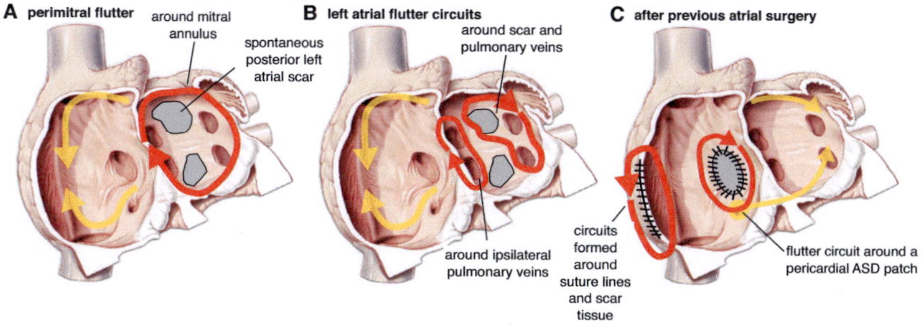

Figure 2.6: Atypical flutter circuits. Red arrows indicate the driving circuit whereas the remaining myocardium is activated via pathways indicated by yellow arrows. Gray areas indicate non-excitable scar tissue. Perimitral flutter is sustained around the MV annulus (A), whereas the flutter circuits in (B) and (C) anchor around smaller obstacles formed by the PVs, scar tissue, surgical suture lines, or patches covering atrial septal defects (ASD). Reproduced from [62] with permission from the publisher.

Atypical AFlut develops often after corrective atrial surgery (congenital and valvular heart disease) and atrial fibrillation (AF) ablation [8, 65–68] with the driving reentry circuit determined by the lesions (Figure 2.6C). However, it can also occur without previous surgery driven by various reentry circuits. The dominant paths in the RA include the lateral wall (*free wall flutter*), and the IVC (*lower loop reentry*, Figure 2.5B). In the LA, AFlut is mostly observed in patients with enlarged atria [69]. Areas of fibrotic tissue, e.g. induced by chronic dilation, serve as stabilizers of the reentry due to the slowed conduction. Driving circuits are found around the MV (*perimitral flutter*, Figure 2.6A) or the PVs (Figure 2.6B).
The incidence of AFlut in the general population is 88/100,000 person-years and significantly higher for elderly (587/100,000 person-years in subjects older than 80 years) [70]. AFlut is associated with a significantly increased risk for stroke and other negative events with a comparable risk scenario as AF [1], which is described in more detail below. AFlut can be approached with antiarrhythmic drugs. However, pharmacological therapy is often ineffective and more than half of the patients are treated with rate-control strategies due to the failure to maintain sinus rhythm [71]. Catheter ablation (see Section 7.3) is recommended for patients with a first episode of typical AFlut and for flutter appearing after antiarrhythmic treatment of AF [62].

2.3 Atrial Fibrillation

AF is the most common sustained arrhythmia affecting over 8 million people in the European Union [72]. It is characterized by irregular and rapid excitation patterns with frequencies above 300 bpm [1] caused by the interplay of a vulnerable substrate and at least one initiating trigger. AF has a prevalance of 2% to 3% of the general population [73] and is associated with a significantly higher mortality and five-fold increase of the risk of stroke [72] accounting for 25% of all strokes in the general population [2]. Moreover, AF impairs LV function severely even though the AV node prevents the tachyarrhythmia from affecting the ventricles directly [74, 75]. As AF prevalence increases with age, the number of patients is estimated to double within the next decades due to demographic change [5].

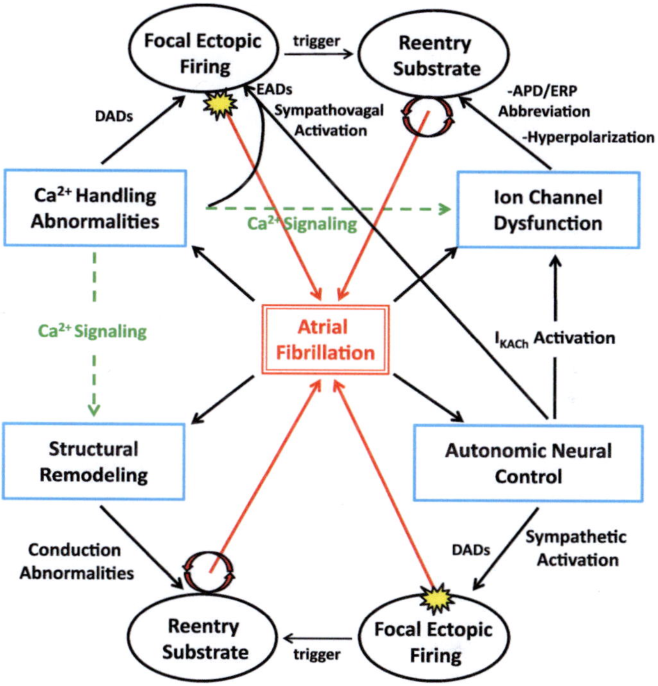

Figure 2.7: Mechanisms contributing to the initiation and perpetuation of AF by affecting the arrhythmia-initiating trigger and the arrhythmia-sustaining substrate. Abbreviations: delayed afterdepolarization (DAD), early afterdepolarization (EAD), action potential duration (APD), effective refractory phase (ERP). Reproduced from [76] with permission from the publisher.

AF is a progressive disease typically starting with short silent paroxysms translating to symptomatic and longer episodes of AF [1, 77]. Clinically, AF is categorized as paroxysmal if episodes are self-terminating within a maximum of 7 days (typically within 48 hours). Persistent AF does not terminate within 7 days without pharmaceutical or electrical cardioversion. AF is categorized as long-lasting persistent if it lasts longer than one year. If no rhythm control strategy is pursued but only the rate is controlled, the term permanent AF is used [1].

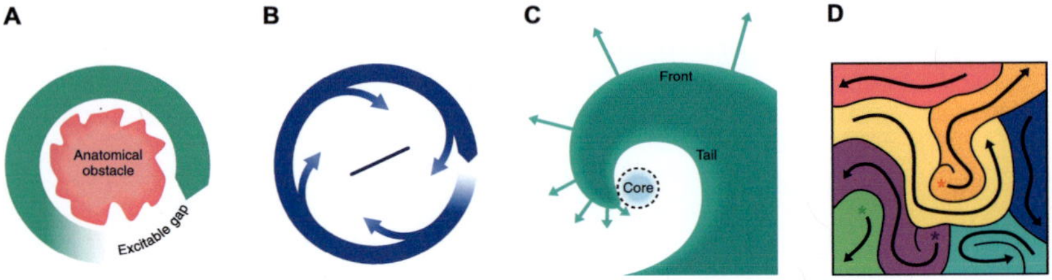

Figure 2.8: Reentry mechanisms: circus movement reentry (A), leading circle concept (B), spiral wave reentry (C), and multiple wavelet hypothesis (D). Reproduced from [77] with permission from the publisher.

The mechanisms initiating and perpetuating AF are far from being understood completely. Despite considerable research efforts, the role of calcium handling, atrial fibrosis, and the drivers of AF are under discussion [76, 78] (Figure 2.7). Regarding the triggers, enhanced and abnormal autorhythmicity particularly in the myocardial sleeves of the PVs are a known contributor [79]. Moreover, triggered activity (early and delayed afterdepolarizations) can elicit excitation [80–82]. Several concepts regarding the perpetuation of fibrillatory activity in the atria (partly complementary, partly contradicting) are being discussed [77, 78, 83].

Reentry around an anatomical obstacle is called *circus movement reentry* (Figure 2.8). A necessary condition is that the wavefront always has some excitable tissue ahead of it. Thus, the waveback has to have regained excitability after the ERP. Hence, low CV and short ERP favor this kind of reentry by widening the excitable gap for a given reentry path. The *leading circle concept* does not require a clearly defined anatomical obstacle. Rather, reentry is sustained around a non-activated center, which shows electrotonic depolarizations, such as a functional line of block (Figure 2.8B). Circus movement reentry and the reentry according to the leading circle concepts are also observed during atrial flutter.

The concept of *spiral wave reentry* was inspired by chemical reactions in excitable media [84]. Today, the term *rotor* is used as well for this kind of functional reentrant activity (Figure 2.8C). While the cells in the core of the rotor are excitable in general, the CV is dramatically reduced from the tip towards the core due to the increasing source-sink imbalance eventually causing conduction block. Reentry can therefore be sustained around the

core. While rotors were observed in human AF during electroanatomical mapping [85], several experimental studies reported multiple unstable excitation patterns supporting the *multiple wavelet hypothesis* (Figure 2.8D) [86–88]. If several fibrillation waves are present and meander through the tissue, continuous wavefront-wavetail interactions cause the generation and termination of wavefronts winding up in a self-sustaining, chaotic pattern [89]. While additional fibrillation waves emerge due to wavebreak, others cease due to block, collision, or fusion of wavefronts.
Dissociation between the endocardial and the epicardial layer and breakthrough from one layer into the other contributes to this phenomenon, as well [90–92]. Short ERP, pronounced heterogeneity of refractoriness, slow CV, and a large substrate favor multiple wavelet reentry [77].
Current state-of-the-art therapies for AF include antiarrhythmic drug therapy (see Section 2.4) and substrate modification by catheter ablation (see Section 2.5).

2.3.1 Remodeling

The rapid excitation rate during AF drives several long-term adaptation mechanisms in the cardiovascular system [93–95]. While these mechanisms partly prevent intracellular Ca^{2+} overload [96 ,97] and allow to minimize the metabolic cost [98], they also promote the perpetuation of the reentry. This so-called *remodeling* process contributes to the progressive nature of AF and coined the term *AF begets AF* [99]. Figure 2.9 summarizes the four main positive-feedback loops driving AF-induced remodeling. In the scope of this thesis, electrical remodeling and structural remodeling (to a lesser extent, though) are in the focus.

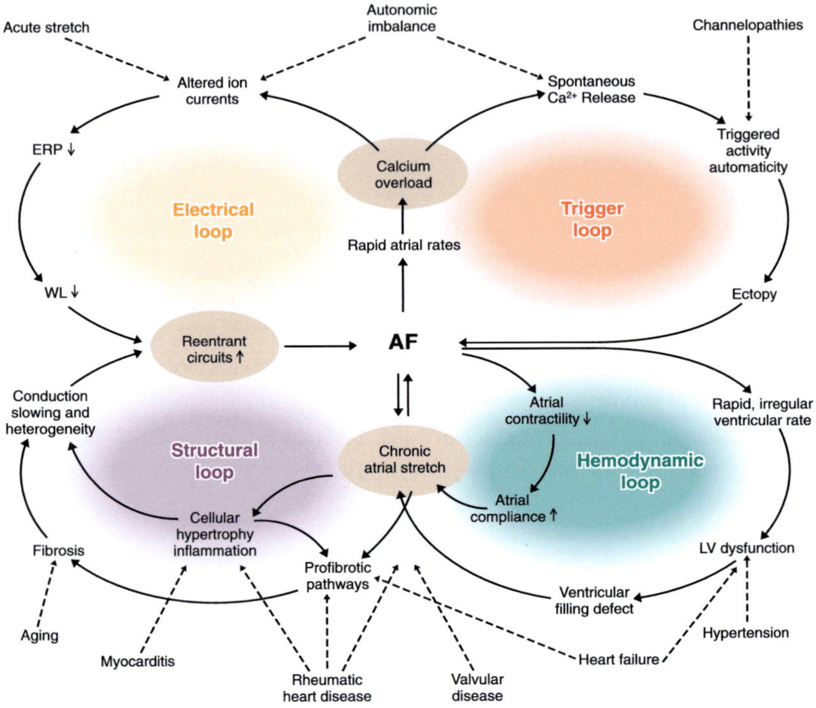

Figure 2.9: Overview of the main driving forces of AF and AF-induced remodeling. Four positive-feedback loops cause the remodeling process. Reproduced from [77] with permission from the publisher.

Electrophysiologically, the main effects are a reduction of $I_{Ca,L}$, I_{to}, and I_{Kur}, as well as an increase of I_{K1}, $I_{K,ACh}$, and I_{Ks} [77]. Table 2.1 gives an overview of experimental data regarding functional reduction and changes in mRNA levels obtained in humans. mRNA levels serve as a surrogate measure for the conductivity but do not allow to draw quantitative conclusions regarding functionality as protein expression and trafficking can be affected as well. No functional data from humans were available for I_{Kr}. However, measurements in dogs revealed no change in maximum conductivity [100, 101]. In combination, the changes of ion channel conductivities lead to a shortening of the ERP.

Table 2.1: Altered maximum conductivity values and mRNA levels due to cAF induced remodeling in humans. Values given are relative changes of measured current amplitudes. Tissue samples were taken from either left (L) or right (R) human atrial appendages (hAA) or unspecified human atrial tissue including the free walls.

Current	Tissue	Change
I_{K1}	hRAA	± 0% [102], + 75% [103], + 75% [104], + 83% [105], + 91% [106], + 100% [107], + 105% [108], + 137% [109]
	hLAA	+ 106% [102]
$I_{Ca,L}$	hRAA	- 73% [108], - 73% [110], -50% [111], - 43% [112], - 42% [113]
	hAA	- 63% [103]
I_{to}	hRAA	- 84% [114], - 83% [108], - 67% [115], - 66% [102], - 65% [103], - 45% [116], - 44% [117]
	hLAA	- 74% [116], - 61% [102]
I_{Kr}	human atria	- 27% mRNA [118]
	hAA	- 34% mRNA [119]
	hRAA	- 30% mRNA [120], ± 0% mRNA [121]
I_{Kur}	hRAA	- 55% [117], - 50% [115], - 25% to - 50% [108], - 25% to - 50% [114], ± 0% [103]
	hLAA	- 53% [102], - 43% [116]
I_{Ks}	hRAA	+ 150% [116], + 56% mRNA [121]
	hLAA	+ 80% [116]
	human atria	- 30% mRNA [118]
I_{Na}	hRAA	± 0% [108]
I_{NaCa}	hRAA	+ 60% [113], + 85% [112], + 43% mRNA [122], + 67% mRNA [123]
I_{leak}	hRAA	+ 50% [113], + 280% [122]
I_{NaK}	hRAA	± 0% [124]

The reported increase of cell capacitance ranged from +5% to +71% [102, 104, 106, 108–111, 114–116, 125]. On the structural level, the increase of interstitial fibrosis [77] and potentially altered connexin connections [126] cause a reduction of CV macroscopically. Through the reduction of the CV and the ERP, the wavelength (WL) as the product of the two measures is affected quadratically. The interested reader is referred to [127] for a detailed literature review of remodeling of ion currents (also concerning gating kinetics), cell capacitance, and connexin expression.

As the different stages of AF are not completely selective and experimental data regarding the remodeling effects of the distinct stages are sparse, the remodeling due to persistent, long-standing persistent, and permanent AF is subsumed as *chronic atrial fibrillation (cAF)* induced remodeling in the remainder of this thesis.

2.4 Atrial Antiarrhythmic Drugs

2.4.1 Amiodarone

Amiodarone is an antiarrhythmic agent classified as class III according to the Vaughan Williams classification [128] due to its pronounced effect on outward potassium currents. However, it exhibits inhibitory effects on other cardiac ion currents, such as I_{Na}, or $I_{Ca,L}$, as well [129]. Thus, it has to be considered a multi-channel blocker. Amiodarone has been used for the treatment of ventricular and supraventricular tachycardia for over 50 years and is still one of the recommended agents for pharmacological AF cardioversion, as well as rate and rhythm control in current guidelines [1, 72, 130].
While exhibiting a high anti-arrhythmic efficacy, amiodarone is associated with several side effects, such as corneal micro-deposits, thyroid dysfunction, and bradycardia [131, 132]. The interested reader is referred to e.g. [133, 134] for a more in-depth description of amiodarone.

2.4.2 Dronedarone

Dronedarone is a benzofuran derivative, structurally related to amiodarone and was designed as a less thyrotoxic alternative to amiodarone [135]. Towards this end, iodine was removed and the lipophilicity was reduced. It has been introduced to the market in 2009 [135]. Despite being classified as class III, it is as well a multi-channel blocker that inhibits sodium, potassium, and calcium channels. Besides certain differences in the inhibitory effects on ion channels, both drugs differ markedly in their pharmacokinetic properties: Amiodarone has a biological half-life of several weeks, caused mainly by accumulation

in a third compartment due to its lipophilic properties [136]. In contrast, dronedarone is less lipophilic and has a much shorter biological half-life of 24 h [136].
Regarding the maintenance of sinus rhythm after AF, dronedarone has proven to be superior to placebo but inferior to amiodarone [72]. In patients with longer lasting AF, dronedarone is not recommended according to current guidelines. However, it is the favorable antiarrhythmic drug for patients with certain structural heart diseases, such as left ventricular hypertrophy in combination with hypertensive heart disease [72]. The interested reader is referred to e.g. [137–139] for more detailed information on dronedarone.

2.4.3 Vernakalant

Vernakalant is a relatively new antiarrhythmic agent and was approved in Europe in 2010 [140]. Because of its effect on cardiac potassium and sodium channels, it is classified as class III and class I according to the Vaughan Williams classification [128]. Due to the pronounced inhibition of the atria-selective I_{Kur}, vernakalant acts preferentially in the atria and is thus less likely to cause ventricular torsade de pointes arrhythmia due to prolonged repolarazi-ation [72].
It proved to be superior to placebo and more effective than amiodarone regarding the conversion of recent onset AF. Patients were 8.4× more likely to convert to sinus rhythm within 90 minutes after intravenous infusion of vernakalant than after infusion of amiodarone or a placebo without increased risk of severe adverse events [141]. AF after cardiac surgery was converted in 47% of patients using vernakalant compared to 14% converting spontaneously [142]. However, vernakalant was ineffective in converting AF of more than 7 days duration and typical atrial flutter in several studies [143–145]. Vernakalant has an elimination half-life of 3 to 5 hours [72]. The interested reader is referred to [72, 146] for more information regarding vernakalant.

2.5 Ablation Therapy

In patients with recurrent AF that are resistant to antiarrhythmic drugs, catheter ablation of atrial tissue is the recommended therapy [1]. Tissue is rendered non-excitable by heating the tissue via radio-frequency currents (*RF ablation*) or cooling it (*cryo ablation*) with comparable success rates [147].
As in the majority of patients, focal discharges from the PVs trigger AF or at least contribute to the initiation, PV isolation is the standard approach since the seminal work of Haïssaguerre et al. almost 20 years ago [79]. Many paroxysmal AF patients maintain sinus rhythm and are free from arrhythmic episodes after PV isolation. The AF recurrence rate is up to 60% in patients with persistent and long-standing persistent AF [6] and was recently reported to be 45% within one year in 2306 paroxysmal AF patients in Germany [7]. Therefore, several other strategies aiming at a modification of the atrial substrate have been proposed [148]: isolation of the LA posterior wall, ablation of sites exhibiting complex fractionated atrial electrograms (CFAEs) or signals of low voltage, ablation of ganglionated plexuses where the adrenergic fibers from the central nervous system end, ablation of sites exhibiting a high dominant frequency, as well as most recently ablation of rotors identified through panoramic mapping or non-invasive electrocardiographic imaging (ECGI). However, the success rates of PV isolation in persistent AF patients could not be increased by additional CFAE ablation as well as linear lesions in a big randomized multi-center study [149]. Therefore, a controversial discussion regarding the optimal strategy in different patient population is ongoing and was fueled by recently reported remarkable success rates of rotor ablation that remain to be reproduced [150, 151].
The interested reader is referred to e.g. [148] for a review of current ablation strategies.

CHAPTER 3

Computational Cardiac Modeling

In this chapter, the basic concepts of computational models of cardiac electrophysiology are introduced. The mathematical formulations range from the single ion channel level via integrated cell models and excitation propagation in tissue up to the electric fields on the whole body scale.

3.1 Electrophysiological Modeling

Hodgkin and Huxley were the first to describe ionic membrane currents by a mathematical model in their seminal work from 1952 [152]. They represented the membrane of giant squid axons by an equivalent electric circuit (Figure 3.1).

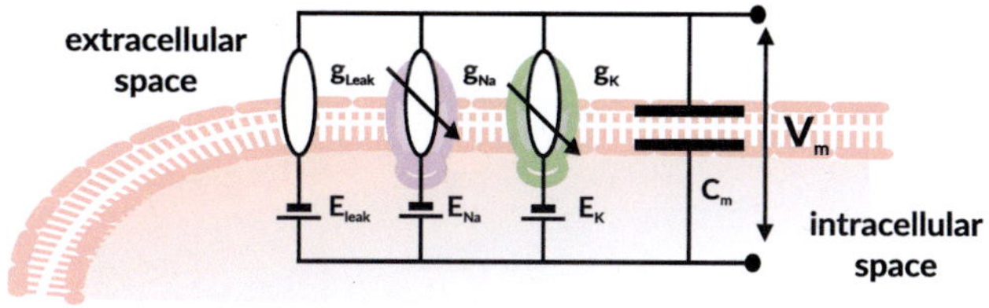

Figure 3.1: Equivalent electric circuit of a giant squid axon according to Hodgkin and Huxley [152]. Under physiological conditions, the Nernst potential for potassium is negative whereas those for sodium and leak are positive. Adapted from [15] with permission.

The transmembrane voltage V_m is defined as the difference between the intracellular potential Φ_i and the extracellular potential Φ_e. The cell membrane is represented by a capacitor and the different ion channels by variable resistors in line with the respective Nernst voltages E_X represented by voltage sources. Thus, the membrane current is given as the sum of the ionic currents plus the capacitive current resulting in the following ordinary differential equation (ODE) for V_m:

$$\frac{dV_m}{dt} = -\frac{I_{ion} + I_{stim}}{C_m}, \tag{3.1}$$

considering an additional stimulus current I_{stim}, as well. For electrophysiological models, C_m is regularly defined as membrane capacity per unit area in F/m^2 resulting in current densities I_x in A/m^2:

$$I_x = g_x \left(V_m - E_x\right) . \tag{3.2}$$

The conductivity g_x is defined as the product of a maximum conductivity $\hat{g_x}$ of all channels carrying I_x and the open probability of this channel type. The dimensionless open probability of a channel $\in [0,1]$ is determined as the product of all gating variables γ_i involved:

$$g_x = \hat{g_x} \prod_i \gamma_i . \tag{3.3}$$

The evolution of each gating variable γ_i over time is described by the following first order ODE through transition rates α_{γ_i} from the closed to the open state and β_{γ_i} vice versa:

$$\frac{d\gamma_i}{dt} = \alpha_{\gamma_i} (1 - \gamma_i) - \beta_{\gamma_i} \gamma . \tag{3.4}$$

As the rate constants depend on V_m, the channels exhibit a voltage dependency. During steady-state, the derivative equates to zero yielding the steady-state open probability $\gamma_{i,\infty}$:

$$\gamma_{i,\infty} = \frac{\alpha_{\gamma_i}}{\alpha_{\gamma_i} + \beta_{\gamma_i}} . \tag{3.5}$$

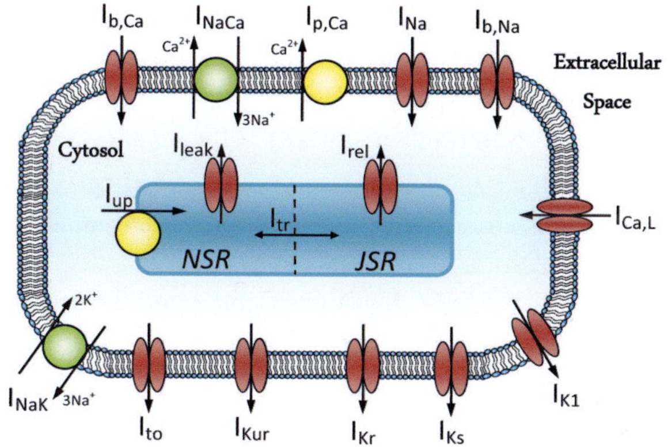

Figure 3.2: Schematic representation of the Courtemanche et al. model of human atrial myocytes [47]. Ion channels (red), pumps (green), and transporters (yellow) allow the exchange of ions between the intracellular space (cytosol), the extracellular space and the calcium subspaces (NSR and JSR). Reproduced from [155] with permission.

Using energy arguments, the steady-state open probability can be described by a Boltzmann equation [153]:

$$\gamma_{i,\infty} = \frac{1}{1 + \exp\left(\frac{V_{1/2,\gamma_i} - V_m}{k_{\gamma_i}}\right)}, \tag{3.6}$$

with $V_{1/2,\gamma_i}$ being the transmembrane voltage at which the gate γ_i exhibits an open probability of 0.5 (the so-called *half-activation voltage*) and k_{γ_i} being the slope at the half-activation voltage. k is determined by the ratio zF/RT, with z being the valency of the gating ion, F being Faraday's constant, R being the gas constant, and T being the absolute temperature.

Discrete further states (e.g. inactive states) and state-dependent transitions can be represented in Markov models with explicit representations of single ion-channel states. The number of gates and the number of states depends on the ion channel being modeled and the degree of complexity desired to cover. The interested reader is referred to e.g. [60, 154] for more detailed information regarding mathematical models of ion channels.

The ion channels present in distinct cells are integrated in computational cell models by coupling the ODEs via the transmembrane voltage and the ion concentrations. Within the scope of this thesis, the Courtemanche et al. model of human atrial myocytes [47] is mainly used as it convinced in a benchmark of the five currently available models of human atrial myocytes [156]. Figure 3.2 gives an overview of the ion channels, transporters, and pumps considered in the Courtemanche et al. model. Besides the extracellular and the intracellular space (*cytosol*), two calcium subspaces in the sarcoplasmic reticulum are represented in the model. The junctional sarcoplasmic reticulum compartment (JSR) releases Ca^{2+} while the network sarcoplasmic reticulum compartment (NSR) is responsible for Ca^{2+} uptake. The intracellular ion concentrations and the Ca^{2+} concentration in the sarcoplasmic reticulum compartments are computed dynamically whereas the extracellular concentrations are assumed to be constant.
While most current formulations in the Courtemanche et al. model are based on human experimental data, the pumps I_{NaCa}, I_{NaK}, $I_{p,Ca}$, the background currents $I_{b,Na}$ and $I_{b,Ca}$, and the intracellular calcium handling build on the Luo-Rudy model representing guinea pig ventricular myocytes [157]. Krueger et al. presented a heterogeneous version of the Courtemanche et al. model comprising 13 distinct regions in the atria [158].

3.2 Simulating Excitation Propagation

As cardiac myocytes form a syncytium as described in Section 2.1.1.2, excitation can propagate through cardiac tissue. To investigate excitation propagation phenomena on the tissue level *in silico*, a mathematical formulation of the coupling between cells is required. Several approaches exist that range from very microscopic descriptions up to macroscopic, phenomenological models. While very low-level descriptions provide the means to cover phenomena on the sub-cellular scale, as e.g. intracellular calcium waves [159], the focus of this thesis is on tissue and organ level phenomena as far as excitation propagation is concerned. For this purpose, the bidomain model and the monodomain model proved to be suitable for complex excitation patterns including e.g. wave break [160]. For simpler activation patterns, the fast marching scheme based on the eikonal equation can provide reasonable activation sequences at significantly reduced computational cost [161, 162].

3.2.1 The Bidomain Model and the Monodomain Simplification

The bidomain model introduced by Tung [163] represents cardiac tissue as a homogeneous medium with two coupled domains: the intracellular and the extracellular space. In this way, the complex microstructure of the cardiac tissue is disregarded and homogenized. The two computational domains coexist and interfere at each point, thus occupying the same geometrical space [164]. A transmembrane current per volume i_m can flow from one domain into the other at each point serving as the source for the current densities $\mathbf{j}_{(\mathbf{i}/\mathbf{e})}$ in the two domains. The potentials in the intracellular and extracellular domain are defined by Poisson's equation of stationary electrical fields:

$$\nabla \cdot \mathbf{j_i} = \nabla \cdot (\sigma_\mathbf{i} \nabla \Phi_i) = i_m \ , \tag{3.7}$$

$$\nabla \cdot \mathbf{j_e} = \nabla \cdot (\sigma_\mathbf{e} \nabla \Phi_e) = -i_m \ , \tag{3.8}$$

with Φ_i being the intracellular potential and Φ_e the extracellular potential, and $\sigma_\mathbf{i}$ and $\sigma_\mathbf{e}$ being the respective conductivity tensors, which are composed of conductivities along ($\sigma_\parallel$) and transversal ($\sigma_\perp$) to the myocardial fibre direction. The ratio $k = \sigma_\parallel / \sigma_\perp$ is called anisotropy ratio (see also Section 3.2.2).
Using the definition of the transmembrane voltage $V_m = \Phi_i - \Phi_e$, transformations on Equation (3.7) and Equation (3.8) [165] yield the following two coupled equations that are called the bidomain equations:

$$\nabla \cdot ((\sigma_\mathbf{i} + \sigma_\mathbf{e}) \nabla \Phi_e) = -\nabla \cdot (\sigma_\mathbf{i} \nabla V_m) \ , \tag{3.9}$$

$$\nabla \cdot (\sigma_\mathbf{i} \nabla V_m) + \nabla \cdot (\sigma_\mathbf{i} \nabla \Phi_e) = i_m \ . \tag{3.10}$$

The transmembrane current density per volume i_m is normally composed of an ionic transmembrane current density (per surface) I_{ion} defined by a cell model (such as the Courtemanche et al. model of human atrial myocytes), a capacitive current density, and an optional external stimulus current density I_{stim}:

$$i_m = \beta \left(C_m \frac{dV_m}{dt} + I_{ion} + I_{stim} \right) , \tag{3.11}$$

with β being the cell surface to volume ratio translating surface current densities to volume current densities.

If the anisotropy ratio k is equal for the intracellular and the extracellular conductivity tensors, $\sigma_\mathbf{i}$ can be expressed as $\kappa\sigma_\mathbf{e}$ and the bidomain formulation can be simplified to the so-called monodomain equation, which is computationally less expensive to solve:

$$\nabla \cdot (\sigma_\mathbf{i} \nabla V_m) = (\kappa + 1)\beta \left(C_m \frac{dV_m}{dt} + I_{ion} + I_{stim} \right) \tag{3.12}$$

The monodomain equation coupled to a membrane model such as the Courtemanche et al. model represents a reaction-diffusion system. By computing the currents flowing within the computational domain explicitly, effects like source-sink balance due to convex or concave wavefronts leading to CV modulation (Figure 3.3), wave break, and conduction block can be considered [165]. Finite difference discretizations of the monodomain equation or finite element schemes with mass lumping do not require to solve systems of linear equations but can be formulated using matrix vector multiplications [166–168].

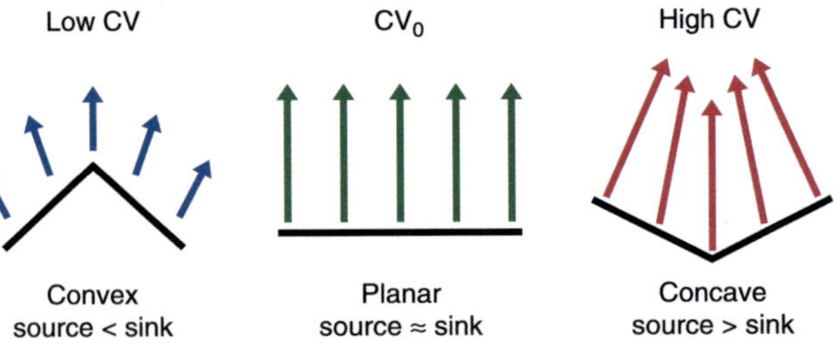

Figure 3.3: Influence of wavefront curvature-based source-sink balance on CV. A convex wavefront represents a smaller source at the tip and leads to low CV whereas the larger source in a concave wavefront results in high CV. A planar wave requires matched source and sink. Reproduced from [77] with permission from the publisher.

As the assumption $\sigma_\mathbf{i} = \kappa\sigma_\mathbf{e}$ holds within the scope of this thesis, all excitation propagation simulations were conducted using the monodomain model. The formulation was implemented at IBT in the parallel modular solver *acCELLerate* [169], which was verified by an N-version benchmark [170].

3.2.2 The Eikonal Equation and the Fast Marching Scheme

While the monodomain reaction-diffusion model provides the means to capture behavior of complex excitation patterns, it is also computationally expensive. Simpler schemes like cellular automata or eikonal-based approaches do not provide the means to reflect the diffusion processes but are suitable to compute the spread of activation for scenarios in which source-sink balance does not play an important role [161].
The eikonal equation governs the spread of an activation wave in a possibly anisotropic medium resulting in a scalar field $t_a(x_i)$ – the activation map:

$$c\sqrt{\nabla t_a \mathbf{G} \nabla t_a} = 1 \ , \tag{3.13}$$

with $c(x_i)$ being the speed function defined for each node x_i, $t_a(x_i)$ being the activation time, and $\mathbf{G}$ being a tensor creating anisotropy. $\mathbf{G}$ provides the means to account for faster conduction along the principal axis of myocytes (cf. Section 2.1.1.2) than perpendicular to it. Towards this end, the euclidean distance $\|\mathbf{d_{iso}}\|_2$ between two points representing the isotropic case is scaled according to the myocyte orientation and the angle between the two points.
A transformation aligning the positive x-axis with the myocyte orientation given by the angles ϕ and θ' can be established using conventional rotation matrices R_y and R_z:

$$R_y(\theta') = \begin{pmatrix} \cos\theta' & 0 & \sin\theta' \\ 0 & 1 & 0 \\ -\sin\theta' & 0 & \cos\theta' \end{pmatrix} , \tag{3.14}$$

$$R_z(\phi) = \begin{pmatrix} \cos\phi & -\sin\phi & 0 \\ \sin\phi & \cos\phi & 0 \\ 0 & 0 & 1 \end{pmatrix} . \tag{3.15}$$

At IBT, $\phi \in [0,\pi]$, is defined as the angle in the x-y-plane with respect to the positive x-axis as we only care about the direction but not the orientation of the myocyte orientation. $\theta \in [0,\pi]$ is defined as the angle with respect to the x-y-plane. Thus, θ' needs to be substituted by $\theta := \theta' + 270°$ to follow the conventional spherical coordinate system defined with respect to the positive z-axis. When only applied within trigonometrical functions, $\theta = \theta' - 90°$ holds, which gives us:

$$R_y(\theta) = \begin{pmatrix} \cos(\theta - 90°) & 0 & \sin(\theta - 90°) \\ 0 & 1 & 0 \\ -\sin(\theta - 90°) & 0 & \cos(\theta - 90°) \end{pmatrix} = \begin{pmatrix} \sin\theta & 0 & -\cos\theta \\ 0 & 1 & 0 \\ \cos\theta & 0 & \sin\theta \end{pmatrix} . \tag{3.16}$$

To align the positive x-axis with the principal myocyte orientation, we need to apply R_y followed by R_z.

$$\mathbf{coords_{local}} = R(\phi, \theta) \cdot \begin{pmatrix} 1 \\ 0 \\ 0 \end{pmatrix} , \tag{3.17}$$

with:

$$R(\phi, \theta) := R_z(\phi) \cdot R_y(\theta) = \begin{pmatrix} \sin\theta\cos\phi & -\sin\phi & -\cos\theta\cos\phi \\ \sin\theta\sin\phi & \cos\phi & -\cos\theta\sin\phi \\ \cos\theta & 0 & \sin\phi \end{pmatrix} . \tag{3.18}$$

If we want to transform from the global coordinate system to the local coordinate system with the fiber direction aligned with the x-axis, we need to apply the inverse operation using the identity $R^{-1} = R^T$. After this transformation is established, appropriate scaling can be applied using the anisotropy factor k. Transformation back to the global coordinate system yields $\mathbf{d_{aniso}}$ with the anisotropic distance measure $\|\mathbf{d_{aniso}}\|_2$:

$$\mathbf{d_{aniso}} = R(\phi, \theta) \begin{pmatrix} k^{-1} & 0 & 0 \\ 0 & 1 & 0 \\ 0 & 0 & 1 \end{pmatrix} R(\phi, \theta)^T \mathbf{d_{iso}} . \tag{3.19}$$

Algorithm 3.1 The fast marching method. $\mathcal{N}(X)$ denotes the neighborhood of X.

```
while TRIAL ≠ ∅ do
    X ← argmin_{X∈TRIAL} {t_a(X)}
    TRIAL ← TRIAL \ {X}
    KNOWN ← KNOWN ∪ {X}
    for all (X_i ∈ N(X)) ∧ (X_i ∉ KNOWN) do
        t_a(X_i) ← update(X_i, X)
        if X_i ∉ TRIAL then
            TRIAL ← TRIAL ∪ {X_i}
        end if
    end for
end while
```

Hence, **G** in Equation (3.13) is defined as:

$$R(\phi,\theta)\begin{pmatrix} k & 0 & 0 \\ 0 & 1 & 0 \\ 0 & 0 & 1 \end{pmatrix} R(\phi,\theta)^T\ . \tag{3.20}$$

The fast marching method is a scheme to solve Equation (3.13) in an efficient way taking advantage of the causality relationship between nodes. Only adjacent nodes with an activation time $t_a(x_j)$ smaller than the current estimate for the node in question $t_a(x_i)$ can influence its activation. In this way, the complexity of the algorithm is reduced to $\mathcal{O}(N \log N)$ with N being the number of nodes compared to $\mathcal{O}(N^2)$ for a naïve Newton method. Algorithm 3.1 gives an overview of the fast marching scheme to solve the eikonal equation Equation (3.13).

Compared to Dijkstra's algorithm [171, 172] and other graph-based methods [161, 173], a different relaxation scheme is used yielding unique solutions that are not necessarily restricted to the edges of the mesh. This is achieved by considering the anisotropic distance measure $\|\mathbf{d_{aniso}}\|_2$ (Equation (3.19), $solve_{1D}$) and quadratically approximating the activation time of nodes for which activation times of several other nodes in the same element are already known ($solve_{2D}$) according to Algorithm 3.2 (Figure 3.4) [174, 175].

Algorithm 3.2 update(X_i, X) for triangular surface meshes. $\mathscr{N}(X)$ denotes the neighborhood of X.

$t_a(X_i) \leftarrow +\infty$
$\Delta_{X_i}^{X} \leftarrow \{Y \mid (Y \in \mathscr{N}(X)) \wedge (Y \in \mathscr{N}(X_i))\}$
for all $Y \in \Delta_{X_i}^{X}$ **do**
  if $Y \in KNOWN$ **then**
    $t_a(X_i) \leftarrow \min\{t_a(X_i), \text{solve}_{2D}(X, X_i, Y)\}$
  else
    $t_a(X_i) \leftarrow \min\{t_a(X_i), \text{solve}_{1D}(X, X_i)\}$
  end if
end for

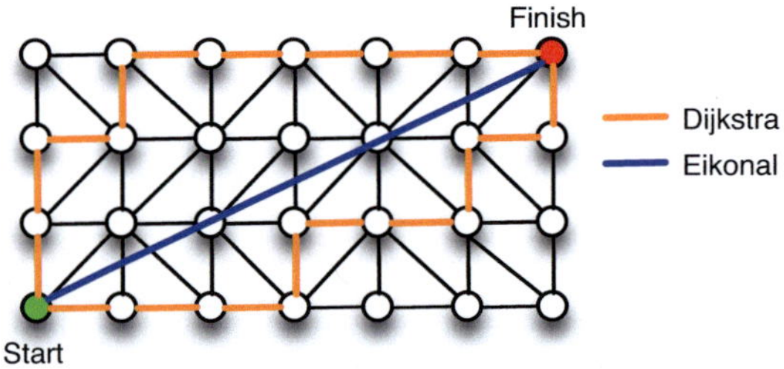

Figure 3.4: Comparison of Dijkstra's algorithm and the solution of the eikonal equation regarding the shortest path between two nodes on a triangular mesh. Dijkstra's algorithm considers only edges of the mesh as segments of the path yielding non-unique results that deviate significantly from the geometrical shortest path between the two nodes. The eikonal approach interpolates activation times considering all adjacent nodes yielding a better result on the same mesh.

Sermesant et al. proposed an extension to the fast marching scheme allowing to include multiple wavefronts [176] (Algorithm 3.3). The extension summarized in Algorithm 3.3 introduces a refractory state in which the nodes remain for the length of the effective refractory period (ERP) after being activated. Moreover, nodes can only activate adjacent nodes within a certain activity period after the activation, which has to be shorter than the ERP. The assignment of the nodes to the classes *REFRACTORY* and *UNKNOWN* is checked and updated after a fixed time step. The simulation runs as long as there are nodes in the *TRIAL* list and the maximum integrated time has not been reached.

Algorithm 3.3 Multifront fast marching. Abbreviations: integrated time (IT), elapsed time (ET), activity period (AcP).

```
IT ← 0.0
while (TRIAL ≠ ∅) ∧ (IT < maxTime) do
    ET ← 0.0
    while (TRIAL ≠ ∅) ∧ (ET < timeStep) do
        X ← argmin_{X∈TRIAL} {t_a(X)}
        TRIAL ← TRIAL \ {X}
        KNOWN ← KNOWN ∪ {X}
        for all (X_i ∈ 𝒩(X)) ∧ (X_i ∈ UNKNOWN) do
            t_a(X_i) ← update(X_i, X)
            if X_i ∉ TRIAL then
                TRIAL ← TRIAL ∪ {X_i}
            end if
            ET ← t_a(X_i) − IT
        end for
    end while
    IT ← IT + timeStep
    for all X ∈ KNOWN do
        if (IT − t_a(X)) > AcP(X) then
            KNOWN ← KNOWN \ {X}
            REFRACTORY ← REFRACTORY ∪ {X}
        end if
    end for
    for all X ∈ REFRACTORY do
        if (IT − t_a(X)) > ERP(X) then
            REFRACTORY ← REFRACTORY \ {X}
            UNKNOWN ← UNKNOWN ∪ {X}
        end if
    end for
end while
```

3.3 Anatomical Modeling

The activation pattern of the atria is strongly dependent on their anatomical properties. Moreover, mechanisms of arrhythmia initiation and perpetuation interfere with the geometrical substrate [9]. Therefore, a realistic model of human atrial anatomy is required to study such phenomena *in silico*. If body surface potentials are of interest (cf. Section 3.4), also a torso model comprising the most important organs is required [177].

While very detailed, microstructure-based models of single regions of the atria are available, organ models on the atrial or whole heart scale represent only their shape normally [9]. The shape can either be composed of simple geometrical bodies (e.g. surfaces of a sphere with holes for the vessel and valve orifices) or derived from segmentations of imaging data. Gadolinium-enhanced magnetic resonance imaging (MRI) is one of the few methods allowing to include information regarding the substrate in models (e.g. the degree of fibrosis) [178–182]. Three-dimensional models of the atria can be divided in volumetric models comprising an atrial wall with a finite thickness and surface models. Another distinguishing feature are the conductive properties of the atrial septum. While it is modeled as a continuous, fully conducting connection in some models, others include an isolating layer, thus allowing interatrial conduction only via well-defined, discrete connections. The interested reader is referred to e.g. [9, 23] for a comprehensive review of available anatomical models and their features.

Within the scope of this thesis, a virtual population of eight heterogeneous torso models presented by Krueger et al. was used [183]. Torso models and atrial models were segmented from MRI data and augmented with a priori knowledge using the approaches presented in Chapter 7. Figure 3.5 shows two examples of torso models comprising several organs. The characteristics of the virtual study population are introduced in more detail in Section 9.1.1.

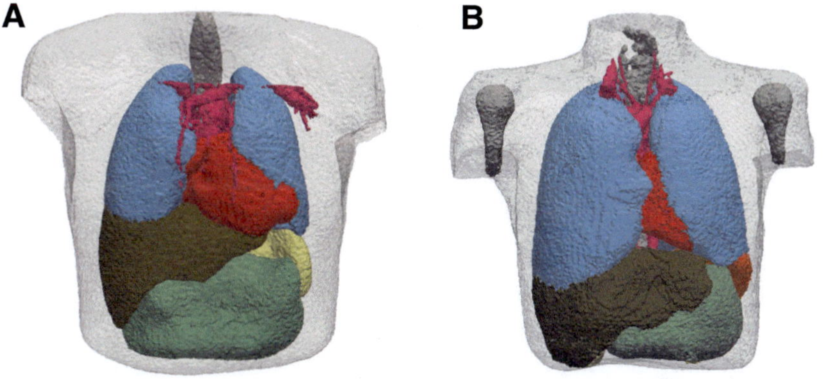

Figure 3.5: Heterogeneous tetrahedral torso meshes of model #5 (A) and model #6 (B). The volumes of the different segmented organs are shown in distinct color: lungs (blue), bone (gray), heart (red), great vessels (pink), liver (brown), kidneys (yellow), intestines (green). Model #6 (B) also comprised a segmented spleen (orange).

3.4 Forward Calculation of the ECG

The spatial gradient of the transmembrane voltages impresses a volume current density i_{imp} on the tissue:

$$i_{imp} = -\nabla \cdot (\sigma_{\mathbf{i}} \nabla V_m) \ . \tag{3.21}$$

This impressed volume current density serves as the source for the extracellular field in the surrounding according to the parabolic part of the bidomain formulation (Equation (3.9)) [184]:

$$\nabla \cdot ((\sigma_{\mathbf{i}} + \sigma_{\mathbf{e}}) \nabla \Phi_e) = i_{imp}. \tag{3.22}$$

Thus, the body surface potentials can be calculated based on the distribution of V_m using this reduced bidomain formulation under the assumption of a passive, purely resistive volume conduction representing the torso [177]. This so-called *forward problem of electrocardiography* is linear and quasi-stationary. A fixed potential at a reference node serves as a Dirichlet boundary condition whereas the thorax-air boundary poses a Neumann boundary condition. Equation (3.22) is usually discretized by finite element or boundary element schemes [9]. While finite element approaches are computationally more expensive, they can handle unequal anisotropy in the volume conductor. The resulting body surface potential maps (BSPMs) can be evaluated for each time instant, as an integral over time [185], or by tracing the potential difference between electrodes over time as performed during electrocardiogram (ECG) recordings.

PART II

MODELING CELLULAR ELECTROPHYSIOLOGY

CHAPTER 4

Parameter Estimation of Ion Current Models

While computational models of cardiac electrophysiology elucidated pathophysiological mechanisms and provided insight into arrhythmogenesis during the last years, most models represent healthy cells. In order to fully leverage the potential of *in silico* cardiology, the models have to be adapted to reflect pathologies, genetic defects (channelopathies), the effects of pharmacological agents, or distinct properties of specific regions of the heart.

Voltage and patch clamp techniques [186, 187] allow to record the response of cells or single channels to a voltage step in terms of current. As the current is proportional to the channel open probability, these experiments allow to assess the channel kinetics, i.e. activation, deactivation and inactivation under specific conditions. The altered gating behavior often translates to counter-intuitive changes on higher levels of integration due to the complex and mostly non-linear structure of the biophysical systems. Thus, an integration of these ion channel data into comprehensive cellular models is imperative for a thorough evaluation of the systemic effects (e.g. on the whole cell, tissue, or organ level) of altered gating behavior (see e.g. [188]).

A common approach is to reparameterize established models (see Section 3.1) while leaving their structure unaltered. The parameter estimation aims to minimize the difference between the model output and the measured data, thus at a model parameter set optimally reflecting the data. This process can be

computationally expensive and time-consuming depending on the complexity of the model, the number of parameters to estimate, and the abundance of measurement data. Particularly the high-dimensional, highly non-linear, and often non-convex nature of the problem renders this a challenging task.
The advent of automated high-throughput patch clamping techniques [189] led to a significant increase of the amount of available ion channel data. In many cases, experimental data are available on very low levels of integration (e.g. ion currents) and very high levels of integration (e.g. the body surface electrocardiogram (ECG)). Multi-scale simulations can aid to bridge the gap of missing links on intermediate levels arising from a lack of data. In this way, model-based approaches can foster our understanding of patho-mechanisms and pave the way for the development of tailored therapeutic approaches. Thus, there is a need for automated, accurate, efficient, and robust parameter estimation techniques.
In this chapter, two algorithms from different families are evaluated regarding their suitability for the scenario sketched above. First, optimization-based approaches are evaluated and advanced in Section 4.1. Then, an approach based on multivariate metamodeling is evaluated in Section 4.2.

4.1 Hybrid Optimization

Besides classical gradient-based optimization approaches, derivative-free algorithms have been proposed to tackle high-dimensional, non-linear, and non-convex minimization problems. In this study, gradient-based trust-region-reflective (TRR) optimization [190] and derivative-free, population-based particle swarm optimization (PSO) are evaluated. Using idealized synthetic input data as well as measured current data, the shortcomings of each of the approaches when being applied to different cardiac ion currents are identified. Thus, a new hybrid approach coupling PSO and TRR is proposed aiming at an optimization scheme being minimally dependent on the initial parameter guess.
Previous work by other authors suggested different algorithms to estimate parameters of ion current formulations or whole cell models to reproduce measured currents, action potentials or restitution curves (e.g. [191, 192]). Also derivative-free metaheuristic algorithms were used in the field of cardiac

electrophysiology: e.g. particle swarm optimization (PSO) in [193, 194] and a genetic algorithm in [195–197]. However, the study presented here is the first to combine the two approaches in a coupled hybrid scheme [198, 199] for this purpose to the best of my knowledge.
Parts of this study have been published as a journal article [200] as well as conference contributions [201–203] and are based on earlier work [127, 204, 205].

4.1.1 Methods

4.1.1.1 Ion Current Formulations

The parameter estimation algorithms were evaluated using ion current formulations from the Courtemanche et al. human atrial cell model (see Section 3.1). The currents are formulated using Hodgkin-Huxley type equations [152]:

$$I_X = \hat{g_X} x (V_m - E_X) \tag{4.1}$$

with $\hat{g_X}$ being the maximum conductance of all channels conducting the current I_X, x being the open probability of the channels, and E_X being the Nernst potential of the ion type carrying the current I_X. Based on pilot studies, the parameters of the rapid delayed rectifier potassium current I_{Kr}, the ultra-rapid delayed rectifier potassium current I_{Kur}, and the slow delayed rectifier potassium current I_{Ks} were chosen to be estimated because they span a wide range of characteristics (e.g. fast I_{Kur} kinetics compared to I_{Kr}).
For I_{Kr}, the Courtemanche et al. formulation [47] being used was:

$$I_{Kr} = g_{Kr} x_r (V_m - E_K) \frac{1}{1 + \exp\left(\frac{V_m + 15}{22.4}\right)}, \tag{4.2}$$

with g_{Kr} being the maximal conductance, x_r the activation gating variable, and E_K the potassium Nernst voltage, and V_m the transmembrane voltage in mV. Besides the instantaneous inactivation gate represented by the fraction in Equation (4.2), the formulation comprises the time-dependent gating variable x_r governed by the following ordinary differential equation (ODE):

$$\frac{dx_r}{dt} = \frac{x_{r\infty} - x_r}{\tau_{x_r}}, \tag{4.3}$$

with $x_{r\infty}$ being the steady-state value and τ_{x_r} the time constant of the gating variable x_r. These two parameters depend on V_m again:

$$x_{r\infty} = \frac{1}{1+\exp\left(-\frac{V_m+14.1}{6.5}\right)} , \tag{4.4}$$

$$\tau_{x_r} = \frac{1}{\alpha_{x_r}+\beta_{x_r}} . \tag{4.5}$$

The rate constants α_{x_r} and β_{x_r} are defined as a function of V_m as well:

$$\alpha_{x_r} = 0.0003\frac{V_m+14.1}{1-\exp\left(-\frac{V_m+14.1}{5}\right)} , \tag{4.6}$$

$$\beta_{x_r} = 7.3898\times 10^{-5}\frac{V_m-3.3328}{\exp\left(\frac{V_m-3.3328}{5.1237}\right)-1} . \tag{4.7}$$

For each current, the parameters to be estimated were identified and classified as additive or multiplicative depending on whether they enter the equation in a sum or a product. Maximum conductances are an example for multiplicative parameters whereas half-activation voltages are an example for additive parameters (cf. Section 3.1). For I_{Kr}, 12 parameters were estimated. The complete set of equations for I_{Kr}, I_{Kur}, and I_{Ks} together with the estimated parameters, their original Courtemanche et al. values, and their classification as additive or multiplicative are given in Section A.1.
The gating ODEs as e.g. Equation (4.3) are normally solved numerically in computational cardiology. This is necessary as the steady-state value $x_{r\infty}$ and the time constant τ_{x_r} are voltage-dependent and change during the cardiac cycle. Thus, no closed analytical solution can be obtained. During clamp experiments with classical voltage protocols however, V_m is a piecewise constant function. Therefore, an analytical solution for Equation (4.3) can be derived [206]:

$$x_r(t-t_0) = x_{r\infty} + (x_{r0}-x_{r\infty})\exp\left(-\frac{t-t_0}{\tau_{x_r}}\right) , \tag{4.8}$$

with t_0 being the time of a step of V_m and x_{r0} the corresponding initial value at that time. Using the analytical solution, the calculation of the current is computationally far less expensive as compared to numerical approximation.

All current formulations were implemented in *Matlab (R2015a, The MathWorks, Natick, MA, USA)*.

4.1.1.2 Voltage Clamp Data

For the evaluation of the algorithms, two sets of data were used: synthetic and measured currents. Synthetic data were generated using the original formulations and parameters from Courtemanche et al. [47]. These synthetic data had the advantage that it was known that a parameter set exists which exactly reproduces the input data allowing to optimally assess the accuracy of the estimation. Moreover, the parameter values used to generate the input data were available for comparison of the estimated parameters even though the optimization algorithm was blinded to these values. This allowed to assess parameter identifiability. In addition, noise was added to the synthetic signals to evaluate the robustness regarding the influence of noise under controlled conditions. Synthetic data were generated for I_{Kr} which was identified as rather easy to fit in a pilot study and for I_{Kur} which was identified as hard to fit. The voltage protocol is shown in Figure 4.1 and was composed of 13 traces consisting of 20 ms at –80 mV resting voltage, 400 ms at the respective step voltage ranging from –70 mV to +50 mV in steps of 10 mV, and 400 ms at –110 mV resulting in a total length of 10.66 s. The resulting currents were sampled every 2 ms. For the sensitivity analysis regarding noise, the non-noisy signals were corrupted with additive white Gaussian noise resulting in signal to noise ratios (SNRs) of 10, 20, 35, and 65 dB.
The study also comprised a second set of data which were acquired in wet-lab experiments. Measured data pose additional challenges in terms of noise and other artifacts. Moreover, the biophysical entity being measured will not be perfectly replicated by the model as opposed to synthetic data. The investigation performed in the group of Eberhard Scholz at University Hospital Heidelberg conformed to the "Guide for the Care and Use of Laboratory Animals" published by the US National Institutes of Health (NIH publication No 85-23, revised 1996) and was approved by the regional administrative council (Regierungspräsidium Karlsruhe, Karlsruhe, Germany, application number G-221/12). The details of the acquisition procedures for the human ether-à-go-go-related gene (hERG) (I_{Kr}), KCNA5 (I_{Kur}), and KCNQ1+KCNE1 (I_{Ks}) are given in Section A.2.

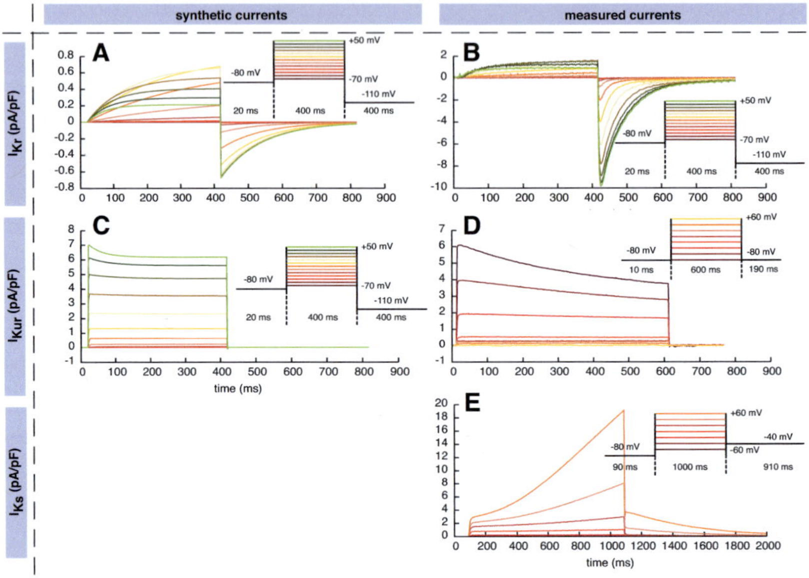

Figure 4.1: Synthetic ((A) and (C)) and measured ((B), (D), and (E)) input current data used to estimate parameters together with the corresponding voltage protocols. (A) and (B) show I_{Kr}, (C) and (D) show I_{Kur}, (E) shows I_{Ks}.

4.1.1.3 Optimization Algorithms

In this study, the estimation of model parameters was treated as a minimization problem aiming at an optimal fit of the model output to the input data. Therefore, the following cost function was used:

$$\min_{\mathbf{p}} \left(\sum_{\mathrm{j}}^{\mathrm{M}} \sum_{\mathrm{i}}^{\mathrm{N}} \left(I\left(t_{\mathrm{i}}, V_{\mathrm{j}}\left(t_{\mathrm{i}}\right), \mathbf{p}\right) - I^{*}\left(t_{\mathrm{i}}, V_{\mathrm{j}}\left(t_{\mathrm{i}}\right)\right)\right)^{2} \right), \tag{4.9}$$

with I being the output of the ion current model using the vector of adjustable parameters $\mathbf{p}$ aiming to match the measured current I^{*}, t_{i} being a discrete time, and V_{j} the transmembrane voltage trace, which is described by a piecewise constant function for each step voltage. Thus i covered all N time instants for which samples were considered and j covered all M step voltages.

The parameter search spaces were restricted. Two sets of ranges were evaluated. For the "narrow" range, additive values were allowed to vary between –60 and +60 of their standard Courtemanche et al. values [47] in the unit of the standard value. Multiplicative values were restricted to the interval of 0.1 and 10 times their standard value in the "narrow" case. For the "wide" range, limits were ± 120 and $0.01..100\times$, respectively. All optimization code was implemented in *Matlab (R2015a, The MathWorks, Natick, MA, USA)*. In order to obtain statistics regarding the dependency on the parameter vector used to initialize the optimization ("initial guess"), all experiments were run 25 times with uniformly distributed random initial values.

Trust-Region-Reflective The TRR optimization algorithm is a second order scheme, which approximates the function $f(\mathbf{p})$ quadratically as $q_i(\mathbf{p})$. Thus, it requires the values of the first and the second derivative in the current parameter vector $\mathbf{p_i}$. The quadratic approximation is considered within a region of trust around that point:

$$q_i(\mathbf{p}) = f(\mathbf{p_i}) + \nabla f(\mathbf{p_i})^T (\mathbf{p} - \mathbf{p_i}) + \frac{1}{2} (\mathbf{p} - \mathbf{p_i})^T \nabla^2 f(\mathbf{p_i}) (\mathbf{p} - \mathbf{p_i}) \; , \qquad (4.10)$$

$$\min_{\|\mathbf{s}\|_2 \leq r_\Delta} q_i(\mathbf{p_i} + \mathbf{s}) \; . \qquad (4.11)$$

The size of the region of trust r_Δ is varied depending on the quality of the second order approximation. The more accurate the approximation was in the current iteration, the larger r_Δ will be in the next iteration. TRR is provided by the *Matlab* function *lsqnonlin* and can terminate due to several criteria. The minimum change of the norm of the parameter vector $\mathbf{p}$ (*pTol*) and the minimum change of the cost function value (*fTol*) were set to 1×10^{-11} (pA/pF)^2. The number of iterations (*maxIter*) was limited to 1×10^5 and the number of cost function evaluations (*maxFunEval*) to 5×10^5. Each TRR experiment comprised 22 parallel instantiations with random start vectors.

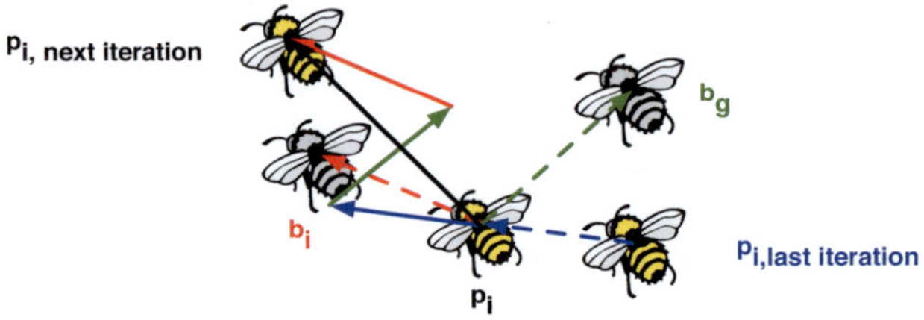

Figure 4.2: Basic principle of the PSO. Each particle with its position $\mathbf{p_i}$ experiences attracting forces towards the best position found so far by the entire swarm $\mathbf{b_g}$, the best position found so far by itself $\mathbf{b_i}$, and an inertia force defined by the difference between the current position $\mathbf{p_i}$ and the one in the last iteration $\mathbf{p_{i,last\ iteration}}$. These three forces are weighted using uniformly distributed numbers $\in [0,1]$ and added vectorially to obtain the position for the next iteration ($\mathbf{p_{i,next\ iteration}}$).

Particle Swarm Optimization Derivative-based algorithms such as TRR introduced above are prone to get stuck in local minima as shown in [201]. As a consequence, the result is sensitive to the choice of the initial parameter vector, which is undesirable. Thus, a population-based algorithm, which does not use gradient information, was implemented in addition. PSO is inspired by the swarming behavior observed in nature as e.g. flocking birds or fish schools [207]. A population of "particles" swarms through the parameter space searching for the globally best solution. Each particle i knows about the best position it has found so far itself ($\mathbf{b_i}$) and the best position found so far by the entire swarm ($\mathbf{b_g}$). The particles experience attracting forces towards $\mathbf{b_i}$ and $\mathbf{b_g}$ with random weights. Moreover, inertia tries to keep particles moving in a similar direction as before as shown e.g. in [208]. Thus, the parameter vectors are updated as follows in each iteration:

$$\mathbf{v}_i \leftarrow \chi(\mathbf{v}_i + \mathbf{U}(0,\phi_1) \otimes (\mathbf{b}_i - \mathbf{p}_i) + \mathbf{U}(0,\phi_2) \otimes (\mathbf{b}_g - \mathbf{p}_i)) \ , \tag{4.12}$$

$$\mathbf{p}_i \leftarrow \mathbf{p}_i + \mathbf{v}_i \ , \tag{4.13}$$

with $\mathbf{U}(0,\phi_1)$ and $\mathbf{U}(0,\phi_2)$ being vectors of the same length as $\mathbf{p}$ of uniformly distributed random numbers (between 0 and ϕ_1 or ϕ_2) and $\otimes$ being a component-wise multiplication. Clerc and Kennedy showed that a choice of $\phi_1 = \phi_2 = 2.05$ is optimal together with the following definition of the constriction coefficient χ:

$$\chi = \frac{2}{\phi - 2 + \sqrt{\phi^2 - 4\phi}} \approx 0.73 , \qquad (4.14)$$

with $\phi = \phi_1 + \phi_2$ [209].
In this study, PSO was adjusted in order to handle restricted search spaces. If one of the parameters was out of the prescribed ranges after the update step Equation (4.13), a correction step was performed. The particular elements of p which crossed a boundary were placed randomly within a 25% margin starting at this boundary.
The number of particles N was varied between 24 and 12,288 with the number being doubled from one setup to the next. The algorithm was run for a fixed number of iterations L. The approach was implemented in *Matlab* with parallelized computation of the cost function across the particles.

Combination of Algorithms As it turned out that none of the algorithms alone performed satisfactory for all investigated currents (see Section 4.1.2.1), combinations were evaluated. In the *"two-stage PSO+TRR"* approach, the algorithms were combined in a sequential manner. Motivated by the fact that TRR was sensitive to the initial guess and thus dependent on a good start vector, the best $M = 12$ parameter vectors yielded by PSO were used as initial guesses for subsequent TRR optimization as shown in Figure 4.3A.
The *"two-stage PSO+TRR"* approach was not superior compared to pure PSO or pure TRR for some of the current formulations and the resulting error using the synthetic data deviated significantly from zero (see Section 4.1.2.1). Thus, a hybrid approach coupling TRR and PSO in each PSO iteration was developed and implemented as shown in Figure 4.3B and detailed in Algorithm 4.1. After each PSO update step Equation (4.13), each of the N particles with their respective parameter vectors were subject to a fixed number of K TRR iterations. This approach is being referred to as *"hybrid (PSO+TRR)"*. For *"hybrid (PSO+TRR)+TRR"*, TRR was additionally run until convergence for the best $M = 12$ particles after PSO termination. Three different combinations of the number of TRR iterations in each PSO iteration K, the number of PSO iterations L, and the number of particles N were evaluated: *"low"* ($K = 5$, $L = 250$, $N = 96$), *"medium"* ($K = 10$, $L = 500$, $N = 192$), and *"high"* ($K = 20$, $L = 1000$, $N = 384$).

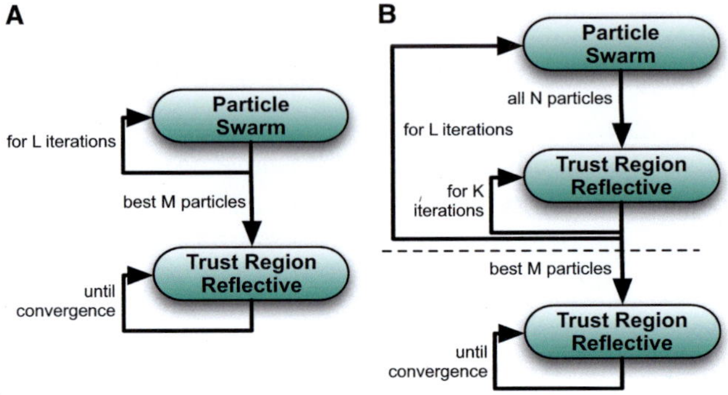

Figure 4.3: Flow chart of the *two-stage PSO+TRR* algorithm (A) and the *hybrid (PSO+TRR)+TRR* algorithm (B). The steps above the horizontal, dashed line in (B) are referred to as *hybrid (PSO+TRR)*.

Algorithm 4.1 "hybrid (PSO+TRR)+TRR" optimization approach

> **for** $itPSO < L$ **do**
>   **for** $i < N$ **do**
> $\mathbf{v}_i \leftarrow \chi(\mathbf{v}_i + \mathbf{U}(0,\phi_1) \otimes (\mathbf{b}_i - \mathbf{p}_i) + \mathbf{U}(0,\phi_2) \otimes (\mathbf{b}_g - \mathbf{p}_i))$
> $\tilde{\mathbf{p}}_\mathbf{i} \leftarrow \mathbf{p}_\mathbf{i} + \mathbf{v}_\mathbf{i}$
>   enforce boundary constraints on $\tilde{\mathbf{p}}_\mathbf{i}$
>   **for** $itTRR < K$ **do**
>   perform TRR iteration on $\tilde{\mathbf{p}}_\mathbf{i}$
>   **end for**
> $\mathbf{v}_\mathbf{i} \leftarrow \tilde{\mathbf{p}}_\mathbf{i} - \mathbf{p}_\mathbf{i}$
> $\mathbf{p}_\mathbf{i} \leftarrow \mathbf{p}_\mathbf{i} + \mathbf{v}_\mathbf{i}$
>   **end for**
> **end for**
> sort $\mathbf{b}[]$ by ascending squared error
> **for** $i < M$ **do**
>   **while** (not converged) $\wedge$ $(itTRR < maxIter)$ **do**
>   perform TRR iteration on $\mathbf{b}_\mathbf{i}$
>   **end while**
> **end for**

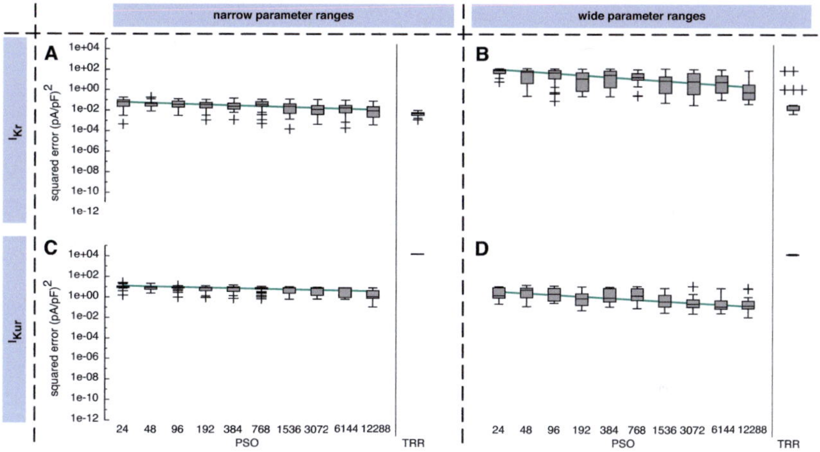

Figure 4.4: Sum of squared errors achieved by pure PSO and pure TRR optimization for synthetic I_{Kr} ((A) and (B)) and I_{Kur} ((C) and (D)) data. The number of particles N for PSO was varied. In (A) and (C), narrow parameter ranges were used whereas in (B) and (D) the search space was wider. Box plots represent 25 experiments each; the green lines indicate linear regressions of the median values in the graph coordinate system.

4.1.2 Results

4.1.2.1 Results Using Synthetic Data

In a first step, the different algorithms and their combinations were evaluated using synthetic input data. For these data, a parameter set yielding an error of exactly zero exists and was available for comparison.

One-Stage Approach Regarding the pure variants of PSO and TRR (one-stage approaches), TRR yielded lower errors and less variance than PSO for I_{Kr}. For I_{Kur} on the other hand, PSO performed better by four orders of magnitude (see Figure 4.4).
The squared errors obtained using pure PSO and the narrow I_{Kr} parameter intervals ranged between 1×10^{-4} (pA/pF)^2 and 0.18 (pA/pF)^2. For higher numbers of particles N, a tendency toward lower errors was observed (median error 6.4×10^{-2} (pA/pF)^2 for $N = 24$ and 9.5×10^{-3} (pA/pF)^2 for $N = 12{,}288$).

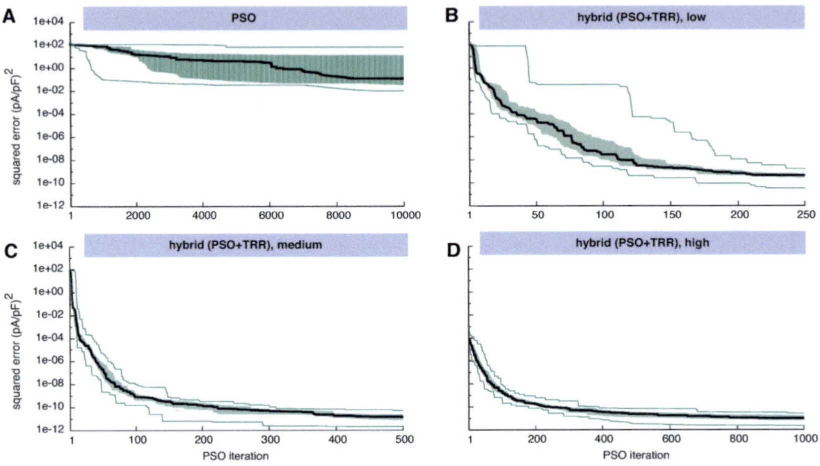

Figure 4.5: Sum of squared errors convergence behavior of pure PSO (A) and *hybrid (PSO+TRR)* (B-D) for synthetic I_{Kr} data. 25 experiments using the wide parameter ranges were performed. The black line indicates the median, the green lines the minimum and the maximum. The green area covers the two central quartiles. The number of particles N, the number of PSO iterations L, and the number of inner TRR iterations K was increased from *low* (B) via *medium* (C) to *high* (D).

The squared errors obtained by pure TRR were lower (5.1×10^{-3}) and showed smaller variance compared to pure PSO in the 25 experiments with random start vectors (see Figure 4.4A). By extending the search space to the wide ranges, the squared error was increased by about three orders of magnitude for pure PSO (see Figure 4.4B). For pure TRR, the median error was unaffected by the wider ranges. However, five of the experiments yielded significantly higher errors (see Figure 4.4B).

The convergence behavior of pure PSO is shown in Figure 4.5A. While the median error decreased until around 8,500 iterations, the maximum error remained almost unchanged after the very first iterations. Regarding the TRR convergence criteria introduced in Section 4.1.1.3, the change of the norm of **p** (*pTol*) caused termination for all experiments using the narrow parameter ranges. This criterion was decisive for only 19% of cases using the wide ranges where the norm of the squared error (*fTol*) terminated the remaining cases.

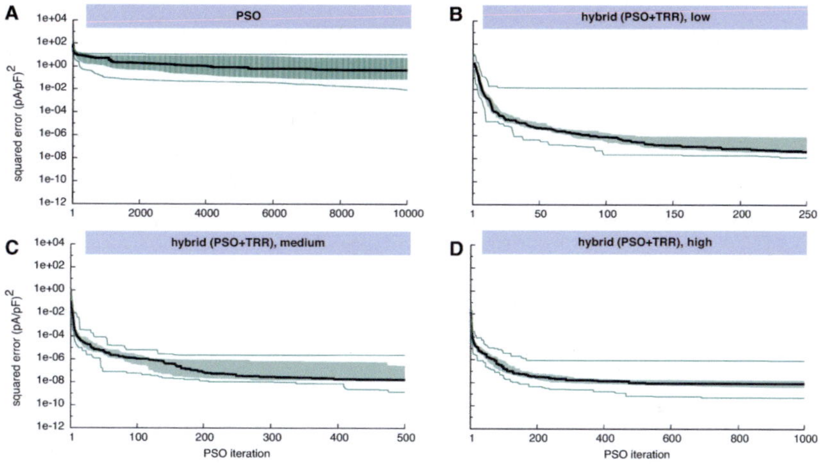

Figure 4.6: Sum of squared errors convergence behavior of pure PSO (A) and *hybrid (PSO+TRR)* (B-D) for synthetic I_{Kur} data. 25 experiments using the wide parameter ranges were performed. The black line indicates the median, the green lines the minimum and the maximum. The green area covers the two central quartiles. The number of particles N, the number of PSO iterations L, and the number of inner TRR iterations K was increased from *low* (B) via *medium* (C) to *high* (D).

Using synthetic I_{Kur} current data as input, two differences were observed compared to I_{Kr}. First, PSO performed better by more than 4 orders of magnitude in terms of squared error (see Figure 4.4C). Second, extending the parameter search space to the wide ranges led to a lower squared error (see Figure 4.4D). Compared to the narrow ranges, the squared error was lower by 80% for PSO ($N = 12{,}288$) and by 12% for TRR.

PSO converged to almost the final value of the cost function within 6,000 iterations (see Figure 4.6A). The maximum error did not decrease significantly after the first 500 iterations as was the case for I_{Kr}. The decisive termination criterion for TRR was *fTol* in 66% of the cases, the number of iterations (*maxIter*) in 31% of the cases, and *pTol* in 3% of the cases using the narrow ranges. For the wide ranges, the distribution was 50/40/10%, respectively.

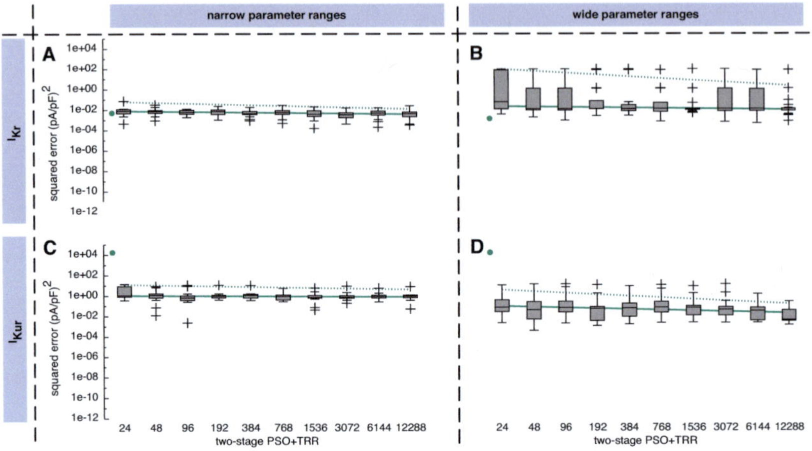

Figure 4.7: Sum of squared errors achieved by *two-stage PSO+TRR* optimization for synthetic I_{Kr} ((A) and (B)) and I_{Kur} ((C) and (D)) data. The number of particles N was varied. In (A) and (C), narrow parameter ranges were used whereas in (B) and (D) the search space was wider. Box plots represent 25 experiments each. The green lines indicate linear regressions of the median values in the graph coordinate system. The green dot on the left of each panel represents the median of pure TRR optimization, the dotted green lines represent linear regressions of the median values of pure PSO (compare Figure 4.4).

Two-Stage PSO+TRR Approach A combination of PSO and TRR in a sequential manner by using the best $M = 12$ particles as start vector for subsequent TRR optimization improved the results compared to pure PSO in all cases and compared to pure TRR in most cases (see Figure 4.7). The advantage of the *two-stage PSO+TRR* approach compared to the one-stage approaches was bigger for I_{Kur} than for I_{Kr} and bigger for the wide parameter ranges than for the narrow ones.

The squared error was reduced by 87% for $N = 24$ and by 56% for $N = 12{,}288$ using the narrow I_{Kr} ranges (see Figure 4.7A). Thus, the median error of the *two-stage PSO+TRR* approach was smaller than for any one-stage approach for $N \geq 1536$. The worst result yielded by pure TRR, however, was better than the worst result obtained using *two-stage PSO+TRR*. Extending the parameter search space to the wide ranges increased the variance of the resulting squared errors accompanied by a slight increase of the median error (1.2×10^{-2} (pA/pF)^2 vs. 4.2×10^{-3} (pA/pF)^2, see Figure 4.7B). This behavior

of the *two-stage PSO+TRR* approach is in contrast to pure PSO for which the median error was significantly increased together with a slight increase of the variance (see Section 4.1.2.1 and Figure 4.4A+B). The TRR step of the *two-stage PSO+TRR* approach was terminated due to *pTol* in all cases using the narrow ranges. For the wide ranges, 16% of the runs were terminated due to *fTol*.
For the I_{Kur} formulation, the improvement of *two-stage PSO+TRR* over the best one-stage approach was 6% for the narrow ranges (see Figure 4.4C) and 88% for the wide ranges (see Figure 4.4D) for N = 12,288. For the wide I_{Kur} parameter ranges, the median error was lower and the variance bigger for *two-stage PSO+TRR* as was the case for pure PSO. The decisive stopping criterion for the TRR step was *maxIter* in 80% of the cases and *pTol* in 20% using the narrow ranges. For the wide ranges, TRR was terminated due to *pTol*, *maxIter*, *fTol* in 51/30/29% of the cases, respectively.

Hybrid Approach The hybrid approach performed best for both I_{Kr} and I_{Kur} synthetic current data irrespective of the parameter ranges used. The improvement compared to the sequential combination of PSO and TRR was more than five orders of magnitude (see Figure 4.8).
Using the *hybrid (PSO+TRR)* approach, median squared error smaller than 1×10^{-9} (pA/pF)^2 for I_{Kr} (see Figure 4.8B) and smaller than 1×10^{-7} (pA/pF)^2 for I_{Kur} (see Figure 4.8D) were obtained. Thus, the results were improved by seven and five orders of magnitude compared to the *two-stage PSO+TRR* approach, respectively. The *low* setup of the hybrid approach comprising the lowest number of particles, the lowest number of PSO iterations, and the lowest number of inner TRR iterations within each PSO iteration yielded a single outlier for I_{Kur}: 1.4×10^{-2} (pA/pF)^2. In this experiment, the value of the cost function remained almost stable after the first 10 iterations indicating a deadlock of the entire swarm in a local minimum. The maximum squared errors obtained using the *medium* and *high* setups of the *hybrid (PSO+TRR)* approach were 5.2×10^{-11} (pA/pF)^2 for I_{Kr} and 2.3×10^{-6} (pA/pF)^2 for I_{Kur}. Restricting the parameters to the narrow ranges did not influence the result in terms of median error and variance significantly for I_{Kr} (see Figure 4.8A).

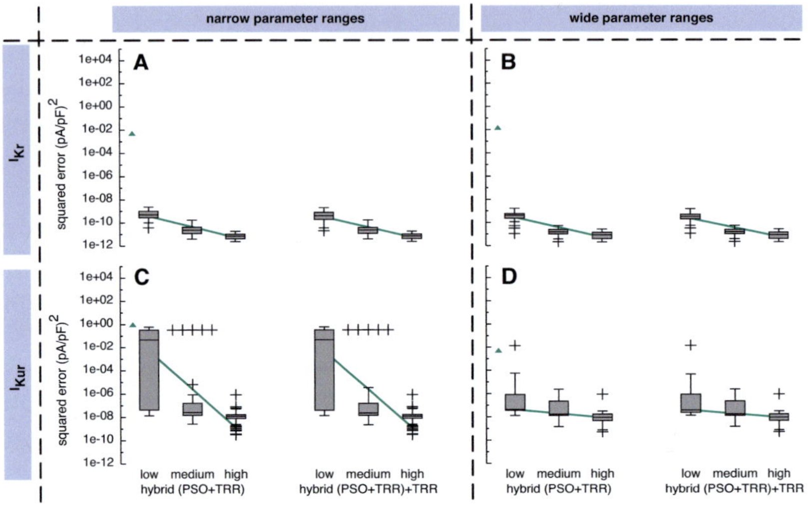

Figure 4.8: Sum of squared errors achieved by *hybrid (PSO+TRR)* and *hybrid (PSO+TRR)+TRR* optimization for synthetic I_{Kr} (A) and I_{Kur} (B) data. Parameter values were restricted to the wide range. The number of particles N, the number of PSO iterations L and the number of inner TRR iterations K was increased from *low* via *medium* to *high*. Box plots represent 25 experiments each; the green lines indicate linear regressions of the median values in the graph coordinate system. The green triangle on the left of each panel represents the median of *two-stage PSO+TRR* for N = 12,288 (compare Figure 4.7).

For I_{Kur}, a similar behavior as for the *two-stage PSO+TRR* approach was observed for *hybrid (PSO+TRR)*: a larger variance of the resulting squared error with several estimates yielding up to 3.5×10^{-1} (pA/pF)^2 for both the *low* and the *medium* setup (see Figure 4.8C).

The convergence of the median error was not highly dependent on the setup being used. It decreased to an interval within one order of magnitude of the final value in 125/217/232 iterations for the *low/medium/high* I_{Kr} setups, respectively (see Figure 4.5B-D). For I_{Kur}, convergence was faster than for I_{Kr} as was the case for pure PSO. A value within one order of magnitude of the final value was reached after 112/167/128 iterations using the *low/medium/high* setups of the *hybrid (PSO+TRR)* approach. Using the *low* setup, however, the maximum error still decreased during the final iterations 200–250.

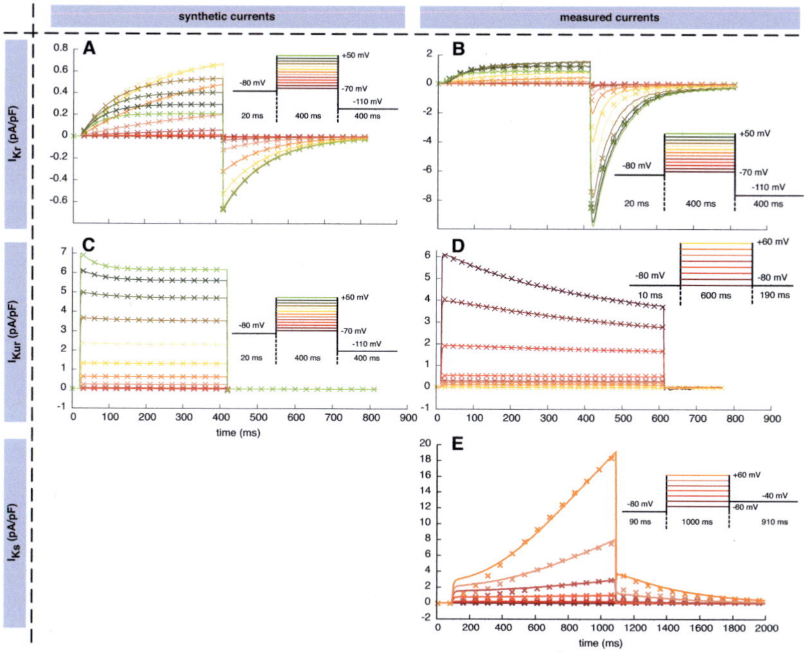

Figure 4.9: Resulting currents using the estimated parameters. Solid lines indicate synthetic ((A) and (C)) and measured ((B), (D), and (E)) input currents used for parameter estimation. Crosses represent the best fit obtained using the *high* setup of the *hybrid (PSO+TRR)+TRR* approach (every 15th sample is shown). (A) and (B) show I_{Kr}, (C) and (D) show I_{Kur}, (E) shows I_{Ks} together with the corresponding voltage protocols.

In the *hybrid (PSO+TRR)+TRR* approach, TRR was run until one of the termination criteria introduced in Section 4.1.1.3 was met. Using this modification, the squared error could only be reduced by <1% (see Figure 4.8). The final TRR step was terminated due to *pTol* in ≈80% of the cases and due to *fTol* in ≈20% irrespective of the current formulation, the parameter ranges, and the algorithm setup being used.

The currents produced by the parameter sets estimated using the high variant of the *hybrid (PSO+TRR)+TRR* approach yielding the highest squared error are shown in Figure 4.9A+C.

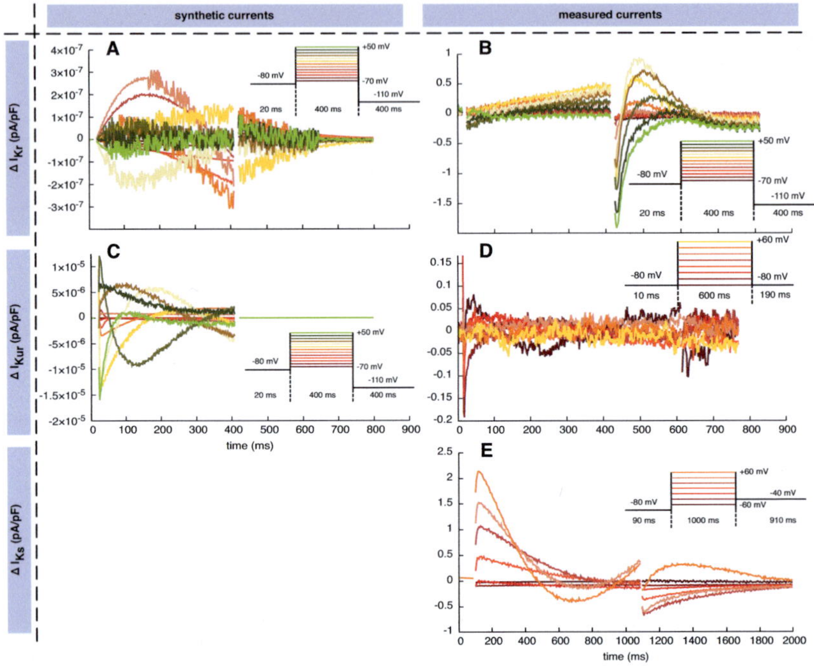

Figure 4.10: Resulting difference between the input currents and the model output using the estimated parameters. The best fit obtained using the *high* setup of the *hybrid (PSO+TRR)+TRR* approach is shown. Samples directly adjacent to voltage steps were ignored in the cost function for the optimization and not plotted. (A) and (B) show I_{Kr}, (C) and (D) show I_{Kur}, (E) shows I_{Ks} together with the corresponding voltage protocols.

For the synthetic data, input and output were visually indistinguishable. Therefore, the magnified difference between the synthetic input data and the model output using the estimated parameters is shown in Figure 4.10A+C. The relative deviation of the estimated parameters from the ground truth parameters used to generate the synthetic input data is shown in Figure 4.11. All twelve I_{Kr} parameters were estimated very accurately with a relative error of <0.1%. For I_{Kur}, some of the 25 parameters deviated significantly. Likely reasons for this observation as well as the offset for g_{Kr} and $u_{i,b2}$ are discussed below (see Section 4.1.3.1).

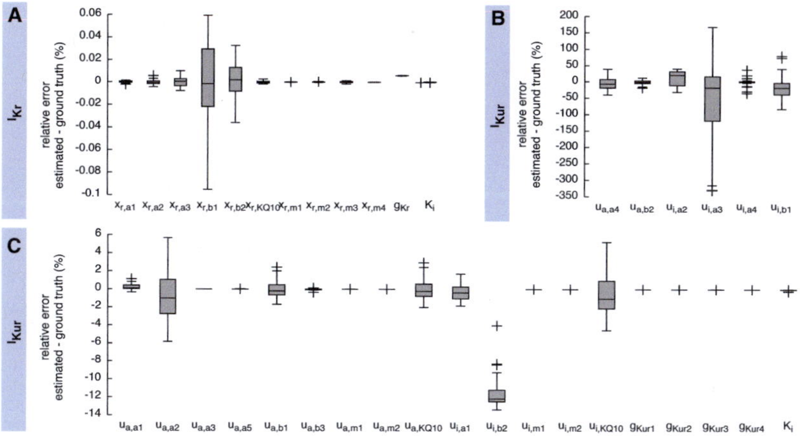

Figure 4.11: Relative error of the estimated parameters using synthetic I_{Kr} (A) and I_{Kur} (B)+(C) data and the *hybrid (PSO+TRR)+TRR* approach in the *high* configuration. Parameter deviations were normalized to their ground truth values. Note the different scales. I_{Kur} parameters were split in high deviation (B) and low deviation (C) groups. Box plots represent 25 experiments.

4.1.2.2 Influence of Noise

The synthetic input data were corrupted with additive white Gaussian noise yielding SNRs of 10, 20, 35, and 60 dB to assess the robustness with respect to noise. The one-stage approaches and the sequential combination of algorithms yielded worse results when raising the SNR to values above 35 dB. The hybrid approach on the other hand proved to be able to cope with data of higher quality as well (see Figure 4.12).

The cost function for the optimization problem was defined as the sum of squared differences between the model output using the estimated parameters and the noisy input data according to Equation (4.9). This metric got worse for signals of poorer quality (increased noise level, thus lower SNR the noise was not reproduced by the model output (see Figure 4.12B+D). The *hybrid (PSO+TRR)* approach yielded better results than simpler approaches for a moderate noise level of 60 dB (2.7×10^{-4} (pA/pF)^2 for *medium* vs. 8.8 10^{-4} (pA/pF)^2 for PSO with N = 12,288).

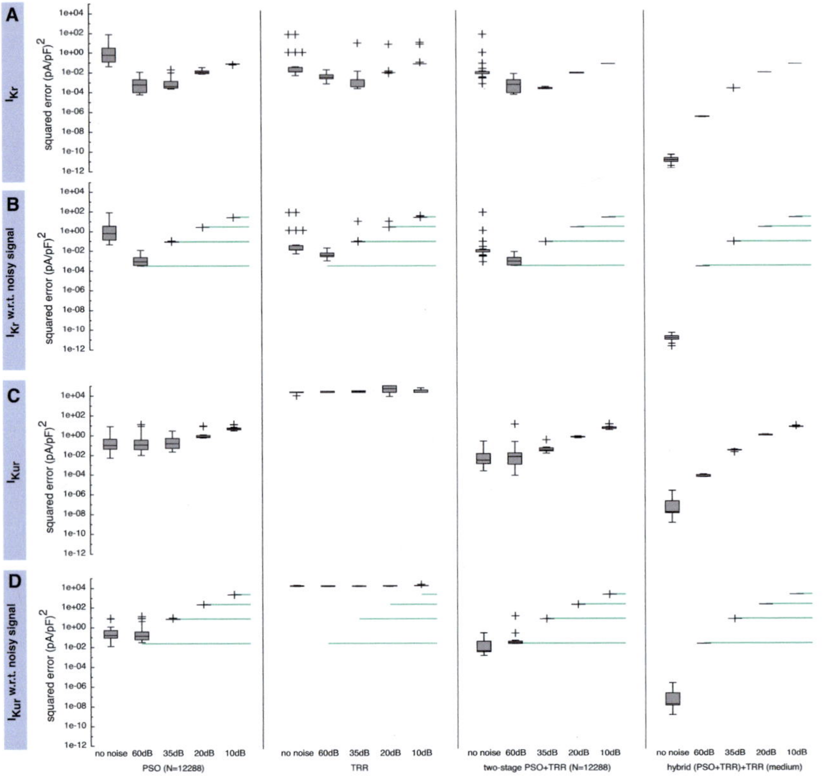

Figure 4.12: Sensitivity of the sum of squared error to noise in synthetic I_{Kr} ((A) and (B)) and I_{Kur} ((C) and (D)) data using pure PSO, pure TRR, *two-stage (PSO+TRR)* and *hybrid (PSO+TRR)+TRR* optimization. The squared error was measured with respect to the original, non-noisy data in (A) and (C). In (B) and (D), the error was measured with respect to the noisy data and the horizontal lines indicate the sum of squared differences between the noisy input data and the ground-truth input data. Parameters were restricted to the wide ranges. Box plots represent 25 experiments.

When increasing the noise level, this difference vanished. For a SNR of 10 dB, all evaluated approaches yielded a sum of squared errors of 2.6×10^1 (pA/pF)^2. For the non-noisy signals of better quality on the other hand, the squared error increased compared to SNR = 60 dB for all but the hybrid approaches. By assuming that the model cannot reproduce the white Gaussian noise, the difference between the noisy and the non-noisy input signal can be considered a lower boundary for the sum of squared errors achieved by the optimization. In this sense, the *hybrid (PSO+TRR)* approach yielded optimal results for all investigated noise levels. While optimal results could be obtained using the PSO and the two-stage PSO+TRR approach for lower quality signals with SNRs below 35 dB as well, they could not cope well with high quality signals. Figure 4.12A+C shows the squared error with respect to the original, non-noisy signal. This is not the cost function which the optimization was subject to. The lower boundary for this metric is zero. The main difference is a lower squared error when relating the model output to the non-noisy signal compared to the corrupted one. For the *hybrid (PSO+TRR)+TRR* approach and a SNR of 60 dB, the squared error was lower by three orders of magnitude. For the one-stage approaches (pure PSO and pure TRR) and *two-stage PSO+TRR*, the squared error was lower for a SNR of 35 dB than for 60 dB. This behavior could not be observed for the hybrid approaches which showed a monotonic increase of error for increasing noise levels also for the quality metric with respect to the ground truth signal.

4.1.2.3 Results Using Measured Data

In contrast to the synthetic input data used in Section 4.1.2.1, measured current data pose additional challenges. In general, a parameter set yielding exactly the input signal as model output does not exist due to noise and other measurement artifacts as well as simplifications in the mathematical models. The best results were obtained using the hybrid approaches for all three investigated currents: I_{Kr}, I_{Kur}, and I_{Ks} (see Figure 4.13). While the choice of the optimization algorithm did not make a significant difference for I_{Kr} (all results within one order of magnitude), the squared error was consistently decreased by one order of magnitude for I_{Kur} by using the hybrid approach. For I_{Ks}, the main advantage of the hybrid approach over the others was reduced variance in the resulting squared error by one order of magnitude.

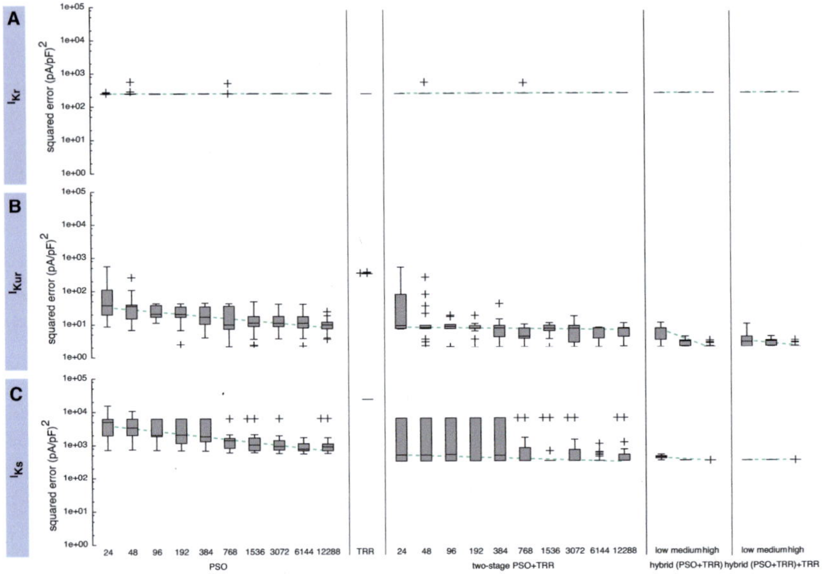

Figure 4.13: Sum of squared errors achieved by pure PSO or TRR, *two-stage PSO+TRR*, *hybrid (PSO+TRR)* and *hybrid (PSO+TRR)+TRR* optimization for measured I_{Kr} (A), I_{Kur} (B) and I_{Ks} (C) data. Parameter values were restricted to the wide range. Note the different scaling compared to Figure 4.4, Figure 4.7, and Figure 4.8. For the one-stage and two-stage PSO approaches the number of particles N was varied. For the hybrid approaches, the number of particles N, the number of PSO iterations L and the number of inner TRR iterations K was increased from *low* via *medium* to *high*. Box plots represent 25 experiments each; the dashed lines indicate linear regressions of the median values in the graph coordinate system.

The slow upstroke following the first voltage step in the measured I_{Kr} current was well reproduced by the model (see Figure 4.9B and Figure 4.10B). The second voltage step down to $-120\,\mathrm{mV}$ caused a fast inward current, which quickly went back to zero again. The Courtemanche et al. current formulation being used in this study could not reproduce this phase well (see Figure 4.9B and Figure 4.10B) because only one gate with a finite time constant is incorporated. The second gate is instantaneous ($\tau = 0\,\mathrm{ms}$), thus forcing the same time constant vs. voltage relation for both step responses. The variance in the resulting squared error was smaller when TRR was incorporated in the optimization (see Figure 4.13A) as was the case for synthetic I_{Kr} input data (see Section 4.1.2.1).

Regarding I_{Kur}, the results using the measured input currents were also comparable to the characteristics observed using the synthetic input data (see Figure 4.13B). First, PSO performed better than TRR (9.4 (pA/pF)^2 for pure PSO with N = 12,288 vs. 3.2$\times$10^2 (pA/pF)^2 for pure TRR). Second, *hybrid (PSO+TRR)* was superior to the sequential combination (*two-stage PSO+TRR*) in terms of both the median and the maximum squared error. The model output currents using the estimated parameters were visually indistinguishable from the input data (see Figure 4.9D). The remaining difference in Figure 4.10D showed no clear pattern which could be traced back to the voltage protocol and was dominated by measurement noise.
The algorithm performance for the Courtemanche et al. I_{Ks} formulation was only assessed using measured data and showed comparable characteristics as were observed for I_{Kur}. PSO performed better than TRR for sufficiently large N (see Figure 4.13C). However, two differences could be observed. First, the variance in the resulting squared error using the *two-stage PSO+TRR* approach was significantly larger for I_{Ks} compared to I_{Kur}, as well as compared to pure PSO. Second, the main advantage of the hybrid over the two-stage approach was a reduced variance in the resulting squared error rather than a reduction of the median error. The resulting current reproduced the steady-state currents well (see Figure 4.9E). The difference signal with respect to the input data (Figure 4.10E) reveals that the biphasic nature of the response to the first voltage step could not be well reproduced. While the slow, exponential increase was covered by the Courtemanche et al. I_{Ks} formulation comprising four identical x_s gates, the almost instantaneous upstroke was not.

4.1.2.4 Computing Times

Table 4.1 gives an overview of the median computing times (n = 25) of the different algorithms. All experiments were performed on Mac Pro machines equipped with two 2.4 GHz *Intel Xeon E5645* processors with six cores each and 64 GB RAM under Mac OS X (*Apple Inc., Cupertino, CA, USA*). PSO was the least computationally expensive algorithm, in general.

Table 4.1: Median computing times in seconds (n = 25) for the parameter estimation using synthetic (s) and measured (m) input data. For pure PSO and *two-stage PSO+TRR*, the number of particles was set to N = 1,536. For *hybrid*, the *medium* setup was used.

	sI_{Kr} (s)	sI_{Kur} (s)	mI_{Kr} (s)	mI_{Kur} (s)	mI_{Ks} (s)
PSO	475	714	839	569	341
TRR	40	2,747	2,763	1,570	599
two-stage PSO+TRR	532	2,096	854	832	361
hybrid (PSO+TRR)	7,392	20,220	8,923	21,840	3,687
hybrid (PSO+TRR)+TRR	7,393	20,225	8,925	21,894	3,692

One exception were the synthetic I_{Kr} data for which TRR was faster than PSO by one order of magnitude. TRR converged faster when particle swarm optimized start vectors were used (*two-stage PSO+TRR*) compared to random initial guesses (pure TRR) even when counting in the time spent for PSO.
For the synthetic data and the hybrid approaches applied to the measured data, I_{Kur} was computationally more expensive than the other two currents. The hybrid approaches took the longest time compared to the one-stage approaches or sequential combination of algorithms (2.5 h for I_{Kr}, 6.1 h for I_{Kur}, and 1.0 h for I_{Ks} using the measured data). In general, synthetic and measured input data did not lead to significantly different computing times. However, TRR was faster using the synthetic data by two orders of magnitude for I_{Kr} and pure TRR as well as *two-stage PSO+TRR* were faster by a factor of $\approx$2 for measured I_{Kur}. The convergence of the final TRR step in the *hybrid (PSO+TRR)+TRR* approach was faster using the synthetic data than using the measured data. For I_{Kr}, it was terminated within 2 s for the synthetic and within 3 s for the measured data in all cases. For I_{Kur}, the maximum times were 20 s and 1167 s. For the measured I_{Ks} data, the final TRR step converged within less than 700 s in all cases.
For all investigated approaches, less than 5% of the time was spent in algorithm-specific code and more than 95% on the evaluation of the cost function Equation (4.9).

4.1.3 Discussion

In the study described in this section, the population-based PSO, the gradient-based TRR algorithm, as well as sequential and tightly coupled combinations of both algorithms were evaluated regarding their performance for parameter estimation of cardiac ion channel formulations. The suitability was assessed in terms of accuracy and robustness with respect to noise and the choice of the initial guess.

4.1.3.1 Algorithm Performance

The type of problem, i.e. the current for which the parameters are estimated, had a huge impact on the performance of the two algorithms being used stand-alone (one-stage approaches). While the results obtained using TRR were significantly better for I_{Kr}, PSO outperformed TRR by orders of magnitude for I_{Kur} data. By combining the two algorithms sequentially (*two-stage PSO+TRR*), the median error could be reduced. This benefit came, however, at the expense of a larger variance, particularly when the search space was extended to the wide parameter ranges. As the performance of the one-after-the-other combination was not satisfactory, the algorithms were coupled in each PSO iteration in the newly proposed *hybrid (PSO+TRR)* approach. This novel scheme yielded consistently low median and maximum squared error values. Thus, the variance for experiments using different initial guesses was minimal. The observed characteristics can be explained by the properties of the different optimization problems. The cost function for I_{Kr} parameter estimation was relatively well fit by the quadratic approximation in TRR. Moreover, the gradient-based TRR approach could overcome local minima due to their relatively low number and shallow nature. The cost function for I_{Kur} on the other hand was characterized by extensive plateaus with narrow and steep minima. Therefore, the random movement of the PSO particles helped to overcome the plateaus. Furthermore, the incorporation of the gradient information in each PSO iteration was needed to identify the actual minima and descend into them. Regarding pure PSO, we showed that the first few iterations are crucial. A high number of iterations did not help to prevent bad results if the swarm moved in a bad direction at the start.

Regarding signal quality and noise conditions, the results got worse when the quality of the input data, thus the noise conditions of the experimental design, were improved for the non-hybrid approaches. This observation can be explained by the accuracy requirements. The fewer noise there is in the signal, the narrower is the margin of parameters yielding the optimal results in the sense of the cost function. Thus, the minima in the cost function are more articulated for less noisy signals and more blurred for signals of lower quality. Hence, the probability to get stuck in a local minimum can be reduced by adding noise to the signal. Conversely, this implies that the parameter estimation approach being used must be capable of handling data of the quality at hand. We showed that the novel hybrid approach proposed in this study is not limited in this respect and is suitable for data of arbitrary high quality. Moreover, the approach yields the optimal result up to the theoretical limit for noisy data.
The accuracy provided by the hybrid approach is probably higher than required for most applications. However, Figure 4.14 shows an example of the physiological relevance of the superiority regarding the quality of fit. While the *two-stage PSO+TRR* approach (Figure 4.14A) failed to reproduce the I_{Kur} dynamics for medium step voltages and yielded almost piece-wise constant current traces, the *hybrid (PSO+TRR)* approach (Figure 4.14B) succeeded to fully capture the gating kinetics resulting in a good reproduction of the current dynamics. Moreover, the hybrid approach estimated the I_{Kr} and most of the I_{Kur} parameters very accurately. For g_{Kr}, a small (0.01%) but consistent offset was observed as well as for $u_{i,b2}$ (Figure 4.11). These offsets can be explained by different implementations used to calculate the currents during the generation of synthetic measurement data (*C++*, intermediate parameter discretized in look up tables) and for the evaluation of the cost function during the optimization (*Matlab*, accurate up to machine precision) and the interface between the two (text files with limited precision). In order to be useful in practical application, the ability to generate reliable estimates in a single run regardless of the initial guess is of great importance. The newly proposed hybrid approach proved to fully meet this requirement as shown particularly for wet-lab I_{Kur} and I_{Ks} data (see Figure 4.13).

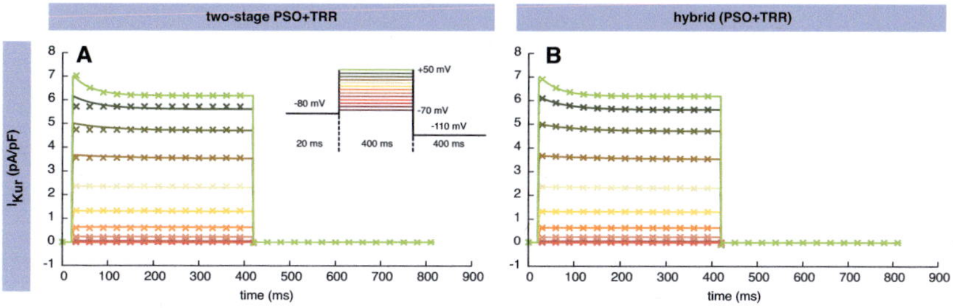

Figure 4.14: Resulting I_{Kur} curves using the parameters estimated by the *two-stage PSO+TRR* (A) and the *hybrid (PSO+TRR)* approach in the *medium* setup (B) together with the corresponding voltage protocols. Solid lines indicate synthetic input currents used for parameter estimation. Crosses represent the worst fit obtained using the respective approach and the wide parameter ranges (every 15th sample is shown). Differences are most pronounced for step voltages between +20 mV and +40 mV.

Regarding the measured data, several reasons are likely to have contributed to the remaining deviation between the input data and the model output using the optimized parameters. First, there are differences between the model and the expression system used to acquire the data. hERG for example only codes for the α-subunit of I_{Kr} while the data used in the original Courtemanche et al. formulation [47] also comprised the β-subunit. Moreover, the measurements were conducted at room temperature rather than at 37° C. Second, measurement noise corrupted the signals. Third, the model formulations being used are simplifications of the actual biophysical systems being analyzed. For I_{Kr}, it has been shown that at least four gates are necessary to fully capture human atrial I_{Kr} [210] while the Courtemanche et al. formulation comprises only one gate with a time constant and a second instantaneous gate. In the I_{Ks} data, there was an almost immediate response to the first voltage step in addition to the commonly observed transient response (see Figure 4.9E). This might be due to the contribution of background currents, which could be addressed and eliminated in a pre-processing step. Fourth, the current traces measured in several cells were averaged to improve the SNR. While this is common practice, it is important to keep the non-linearity of the system in mind. Thus, the model might be able to reproduce the current recorded in each single cell but not the average current.

4.1.3.2 Recommended Approach

The requirements regarding accuracy, robustness and reliability are fully satisfied by the *hybrid (PSO+TRR)+TRR* approach in the *medium* setup as shown by the results in Section 4.1.2. The computing time was below 7 h for one run, thus a good balance between computational cost and quality of fit was achieved. The results regarding the convergence behavior (see Figure 4.5C and Figure 4.6C) suggest that the number of iterations could be lowered to $\approx$300 without a marked loss of quality of the result. The final step of TRR optimization until convergence did not improve the result significantly on the one hand. On the other hand, it did not account for a large share of the computational effort because the algorithm had already almost converged, particularly for synthetic data. While this was also the case for wet-lab I_{Kr} data (being another indicator for the benign nature of this optimization problem), the final TRR step took 35$\times$ longer using measured than using synthetic data for I_{Kur}. This observation fits well with the remarks in Section 4.1.3.1 and can be explained by the absence of a well-defined, convex minimum.
As can be seen in Figure 4.13, the variance in the results is minimal using the *hybrid (PSO+TRR)+TRR* approach in the *medium* setup. Thus, a single run is sufficient to estimate the optimal parameters reliably. This advantage of the hybrid approach outweighs the additional computation time, which was longer by one order of magnitude compared to the two-stage approach. However, the larger variance in the results of the two-stage approach requires several independent runs with different start vectors to reliably obtain a result close to the optimal result possible with this approach, which is still not as good as the result reliably obtained with the newly proposed hybrid approach in a single run. The cost function for each of the particles can be evaluated independently and thus in parallel. Hence, highly parallel hardware architectures, such as graphics processing units (GPUs), could be used to exploit the pronounced parallel nature of the problem and reduce the computation time further.
For the *two-stage PSO+TRR* approach, the parameter search space should be set neither too narrow (compare Figure 4.7C and Figure 4.7D) nor too wide (compare Figure 4.7A and Figure 4.7B). The counter-intuitive observation of lower errors for wider parameter ranges observed for I_{Kur} might be caused by the way the ranges are enforced in the presented variant of the PSO algorithm. When a parameter left the search space, it was randomly placed within a 25%

margin of the size of the allowed parameter interval starting at the border being crossed. Narrowing the 25% range with each iteration during the course of the optimization did not affect the results significantly, however (data not shown). Also in this respect, the hybrid approach proved to be robust and not sensitive to the choice of the parameter ranges advocating its use. In summary, the newly proposed hybrid approach tightly coupling PSO and TRR proved to yield accurate and reliable results for a variety of measured and synthetic currents and regardless of noise conditions and the choice of parameter ranges. Metaheuristic approaches have been proposed earlier for parameter estimation in the field of cardiac electrophysiology: e.g. PSO [193, 194] or genetic algorithms [195–197]. However, this is the first combination of the two approaches in a hybrid scheme [198, 199] for this purpose to the best of my knowledge. The presented results underline that such hybridization is imperative when requiring accurate and reliable parameter estimates. The results of a pilot study suggested genetic algorithm performance to be comparable to PSO (data not shown).

4.1.3.3 Limitations

The parameter estimation pipeline presented in this study can not guarantee that the system being fit is in steady state because only one stimulus is applied during each evaluation of the cost function. However, transient oscillations should not be a problem as the parameters change rather slowly, particularly during later iterations which determine the final result. Furthermore, artifacts stemming from non-steady-state conditions are more of a problem when fitting current densities in a whole-cell model with a complex interplay (see e.g. Section 6.3) than in problems involving only a single current formulation as only the initial values of the gating variables are concerned and ion concentrations etc. do not change. Therefore, the presented approach was chosen based on the balance between runtime and steady-state approximation. Moreover, the stimulus protocol applied during the parameter estimation is equal to the one applied in the wet-lab, thus deviations from steady-state are similar.
All approaches presented in this study cannot provide information on the sensitivity of the system to changes of certain parameters and parameter identifiability. Regression-based algorithms (see e.g. Section 4.2 or [211–213])

or methods based on local sensitivity analysis [214, 215] can in part provide such information in addition to an estimate of the parameters. However, an evaluation of a representative approach of this family of algorithms in Section 4.2 shows that such statistical approaches also struggle with more challenging formulations like I_{Kur}. Future work could combine approaches aiming at a parameter identifiability analysis like proposed in [213, 216] with the hybrid parameter estimation approach presented here. Considering that several I_{Kur} parameters turned out to be hardly identifiable using the voltage protocol employed in this study, a pre-step identifying the set of parameters to be appropriately estimated appears advisable. Then, the hybrid approach could subsequently be applied to actually estimate the values of that subset of parameters.

The assessment of the parameter estimation algorithms in this study was conducted using measured and synthetic data from three different potassium currents. The choice was made based on the range of characteristics being covered (e.g. fast I_{Kur} kinetics vs. rather slow I_{Kr}) and the availability of wet-lab data. The type of ions carrying the current do not make a difference, thus the results should also hold for other currents. Provided that the data are acquired with sufficient temporal resolution, also currents with even faster kinetics (e.g. I_{Na}) can be handled as the algorithm itself is time-agnostic. The current formulations were all taken from the Courtemanche et al. model of human atrial myocytes [47]. This model convinced in a benchmark of different atrial models [156] and is widely used. Despite the choice being made for this study, the presented methods can be applied to other atrial models (like [217–220]), ventricular models (e.g. [221, 222]), or even other types of cells like neurons. The results found in this study should hold for these kinds of models, as well. The method should also be applicable to Markov models of ion channels rather than pure Hodgkin-Huxley type models [216].

4.1.3.4 Outlook and Conclusion

The fact that a number of I_{Kur} parameters were hardly identifiable in this study stems from an insensitivity of the formulation to these parameters with respect to the voltage protocol being used leading to an abundance of local minima.

The voltage protocol did not challenge all mechanisms included in the model comprehensively. Particularly, the second voltage step down to –110 mV did not elicit a current of significant amplitude. A more comprehensive voltage protocol might render the optimization problem a litte more benign. The fact that TRR did often not converge to a solution but was terminated due to the maximum number of iterations shows the challenging nature of the problem in the setting being used in this study. Further contributors to the relatively large differences between the estimated and ground truth I_{Kur} parameters (see Figure 4.11B) are dependencies between the parameters and model sloppiness [213].

The population-based approaches employed in this study were feasible because the ODEs underlying the ion current formulations were solved analytically and thus drastically faster than would have been the case using numerical solvers. The fact that over 95% of the computation time was spent for the repeated evaluation of the cost function highlights the importance of a streamlined cost function implementation. While the analytic solution is faster by a factor of ≈1000 compared to numerical approximation [201], the voltage protocols are restricted to piecewise constant functions in this case. On the other hand, parameter identifiability can be improved by employing more complex voltage protocols [216, 223], which can comprise non-piecewise constant functions [224, 225]. Whether the additional computational effort for a single cost function evaluation is outbalanced by improved parameter identifiability and potentially faster convergence has to be assessed for each problem individually.

The definition of the cost function is a potential field for advancement of the presented method. Phases considered to be more important, e.g. highly dynamic phases elicited by a voltage step or elicited by steps to voltages considered to be physiologically more relevant, could be assigned higher weights. Furthermore, traces with bad SNR could be neglected. An alternative to the sum of squared errors employed in this study (see Equation (4.9)) is to incorporate *a priori* knowledge about the signal morphology. For typical cardiac ion currents, the coefficients of mono- or bi-exponential functions could be determined through curve fitting (see Section 4.2.1). The (potentially weighted) difference of the coefficients obtained for the input data and model output could then be used as the cost function.

The methods presented in this section, particularly the newly proposed hybrid scheme, allow to incorporate altered ion channel behavior caused by genetic mutations or the influence of pharmacological agents into mathematical models routinely. As these models are often embedded in multi-scale simulation environments, the effect of changes on the ion channel level on higher levels of integration can be assessed comprehensively. Section 5.1 gives an example of how changes in hERG translate to altered behavior in the whole-cell, the tissue, and the (pseudo) ECG level. The novel hybrid strategy comprising population-based PSO and gradient-based TRR facilitates parameter estimation of ion current formulation by providing very accurate, reliable and robust results. Using this method, experimental data can be transferred into computational models in a single run, thus it is an important tool to exploit and leverage today's and tomorrow's high-throughput patch clamp methods. A comprehensive multi-scale assessment of the effect of changes on the ion channel is imperative as the biophysical systems of interest are mostly complex and non-linear. Hence, changes on a lower level often translate to counter-intuitive effects on higher levels of integration. In Section 5.1, two hERG mutations are assessed using such methodology.

4.2 Multivariate Metamodeling

The results presented and discussed in the section above give a nice example of how some parameters of ion current formulations are hardly identifiable. This effect could be shown for the combination of the I_{Kur} formulation and the voltage protocol presented in Section 4.1.1 for the special case of synthetically generated input data with known ground truth parameter values. However, in practical parameter estimation applications, the ground truth is not available as a matter of course. Therefore, some algorithms aim to provide information on identifiability of and sensitivity to the parameters besides an estimate of their value. Tøndel et al. presented a comprehensive parameter fitting framework recently [213] and used it to quantify interspecies differences in contractile function [226]. In this section, the method is adapted for the voltage clamp ion current application introduced in Section 4.1 and evaluated.
Parts of this study have been conducted in a supervised student's project [227].

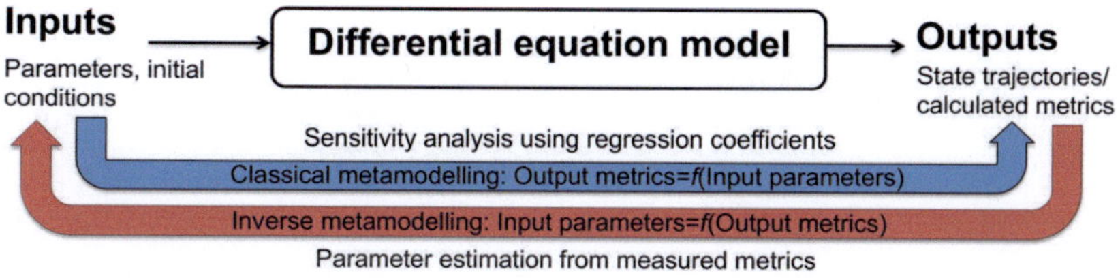

Figure 4.15: Basic concept of classical and inverse metamodeling. Classical (forward) metamodeling predicts the output of the detailed differential equation model using the input parameters aiming at a sensitivity analysis based on the regression coefficients of the metamodel. Inverse metamodeling on the other hand estimates the input parameters based on the output. In this case, the input is composed of the parameters of the detailed model and the output is represented by the measurements. Figure from [213].

4.2.1 Methods

Voltage protocols applied to ion current formulations link a set of model parameters $\mathbf{X}$ to a set of output metrics $\mathbf{Y}$:

$$\mathbf{X} \xrightarrow[voltage\ protocol]{ion\ current\ formulation} \mathbf{Y}\,. \tag{4.15}$$

$\mathbf{X}$ is of size $n \times m$, with n being the number of instantiations, so-called *experimental designs*, and m being the number of model parameters. Thus, $\mathbf{X}$ is a set of parameter vectors like the ones used for PSO. $\mathbf{Y}$ is of size $n \times k$ with k being the number of output metrics.

4.2.1.1 State of the Art

The approach presented in this section is composed of two metamodeling steps. Figure 4.15 illustrates the basic concept of classical and inverse metamodeling. The classical metamodel is built by a partial least squares regression (PLSR) [228–230] of the model output $\mathbf{Y}$ (features describing the current traces) based on the model parameters $\mathbf{X}$:

$$\hat{\mathbf{Y}} = \mathbf{X}\mathbf{b}\,. \tag{4.16}$$

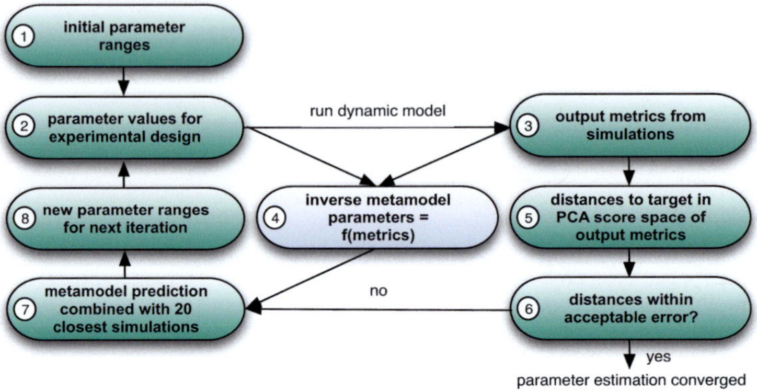

Figure 4.16: Multivariate metamodeling pipeline. After the initial parameter ranges are set in step 1, steps 2-8 are iteratively repeated until the termination criterion in step 6 is met. Step 8 zooms successively into interesting parameter ranges. Figure concept from [213].

The regression coefficients in $\mathbf{b}$ provide information on the sensitivity of the model output $\mathbf{Y}$ to the model parameters $\mathbf{X}$, as well as coupling between model parameters. The inverse metamodel on the other hand is used to analyze parameter identifiability and to estimate the values of the model parameters $\mathbf{X}$ given a set of output metrics $\mathbf{Y}$, which is normally a more ill-posed problem than model output prediction [213]. Towards this end, a non-linear extension of the PLSR method is employed: hierarchical cluster-based partial least squares regression (HC-PLSR) [231, 232]. The sets of measurement data which are compared to the model output are called *observations* and are separated into groups by HC-PLSR using fuzzy C-means clustering [233–236]. The fuzzy C-means clustering is performed on the latent variables of a global PLSR model. Within each cluster, the method builds linear local PLSR models. The output is then predicted using a weighted sum of the local models. This approach has proven to be well suited for highly non-linear input-output relationships [213]. In order to handle values of different magnitudes and compensate for offsets, both the input parameters and the output metrics were centered and normalized by the standard deviation before the regression.

Figure 4.16 gives an overview of the automatic parameter fitting pipeline. In each iteration, n sets of parameter values (experimental designs) are drawn randomly from the parameter search space using latin hypercube sampling (LHS) and assembled in **X** (step 2 in Figure 4.16). LHS is a method to generate a collection of parameter value sets from a multidimensional distribution [237]. For the ion current formulation application, the dimensionality was given by the number of parameters to estimate. LHS divides the search space into hypercubes equidistantly along each parameter axis and samples randomly within each hypercube. In this way, it is guaranteed that each segment of a parameter axis is sampled while retaining random sampling. Then, the ion current model output is computed for each of the n experimental designs. Output metrics are calculated for each model output, assembled in **Y**, and compared to the metrics of the input data (measurements) (step 3 in Figure 4.16). In general, any output metric can be used. The particular metrics being used in this study for the ion current application are outlined below.

The comparison is not conducted directly on the output metrics but after transformation using principal component analysis (PCA) (step 5 in Figure 4.16). Thus, the root mean square differences (RMSDs) of the output metrics yielded by the experimental designs and the target output is computed using the PCA scores. The minimal number of principal components explaining 99% of the variance in the output metrics are considered for the distance calculation. Thus, the PCA approach reduces the dimensionality of the problem and inherently weighs the metrics according to their contribution to the variation in the output metrics. If the RMSDs obtained using the experimental designs are within the predefined tolerable error margins, the algorithm terminates (step 6 in Figure 4.16). If this is not the case, the next iteration is initiated by combining the 20 experimental designs with the best output metrics and the parameter set yielded by HC-PLSR in the inverse metamodel (step 4 in Figure 4.16). The output of the metamodel was only considered for the parameters yielding a prediction accuracy of >70%. The prediction accuracy was determined with the Pearson product-moment correlation coefficient R^2 [238] using a test set validation. Only two thirds of the experimental designs were used for the calibration of the inverse metamodel while the remaining third was used as the test set. The correlation related the input and the predicted values. The set of 21 experimental setups in step 7 in Figure 4.16 is called the *guideline set* $\mathbf{X}_{\mathbf{guideline}}$.

The parameter ranges are adjusted in each iteration depending on the performance of the current set of experimental designs and the range spanned by the guideline set (step 8 in Figure 4.16):

$$upperBound_j \leftarrow \max\left(\mathbf{X_{guideline,j}}\right) + \left|\frac{\overline{\mathbf{X_{guideline,j}}}}{stepsize}\right|, \tag{4.17}$$

$$lowerBound_j \leftarrow \min\left(\mathbf{X_{guideline,j}}\right) - \left|\frac{\overline{\mathbf{X_{guideline,j}}}}{stepsize}\right|, \tag{4.18}$$

with j being the index of the parameter $\in [1,m]$, $\overline{\mathbf{X_{guideline,j}}}$ being the mean value of the parameter with the index j with respect to the guideline set, and *stepsize* being a parameter controlling the zooming into the parameter space. Depending on the proximity of the model output using the current estimates to the target outputs, *stepsize* is adjusted. Starting from an initial value of 4, it is increased by 2 if the minimum RMSD in the PCA score space has decreased in the current iteration. Thus, the search space gets more constrained, the closer the distance to the target output metrics gets. The maximum allowed value is 20. If it is reached without meeting the termination criteria, it is decreased by 2 for the next iteration. Using the new parameter ranges, the experimental designs for the next iteration are again determined using LHS.

4.2.1.2 Extension of the Parameter Estimation Pipeline

Below, the modifications and extensions of the parameter fitting pipeline by Tøndel et al. [213] performed during the scope of this work in order to allow for estimation of ion current formulation parameters are described. As outlined in Section 4.1.1.1, the response of most ion current models to a piecewise constant voltage protocol can be modeled as a series of exponential functions. Starting with Equation (4.2) and Equation (4.8), the following transformations can be established exemplary for the I_{Kr} gate x_r:

$$I_{Kr} = \underbrace{g_{Kr}\frac{V_m - E_K}{1+\exp\left(\frac{V_m + x_{r,m1}}{x_{r,m2}}\right)}}_{a} \cdot \left(\underbrace{x_{r\infty}}_{b} - \left(x_{r\infty} - \underbrace{x_{r0}}_{c}\right) \cdot \exp\left(\frac{\overbrace{t_0}^{d} - t}{\tau}\right)\right) \tag{4.19}$$

$$I_{Kr} = \underbrace{(a \cdot b)}_{\text{A}} + \underbrace{a(c-b) \cdot \exp\left(\frac{d}{\tau}\right)}_{\text{B}} \cdot \exp\left(-\frac{t}{\tau}\right) \tag{4.20}$$

$$= A + B \cdot \exp\left(-\frac{t}{\tau}\right) \tag{4.21}$$

The parameters A, B, and τ can be estimated for each phase of measured or synthetic current traces using standard curve fitting tools provided by *Matlab*. Thus, besides the squared error used in Section 4.1, an alternative way to quantify the quality of the cell model's adaption to measured current data is to compare A, B, and τ for each phase of the current traces. One phase was defined for each voltage step of each voltage trace. I_{Kr} traces were fitted using mono-exponential functions, whereas bi-exponential functions were required to fit I_{Kur} traces. While the Courtemanche et al. I_{Ks} formulation comprising four identical x_s gates requires higher order functions in theory, the voltage protocols being used in this study did only elicit currents that could be well fitted by mono-exponential functions. The coefficients of the exponential functions were used as output metrics for this study. As three coefficients were required for mono-exponential functions, k (the number of output metrics) was $3 \times l \times p$ for I_{Kr} and I_{Ks} with l being the number of voltage traces and p being the number of phases (voltage steps) in each trace resulting in $k \in [66,99]$. For the I_{Kr} voltage protocols with 13 different step voltages and 2 phases, this equates to 78 output metrics. All output metrics were equally weighted.

4.2.1.3 Test Cases

The initial parameter search space was set according to the *wide* ranges in Table A.1, Table A.2, and Table A.3. n, the number of experimental designs, was set to 500 and the number of clusters in the HC-PLSR method was set to eight for all experiments described below. The acceptable error margins of the output metrics used as the termination criterion in step 6 in Figure 4.16 were set to $\pm 10\%$ of the target exponential coefficients. All code was implemented in *Matlab* with parallel computation of the model output for the n experimental designs.

The approach introduced above was evaluated using synthetic and measured current data. The first voltage protocol (referred to as "*protocol A*"), was similar to the one used for the synthetic data in Section 4.1.1 and used for I_{Kr} and I_{Kur}. *Protocol A* was composed of 13 traces consisting of 20 ms at –80 mV resting voltage, 380 ms at the respective step voltage ranging from –70 mV to +50 mV in steps of 10 mV, and 400 ms at –110 mV (see Figure 4.17A and Figure 4.21B). *Protocol B* started at –80 mV for 20 ms followed by a 500 ms conditioning pulse to +40 mV and 5 s test pulses to eleven different voltages between –100 mV and 0 mV in steps of 10 mV. Each trace was ended with 500 ms at –80 mV. *Protocol B* was designed to obtain the properties of the fully activated I_{Kr} [239] and is shown in Figure 4.17B. *Protocol C* challenging the I_{Kr} tail currents [239] started with 20 ms at –80 mV followed by 2 s test pulses to eleven different voltages between –40 mV and +60 mV in steps of 10 mV and finished with 6 s at –40 mV (see Figure 4.17C). For I_{Ks}, *protocol D* was used [240], which was composed of 50 ms at –80 mV followed by 2 s test pulses to voltages between –100 mV and +100 mV in steps of 20 mV. Each trace was closed by a 0.95 s step back to –50 mV (see Figure 4.21B). The resulting currents were sampled every 2 ms.

4.2.2 Results

4.2.2.1 Rapid Delayed Rectifier Potassium Current I_{Kr}

The multivariate metamodeling approach was evaluated for the Courtemanche et al. I_{Kr} formulation by impressing the three voltage protocols *A*, *B*, and *C*. The resulting currents are shown in Figure 4.17. While the model output using the estimated parameters was visually close to the synthetic input data for voltage protocol *A* (Figure 4.17A), quantitative analysis revealed a sum of squared differences of 46 (pA/pF)^2. Using protocols *B* and *C* on the other hand, marked differences were observed. For voltage protocol *B*, the steady state values at the end of the second phase deviated for higher step voltages (Figure 4.17B). The same behavior was observed for the first phase of voltage protocol *C* (Figure 4.17C).

A sensitivity analysis of the output variables (exponential coefficients) to the model parameters was conducted by using the regression coefficients of the PLSR-based classical metamodel as sensitivity measures. Figure 4.18A shows the most sensitive output variables for voltage protocol A. The cumulative sensitivity with respect to all model parameters was used to select the most interesting output variables. 41 of the 78 variables were less sensitive than 70% of the maximum cumulative sensitivity and thus not plotted. Some input parameters were reflected in output variables belonging to certain step voltages.

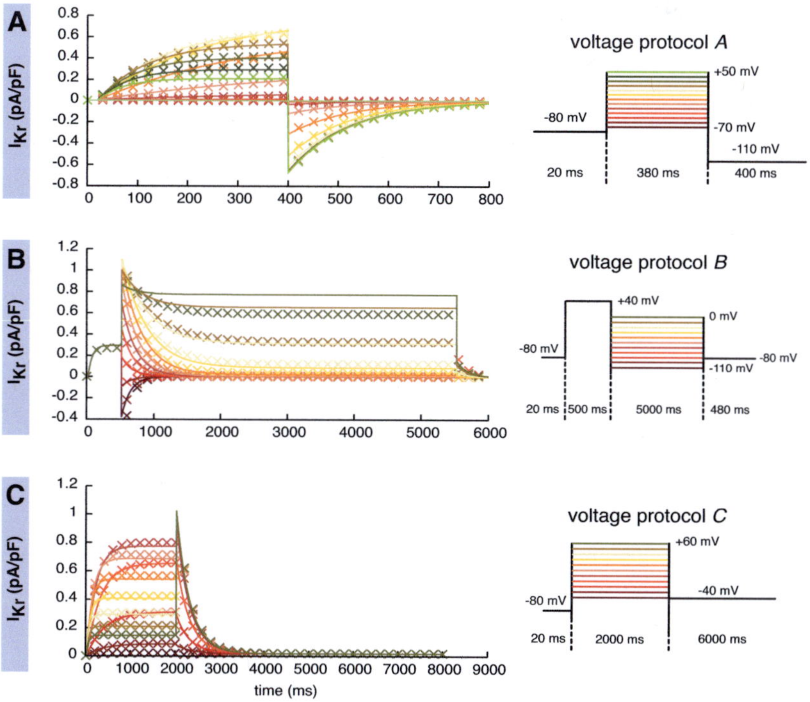

Figure 4.17: Resulting currents using the parameters estimated by the multivariate metamodeling approach. Solid lines indicate synthetic I_{Kr} input currents used for parameter estimation. Crosses represent the best fit obtained (not every sample shown for clarity reasons). The voltage protocols used to generate the input data and to challenge the ion current model are shown on the right part of each panel.

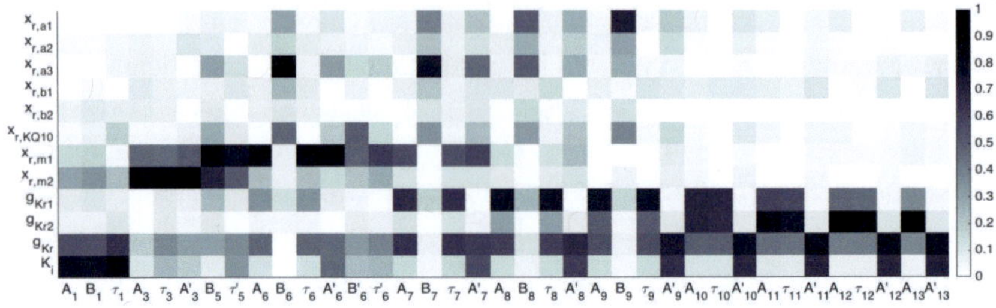

Figure 4.18: Sensitivity of output variables to the parameters of the Courtemanche et al. I_{Kr} formulation and voltage protocol *A* in terms of regression coefficients. A threshold of 70% of the maximum value selected 37 of the 78 output variables. The subscript of the output variable refers to the voltage trace. A, B, and τ are the exponential coefficients determined for the first phase of each voltage trace, whereas A', B', and τ' represent the second phase. Output variables were selected based on the cumulated sensitivity with respect to all model parameters.

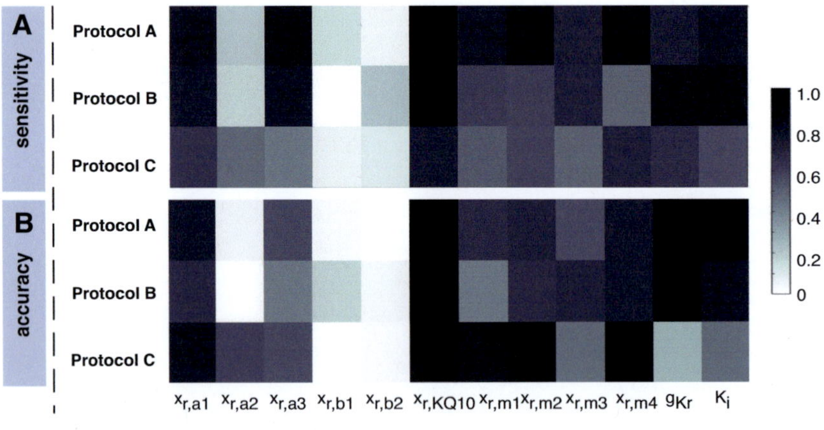

Figure 4.19: Maximum sensitivity (regression coefficients) across the 78 output variables to the parameters of the Courtemanche et al. I_{Kr} formulation (A) as well as parameter prediction accuracy (R^2) in (B) using different voltage protocols (see Figure 4.17).

The intracellular potassium concentration K_i, e.g., translated to changes in all three exponential coefficients defining the first phase (the voltage step) of the trace with a step voltage of –70 mV. Changes in $x_{r,m2}$ translated mostly to changes in the voltage trace with a step voltage of –50 mV. Changes of other parameters like $x_{r,b1}$ and $x_{r,b2}$ were not significantly reflected in the output variables.

The overall sensitivity of the output variables to the model parameters for the different voltage protocols A, B, and C is shown in Figure 4.19A in terms of the maximum sensitivity across all output variables. While the gross pattern is consistent across the three protocols, changes of certain model parameters did translate to markedly more pronounced changes for some protocols than for others. The sensitivity of the output variables to $x_{r,a1}$ for example was higher for protocol C than for the others. The Courtemanche et al. I_{Kr} formulation was hardly sensitive to $x_{r,b1}$ and $x_{r,b2}$ for all investigated voltage protocols, though.

The accuracy of the parameter estimation was assessed by correlating the simulated and the predicted values using the test set in the inverse metamodel. The overall pattern of parameter prediction accuracy (Figure 4.19B) matches that of the sensitivity of the output variables to these parameters (Figure 4.19A). This shows on the one hand that the inverse metamodel does its job of estimating the parameters well, in general. On the other hand, this observation confirms that model parameters that hardly translate into changes of the output variables cannot be estimated well.

While the patterns of sensitivity and accuracy show gross correspondence, differences were observed as well. The achieved accuracy to $x_{r,a2}$ for example was lower than the sensitivity for voltage protocols A and B. Moreover, the performance of the three protocols differed. While protocol B yielded the lowest sensitivity to $x_{r,b1}$, it performed best in terms of accuracy. The differences were not very pronounced and revealed no consistent pattern, though.

Comparing the differences between the estimated parameters and the parameter set used to generate the synthetic input data (ground truth) yielded results corresponding to the sensitivity and accuracy analysis. The algorithm was blinded to the ground truth values as a matter of course. Figure 4.20 shows the distribution of relative errors considering the three voltage protocols. The minimum error was high for parameters yielding low sensitivity and accuracy values ($x_{r,b1}$, $x_{r,b2}$) and low for parameters performing well in terms of sensitivity and accuracy ($x_{r,KQ10}$ to K_i). Interestingly, the intermediate sensitivity and accuracy values observed for $x_{r,a2}$ and $x_{r,a3}$ translated to high errors with a comparable amplitude like $x_{r,b1}$ and $x_{r,b2}$.

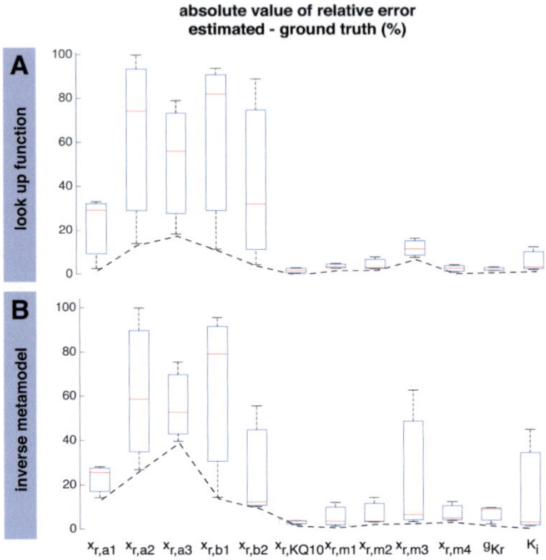

Figure 4.20: Distribution of the relative error of the estimated parameters for the three voltage protocols *A*, *B*, and *C* and the I_{Kr} input data. (A) shows the results obtained by the look up function, whereas (B) shows the results yielded by the inverse metamodel. The dashed line interpolates the minimum values linearly.

Comparing the relative errors of the parameter sets yielded by only considering the forward model (*look up function*, Figure 4.20A, step 3 in Figure 4.16) and including the inverse metamodel (Figure 4.20B, step 4 in Figure 4.16) reveals that the minimum error values for parameters associated with high errors in general ($x_{r,a2}$ to $x_{r,b1}$) were lower for the look up function than for the inverse metamodel. Moreover, the spread between the voltage protocols was lower for the results obtained through the look up function.

The inverse metamodel and the look up function were compared in terms of output current deviation by considering the average squared error in order to compensate for the different duration of the voltage protocols *A*, *B*, and *C*. The parameters estimated by the look up function yielded average squared errors of 1.02×10^{-4} (pA/pF)^2 for protocol *A*, 3.93×10^{-4} (pA/pF)^2 for protocol *B*, and 1.94×10^{-4} (pA/pF)^2 for protocol *C*. The parameter set obtained through the inverse metamodel (weighted sum of the clusters) yielded 4.11×10^{-5} (pA/pF)^2, 7.95×10^{-4} (pA/pF)^2, and 5.85×10^{-4} (pA/pF)^2, respectively.

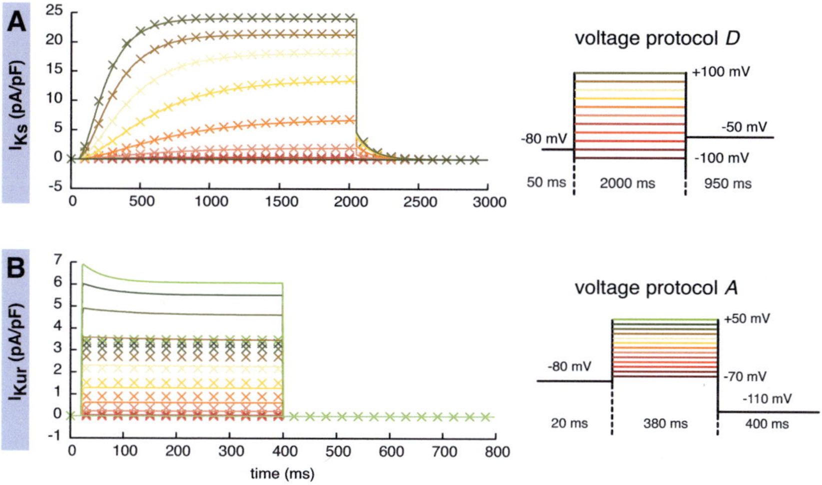

Figure 4.21: Resulting currents using the parameters estimated by the multivariate metamodeling approach. Solid lines indicate synthetic I_{Ks} (A) and I_{Kur} (B) input currents used for parameter estimation. Crosses represent the best fit obtained (not every sample shown for clarity reasons). The voltage protocols used to generate the input data and to challenge the ion current model are shown on the right part of each panel.

Thus, the two methods incorporated in the approach showed comparable performance with no clear advantage of one method over the other as expected for a coupled approach.

4.2.2.2 Slow Delayed Rectifier Potassium Current I_{Ks}

Figure 4.21A shows the best fit obtained through the look up function for the I_{Ks} formulation and voltage protocol D. The average squared error was 5.0×10^{-3} (pA/pF)^2 while the inverse metamodel yielded higher average squared errors of 1.42×10^{-1} (pA/pF)^2 for the weighted sum of HC-PLSR clusters and 21.59 (pA/pF)^2 for a single cluster.
The model parameters influencing the voltage dependence of the rate constants ($x_{s,a1}$, $x_{s,a2}$, $x_{s,a3}$, $x_{s,b1}$, $x_{s,b2}$) were not accurately estimated in terms of the correlation coefficient between the calibration set and the test set used for the inverse metamodel (R^2 <0.44, Figure 4.22B). This behavior was also reflected in the relative error measure (Figure 4.22C). However, these observations could

not be explained by the sensitivity of the output variables to the model parameters, as the regression coefficients were larger than 0.65 for all parameters except $x_{s,b1}$ Figure 4.22A). The reason is rather model sloppiness meaning that while the model output is sensitive to changes in a particular parameter (e.g. $x_{s,b2}$), the effect can be compensated by another model parameter or a set of parameters. Thus, the exact value cannot be identified even though the model is sensitive to the parameter [213]. In such scenarios, the look up function can be superior to the inverse metamodel (see e.g. $x_{s,b1}$ in Figure 4.22).

4.2.2.3 Ultra-Rapid Delayed Rectifier Potassium Current I_{Kur}

The Courtemanche et al. I_{Kur} formulation could not be well parametrized using input data generated with voltage protocol A by the multivariate metamodeling approach. Figure 4.21B shows that neither the step currents nor the exponential decay for high step voltages could be reproduced by the estimated parameters. The sum of squared errors was $6.30\times10^3(\mathrm{pA/pF})^2$ for the best fit obtained using the look up function.

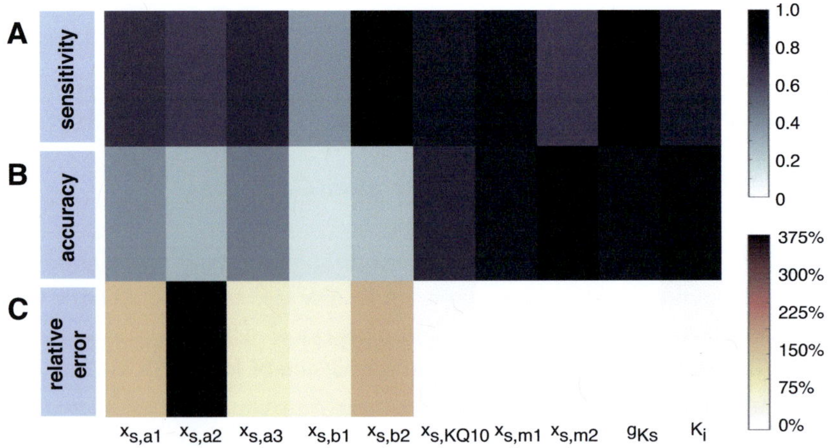

Figure 4.22: Maximum sensitivity (regression coefficients) across the 66 output variables to the parameters of the Courtemanche et al. I_{Ks} formulation (A) as well as parameter prediction accuracy (R^2) in (B) using voltage protocol D (see Figure 4.21A). (C) shows the absolute value of the relative error between the estimated and the ground truth parameters for the results yielded by the look up function.

4.2.3 Discussion

In this chapter, a recently presented multivariate inverse metamodeling approach for parameter estimation was extended and adapted for the application of ion current formulations. The approach has the advantage that it can provide information on the sensitivity of the output variables to the model parameters via PLSR analysis, as well as information regarding parameter identifiability via correlation of a calibration set and a test set in the inverse metamodeling phase.

Using this information, it could be shown that the set of parameters that can be estimated in a meaningful way in terms of accuracy is dependent on the voltage protocol being used (see e.g. Figure 4.19). While this finding is neither new nor surprising, the good correlation between the accuracy determined through the inverse metamodel and the relative parameter deviation with respect to the ground truth values is indeed exciting and good news. In real life parameter estimation scenarios, a ground truth reference, which could be used to identify the subset of parameters that are sensible to estimate, is not available as a matter of course. However, the multivariate metamodeling approach provides the accuracy measure that turned out to be a good surrogate for the relative error. Moreover, discrepancies between sensitivity and accuracy can reveal model sloppiness as observed for the parameters determining the voltage dependency of the rate constants for the Courtemanche et al. x_s gate.

The performance of the approach presented in this section was inferior to the optimization-based approaches presented in Section 4.1. Using the same voltage protocols and current formulations, the squared error was higher by eleven orders of magnitude for I_{Kr} and by nine orders of magnitude for I_{Kur}. Considering the absolute value of the differences observed for I_{Kr} (Figure 4.17A vs. Figure 4.9A), the relative weakness of the multivariate approach might not be relevant for input data of medium to low quality. For I_{Kur}, which turned out to be hard to fit in Section 4.1, the multivariate approach failed to reproduce the physiological behavior of the current (Figure 4.21B vs. Figure 4.9C). Considering the relative error between the estimated parameters and the ground truth parameters used to generate the synthetic input data also showed a superiority by two to three orders of magnitude of the hybrid approach (Figure 4.20 vs. Figure 4.11A).

When comparing the hybrid optimization-based and the multivariate approach, one should keep in mind the differing cost function definitions, though. While the hybrid approach used the scalar-valued sum of squared differences between the input data and the model output obtained using the current parameter set, the multivariate approach operated on a set of differences between exponential coefficients of size 66 to 78 representing the input and output current traces. The definition of the cost function leaves room for future improvement of the method. On the one hand, the parameters of the exponential functions describing the different phases of the current traces could be constrained in an improved way that incorporates a priori knowledge. The first phase of the I_{Kr}, as well as the I_{Ks} traces used in this work did all start at an initial value of zero. Thus, only the time constants and the terminal (close to steady-state) values for the different traces would need to be estimated leaving less room for ambiguity in this step of the approach. Moreover, the coefficients representing the different phases and different step voltages could be weighted according to their amplitude, physiological relevance, or other measures.

The advancements discussed above are currently implemented in a joint follow-up project with Kristin Tøndel, who presented the multivariate inverese meta-modeling approach in [213]. As part of this project, the multivariate metamodeling approach will be compared with the hybrid optimization-based approach developed within the scope of this thesis and presented in Section 4.1, which will be adapted to use the same cost function. The comparison will comprise both synthetic and wet-lab data, a noise sensitivity analysis, and different ionic currents as presented in Section 4.1.

Considering the results of the first evaluation of the multivariate inverse meta-modeling approach for ion current parameter estimation presented in this section and the experience regarding the different currents gained in the previous section, it is unlikely that the metamodeling approach will estimate the parameters in an optimal way, particularly for I_{Kur}. Therefore, a combination of both approaches appears suitable: the accuracy measure provided by the inverse metamodel would identify the subset of parameters that can be identified given a particular set of input data while the hybrid optimization approach would be used to actually estimate the value of these parameters.

CHAPTER 5

Modeling Atrial Substrates

Atrial rhythm disorders, such as atrial fibrillation (AF) and atrial flutter (AFlut), are caused by an interaction of stimuli triggering the arrhythmia and a vulnerable atrial substrate maintaining the reentry. Most of the triggers originate from the pulmonary veins (PVs) and have been in the focus of AF research since the seminal work by Haïssaguerre et al. suggesting electrical isolation of the PV ostia by ablation [79]. Despite high success rates of more than 70% in patients with new onset AF, only one third of patients with persistent AF remains in sinus rhythm in the long run after catheter ablation [241–243]. Considering that AF is a progressive disease, which causes remodeling of the substrate itself, the reduced responder rates in patients with longer lasting AF suggest a more momentous role of the arrhythmia-sustaining substrate in these patients. Therefore, a remodeled substrate due to chronic atrial fibrillation (cAF) (Section 5.2) and substrates of familial AF caused by two gene mutations (Section 5.1) are represented by newly developed models and evaluated in this chapter.

5.1 Genetic Defects in hERG

AF is a progressive disease with increasing incidence levels for populations of higher age and often accompanied by other cardiovascular diseases. However, AF is also observed in young patients in absence of comorbidities. In this case, the term *lone AF* is used. It has been shown that genetic predisposition to AF plays a role [244–247] and led to the formulation of the *second hit model* postulating that a genetic defect is unmasked by a second factor, such as atrial stretch [248].

While mutations in some genes or transcription factors affect the cardiovascular system in a complex way, other mutations translate to effects restricted to certain ion channel proteins. These genetic defects are called *channelopathies* [245] and are in the focus of the study presented in this section. The effect of the mutations on the ionic currents conducted via the mutated proteins can be assessed via patch clamp measurements in an expression system. However, the consequences of a mutation on the cardiovascular system, particularly the vulnerability to AF, is non-trivial to infer from changes measured on the ion channel level due to the often counter-intuitive changes on higher levels of integration caused by the complexity and non-linearity of the system. Assessment of the tissue level effects of certain mutations through computational modeling provides the means to characterize the genetic defects more comprehensively and forms the basis for personalized approaches for AF risk stratification, geno-type guided preventive strategies, and group-specific pharmaceutical therapy.

In this study, experimental data of two human ether-à-go-go-related gene (hERG) missense mutations were integrated into the Courtemanche et al. model of human atrial electrophysiology [249] using the techniques described in Section 4.1. hERG (alternative nomenclature: KCNH2) codes for Kv11.1 forming the α-subunit of the channel conducting the cardiac I_{Kr} current, which plays an important role regarding the delicate balance of inward and outward currents during atrial repolarization [250]. Mutation N588K replaces the uncharged amino acid aspargine (N) by the positively charged lysine (K) at residue N588. N588 is located in the S5 domain in the outer mouth of the channel and has been associated with AF [251]. The second mutation affects residue L532 residing in the S4 domain forming the voltage sensor. Leucine (L) is replaced by proline (P) by mutation L532P. A homologous mutant expressed in zebrafish (zERG L499P) displayed a distinct phenotype of intermittent AF and became known as *reggae mutation* [252]. Previously published experimental data describing the effects of these gain-of-function mutations on I_{Kr} were integrated into a multi-scale computational model. The model was then used to identify mechanisms favoring AF by analysis of the

duration of the effective refractory period (ERP), conduction velocity (CV), reentry wavelength (WL), duration of the vulnerable window (VW), and the restitution of these markers, as well as the inducability and persistence of spiral reentry waves in a two-dimensional tissue patch.
Parts of this work have been published as a journal article [188].

5.1.1 State of the Art

Several *in silico* studies investigated the effect of other genetic mutations on ventricular myocytes [253–255]. Also, a sensitivity analysis of parameters that could be affected by hypothetic mutations was presented [256]. Two studies investigated the effect of N588K on ventricular myocytes [257, 258] using the Luo-Rudy cell model [157]. The effects of the N588K mutation on atrial myocytes was investigated in an AP clamp study [259] and in earlier work by our group using a parameter estimation approach in a premature stage [260, 261]. A comprehensive and detailed analysis of the dynamic behavior of spiral waves for genetically modified atrial substrates was not presented before. An exception is work by Hancox et al. investigating the KCNQ1 mutation S140G [262] affecting atrial I_{Ks} and by Imaniastuti et al. regarding mutation V241F in the same gene [263]. However, their works were published after the results of the study presented in this section were submitted as a journal publication [188]. The hERG mutation L532P was not assessed besides simulations on the cellular level in the original publication describing the mutation [252].

5.1.2 Methods

5.1.2.1 Adaptation of the Cell Model

hERG wild-type (WT) and L532P measurements were conducted in *Xenopus laevis* oocytes in the group of Eberhard Scholz at University Hospital Heidelberg as described in [252]. In brief, double-electrode voltage clamp experiments were performed at room temperature using a voltage protocol similar to protocol *A* in Figure 4.17A but a final voltage of –60 mV instead of –110 mV. Data for N588K were extracted from a study published by McPate et al. [239] in which they performed whole cell patch clamp recordings of WT and N588K hERG at 37° C. Chinese hamster ovary cells were used as expression system. The voltage protocol was composed of steps from –80 mV to voltages between –40 mV and +100 mV for 2 s followed by a 4 s return pulse to –40 mV.

Standard *Matlab* curve fitting tools were used to fit exponential curves to the measured hERG traces as introduced in Section 4.2.1.2. In this way, the steady-state amplitude of the step current, the peak amplitude of the tail current, as well as the respective time constants were estimated for each step voltage of both WT and L532P measurements. Moreover, these exponential coefficients were determined for I_{Kr} traces obtained using the original Courtemanche et al. parameters [47] serving as reference coefficients.

The measurement conditions between new WT and mutant experiments and the ones used to formulate and parameterize the original model may vary in terms of temperature, electrolyte concentrations, expression systems, cell types, et cetera.

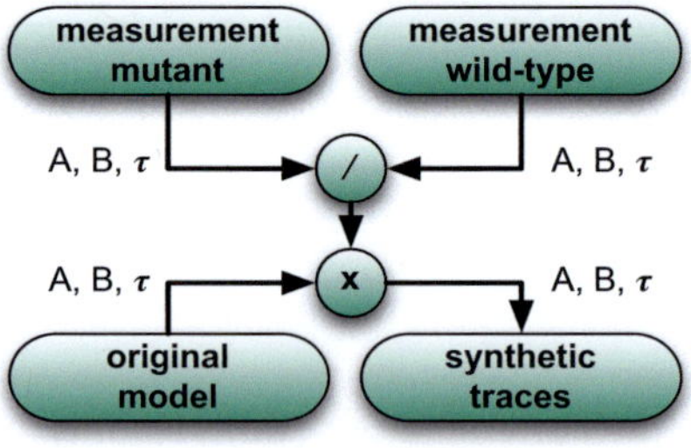

Figure 5.1: Transfer of measured currents into synthetic traces used to estimate parameters. Exponential coefficients were estimated for mutant and WT measured traces, as well as the output of the Courtemanche et al. current formulation using the default parameters [47] and the same voltage protocol as applied during wet-lab experiments. The ratio between mutant and WT coefficients was then multiplied with the coefficients of the original model output in order to generate synthetic traces representing the effect of the mutation in the model environment.

In order to compensate for these influences, only relative differences between WT and mutant data were considered as shown in Figure 5.1: The ratio of the bi-exponential coefficients estimated using the mutant current traces and the WT current traces was computed. This ratio was then applied to the reference coefficients yielded by the standard Courtemanche et al. parameters to obtain synthetic current traces representing the effect of the mutation in the model environment without effects stemming from the different experimental setups. For the step currents, the fast time constant was considered, whereas the slow time constant was considered for the tail currents because of the instantaneous kinetics of the inactivation gate of the Courtemanche et al. I_{Kr} formulation. The synthetic current traces produced in this way were then provided as input to the hybrid optimization approach introduced in Section 4.1 to estimate the values of the I_{Kr} parameters aiming at a minimization of the root mean square error between the model output and the synthetic traces representing the effect of the mutation in the model environment.
For N588K, current data were extracted from literature [239]. The normalized tail current amplitudes were fitted to a Boltzmann function:

$$y_{act} = \frac{1}{1+\exp\left(\frac{V_{1/2}-V_m}{k}\right)}, \tag{5.1}$$

with y_{act} being the level of activation $\in [0,1]$, $V_{1/2}$ being the half-maximal activation potential, and k being the slope factor. Regarding inactivation (y_{inact}), steady-state step current values were normalized to the maximum observed step current and divided by the degree of activation y_{act} for the respective step voltage. $(1-y_{inact})$ represented the level of inactivation and was fitted to a Boltzmann function, as well. Time constants were estimated using exponential curve fitting as introduced above for L532P. In this way, half-maximal inactivation and activation potentials, slope factors, and time constants were obtained for each step voltage of the WT and N588K current traces.
As all wet-lab data were acquired using homozygous expression of the mutation (referred to as *N588K-homo* and *L532P-homo*), heterozygous expression was approximated by averaging homozygous mutant and non-mutant I_{Kr}. Towards this end, an unaltered I_{Kr} with the original Courtemanche et al. parameters was included in the cell model in addition to the mutant I_{Kr} and the maximal conductivity of both formulations was reduced by 50%. Besides this

1:1 mutant to WT ratio (referred to as *N588K* and *L532P*), a 3:1 ratio was assessed on the single cell level (referred to as *N588K-3:1* and *L532P-3:1*), as well.

5.1.2.2 Single Cell Investigations

The I_{Kr} parameterizations representing the two hERG mutations were integrated in the Courtemanche et al. cellular model of human atrial myocytes [47]. Action potentials (APs) were elicited in the cell model by a stimulus current of 1.3 nA being applied for 3 ms at a fixed basic cycle length (BCL) of 1000 ms. Transient oscillations were observed during the first approximately 30 cycles, allowing to assess the steady state properties of the mutant cell models by analyzing the 50th AP in the train. Besides AP amplitude, action potential duration (APD) at 90% repolarization (APD_{90}), APD_{50}, and the maximum diastolic potential (MDP) as a surrogate for the resting membrane voltage $V_{m,rest}$ were determined. A triangulation index (TI) was defined as a measure of linearity of the repolarization, i.e. absence of a plateau, being associated with early afterdepolarizations [264]:

$$TI = 200\% \left(1 - \frac{V_m\left(\frac{APD_{90}}{2}\right) - MDP}{V_m\left(t_{notch}\right) - MDP}\right), \tag{5.2}$$

with $V_m\left(\frac{APD_{90}}{2}\right)$ being the transmembrane voltage after half the APD_{90} had passed, and t_{notch} being defined as the first time step after the upstroke for which the absolute value of the slope dV_m/dt was smaller than 0.4 V/s. If this condition was not fulfilled within the first 50 ms after the upstroke, the time of the peak of V_m was considered.

5.1.2.3 Restitution Analysis

Moving up one scale of integration from the single cell level to a one-dimensional tissue patch composed of coupled cells, not only the electrophysiological properties at a fixed BCL but also their frequency dependence (known as *restitution*) was assessed. The tissue strand was composed of 100 cubic voxels with a side length of 0.1 mm resulting in a total size of

20 mm × 0.1 mm × 0.1 mm. The cell models were initialized for 50 cycles in a single cell environment to let the system adapt to the changed I_{Kr} parameters and varying BCLs to reach steady-state. 20 different BCLs ranging from 300 ms to 1300 ms were distributed equidistantly in the frequency domain. Stimulus currents were applied to the first three voxels for 3 ms with an amplitude of 7 nA in all tissue simulations.

Restitution curves were computed for APD_{90}, the slope of the APD_{90} with respect to the diastolic interval (DI) defined as the difference between BCL and APD_{90}, CV, ERP, and the WL defined as the product of CV and ERP. The ERP was determined through an S1-S2 protocol: after a train of S1 stimuli applied according to the BCL, a premature S2 stimulus was applied for 3 ms with an amplitude of 7 nA at varying S2 times. If the S2 stimulus elicited a wave that propagated along the strand, the ERP was lower than the S2 time. If no excitation wave propagated, S2 was below the ERP. By applying an interval bisection method, the ERP was determined accurately with a residual uncertainty of less than 1 ms.

Besides the markers mentioned above, the duration of the temporal VW was determined in the tissue strand by an S1-S2 protocol as well. Different from S1, the S2 stimulus was applied in the center of the strand and the wave propagation to both sides of the tissue strand was monitored. The S2 time was within the VW if unidirectional block occurred, thus an excitation reached the front of the strand where the S1 stimuli were applied but no wave propagated to the end of the strand. By varying the S2 time, the temporal width of the VW was obtained.

Beat-to-beat alternans was assessed by evaluating the fifth and the sixth beat in the tissue strand.

5.1.2.4 Spiral Wave Analysis

A two-dimensional tissue patch was used to analyze the properties of the mutant cell models regarding the initiation and perpetuation of AF. The homogeneous and isotropic tissue patch was composed of 1000 × 1000 × 1 cubic voxels with a side length of 0.1 mm.

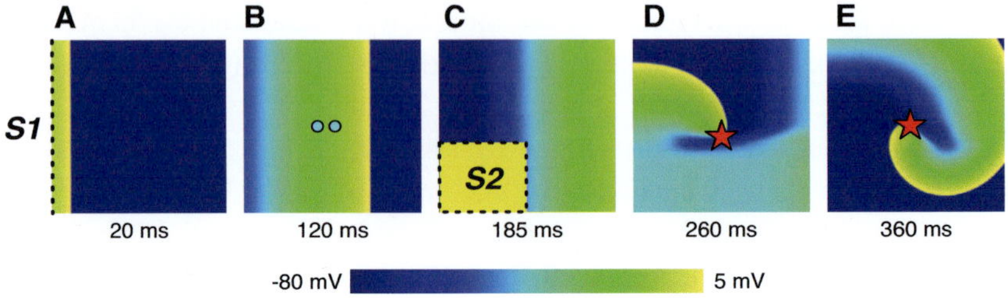

Figure 5.2: S1-S2 cross field protocol used for rotor initiation. After the tissue patch was preconditioned by four stimuli S1 (A) causing planar waves (B), the S2 stimulus in the lower left quadrant (C) initiated spiral wave reentry (D)+(E). The positions of the virtual electrodes for pseudo ECG calculation are depicted by cyan dots in (B). The detected phase singularities at the rotor core are indicate by red stars in (D)+(E).

After initialization in a single cell environment for 50 cycles with a BCL of 350 ms, the tissue was preconditioned by four planar waves with the same BCL (Figure 5.2A+B). Reentry was initiated by a cross-field S1-S2 protocol with the S2 pulse applied to the lower left quadrant of the patch (Figure 5.2C). By default, an area of 50 mm $\times$ 50 mm was stimulated at t = ERP+4 ms meaning that the stimulus was applied 4 ms after the ERP ended at the plane where the S1 stimulus was applied.

Up to 5 s simulation time were covered depending on the lifetime of the spiral wave. The dynamic behavior of the spiral waves was evaluated by tracking their trajectories in time and space using the phase singularities as surrogates for the core of the rotor [265] (Figure 5.2D+E). For this purpose, a transformation from the transmembrane voltage space to phase space was established by point-wise time-delay embedding of V_m with a time delay τ of 1 ms:

$$\phi(\mathbf{r},t) = \operatorname{atan2}\left(V_m(\mathbf{r},t) - V^*, V_m(\mathbf{r},t-\tau) - V^*\right) , \tag{5.3}$$

with $\mathbf{r}$ being the coordinate vector of the point in question, V^* being the activation threshold set to –40 mV, and atan2() being a variant of the arctangent function returning the computed angle in the desired quadrant $\in (-\pi,\pi]$ [266]. The transformation to phase space uniquely defines the temporal position within the reentry cycle and yields independence of amplitude.

The gradient operator ∇ applied on a differentiable scalar field ϕ yields a conservative field $\mathbf{v}$. For a conservative field, the closed loop line integral along the boundary ∂C of arbitrary areas C, for which the field is defined, yields zero:

$$\oint_{\partial C} \mathbf{v} \cdot ds = 0 \,. \tag{5.4}$$

By applying Stoke's theorem, the following transformation can be established:

$$\oint_{\partial C} \mathbf{v} \cdot ds = \oint_{\partial C} \nabla\phi \cdot ds = \iint_C \nabla \times (\nabla\phi) \cdot dC =: n_t \,. \tag{5.5}$$

Thus the curl of the gradient of the phase field can be evaluated to obtain the topological charge n_t. Because the phase field is not well-defined and not differentiable at the point of a phase singularity $\mathbf{r_s}$, n_t does not equate to zero at such points [265–268]. Instead, the topological charge yields an integer value with the sign depending on the chirality of the singularity enclosed by ∂C [269]. By applying the $\mathrm{rot}(\mathrm{grad}(\phi(\mathbf{r},t)))$ operation on every discrete point $\mathbf{r_i}$ of the computational domain for each time step t_i, the spiral core trajectories can thus be determined.

Besides the evaluation of rotor lifetime and trajectories, a pseudo ECG was computed to determine the dominant frequency (DF). The DF has shown to correlate with the persistency of AF indicating that higher DFs are more arrhythmogenic [270–274]. The two-dimensional tissue patch was assumed to be embedded in an infinite homogenous medium for the calculation of the extracellular potential Φ_e at point $\mathbf{r}$ and time t [275]:

$$\Phi_e(\mathbf{r},t) = \frac{1}{4\pi\sigma} \int \frac{\mathbf{I_i}(\mathbf{r}',t)}{|\mathbf{r}-\mathbf{r}'|} d\mathbf{r}' \,, \tag{5.6}$$

with I_i being the intracellular current density yielded by the monodomain model (see Section 3.2.1) and σ being the scalar-valued homogeneous conductivity of the infinite medium. The pseudo ECG was defined as the voltage measured by the potential difference of two virtual unipolar electrodes sensing the extracellular potentials Φ_e. They were placed 5 mm above the patch in z-direction and 5 mm before the center of the patch and 5 mm behind the center in a line aligned with the direction of excitation propagation (x-direction) and centered with respect to the y-axis orthogonal to the excitation wave (Figure 5.2B). The power density spectrum of the signal was obtained as the squared absolute value of the Fourier transform after multiplication with a Hanning window [276] of the same size as the signal and zero padding to achieve a frequency resolution of 0.1 Hz.

Table 5.1: Parameters of the adapted Courtemanche et al. I_{Kr} formulations as well as the control model. Parameter names according to Section A.1.1. The control case was defined by the original values in [47]. For N588K, activation and inactivation characteristics as well as $x_{r,KQ10}$ were extracted from patch clamp measurements by McPate et al. [239]. L532P parameters were obtained through the hybrid optimization approach on synthesized currents based on voltage clamp experiments by Hassel et al. [252].

Parameter	Unit	Control	N588K-homo	L532P-homo
$x_{r,a1}$	1	3×10^{-4}	3×10^{-4}	2.5×10^{-4}
$x_{r,a2}$	mV	14.1	14.1	-196.86
$x_{r,a3}$	mV	-5	-5	-131.36
$x_{r,b1}$	mV	3.3328	3.3328	40.00
$x_{r,b2}$	mV	5.1237	5.1237	3.79×10^{-6}
$x_{r,KQ10}$	1	1.0	2.0	1.0
$x_{r,m1}$	mV	14.1	16.49	-9.88
$x_{r,m2}$	mV	-6.5	-6.76	-22.31
$x_{r,m3}$	mV	15.0	-38.65	-15.54
$x_{r,m4}$	mV	22.4	19.46	24.37
g_{Kr}	nS/pF	0.029412	0.029412	0.091720

5.1.3 Numerical Methods

The ordinary differential equations (ODEs) of the Courtemanche et al. model representing the control and mutant human atrial myocytes were solved with a fixed time step of 10 μs. The Rush-Larsen scheme [206] was applied for the gating variables while a forward Euler scheme was employed to solve for the remaining variables of the cell model. Tissue level simulations were carried out using the monodomain solver *acCELLerate* [169, 170]. The monodomain conductivity was set to an isotropic value of 0.076 S/m yielding a CV of 750 mm/s at a BCL of 1000 ms in the control model.

5.1.4 Results

5.1.4.1 Adaptation of the Cell Model

The resulting parameters of the Courtemanche et al. I_{Kr} formulation representing the homozygous N588K and L532P mutants are given in Table 5.1.

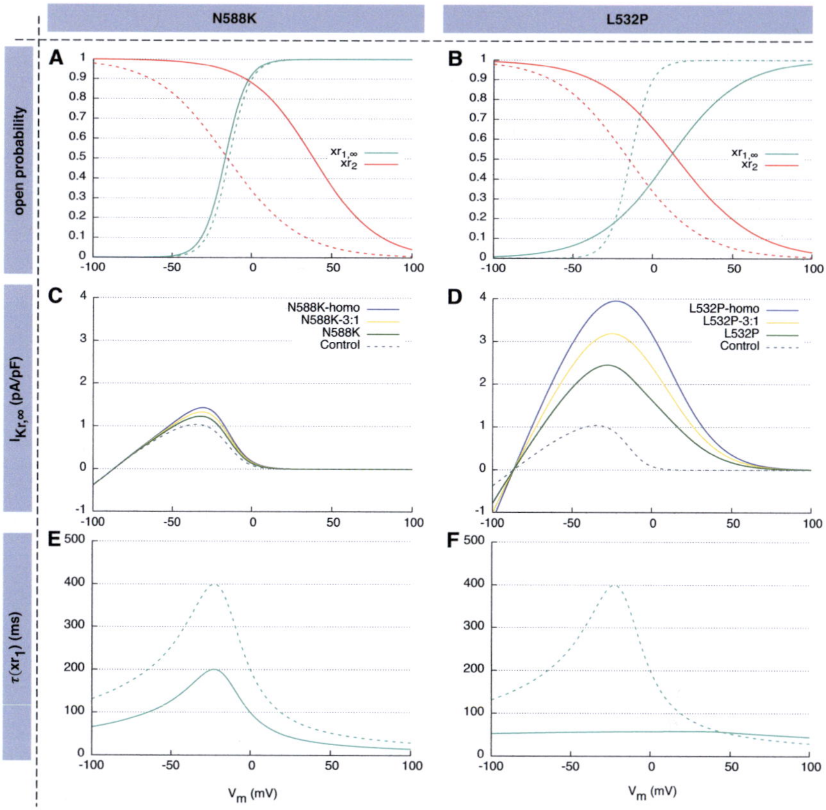

Figure 5.3: Voltage dependency of gate open probabilities of the homozygous mutant model (A)+(B), dashed lines represent the control model. The x_{r1} gate is the classical ODE gate defined by Equation (A.3) to Equation (A.6), while x_{r2} is the instantaneous gate defined in Equation (A.2). Steady-state I_{Kr} of the homozygous and heterozygous mutant models (C)+(D), and time constant τ of the x_{r1} gate of the homozygous model (E)+(F).

For N588K, the half-maximal activation potential was shifted by 2.39 mV towards more negative V_m (Figure 5.3A). Inactivation $V_{1/2}$ was shifted by 53.7 mV in the opposite direction. The respective k values were 6.7 mV and 19.5 mV. The time constant showed an almost constant reduction by a factor of 0.5 for the N588K mutant compared to WT. Therefore, the time constant of the I_{Kr} formulation was reduced to 50% by setting the Q_{10} temperature coefficient to 2 (Figure 5.3E).

Table 5.2: Resulting I_{Kr} parameters in AP clamp and AP stimulation experiments for the control model and the mutant models. The peak current, the time integral of I_{Kr}, and the time of the peak are given. For the AP clamp experiments, the control AP served as the reference.

	AP clamp			AP stimulation		
	$I_{Kr,max}$ (pA/pF)	$\int I_{Kr}dt$ (pC/nF)	$t(I_{Kr,max})$ (ms)	$I_{Kr,max}$ (pA/pF)	$\int I_{Kr}dt$ (pC/nF)	$t(I_{Kr,max})$ (ms)
Control	0.234	51.0	165.0	0.234	51.0	165.0
N588K	0.478	92.5	137.8	0.370	61.7	103.7
N588K-3:1	0.607	113.2	133.5	0.426	63.7	88.0
N588K-homo	0.737	134.1	131.1	0.476	64.6	76.3
L532P	0.726	143.5	128.6	0.537	72.2	71.7
L532P-3:1	0.981	189.7	124.0	0.672	76.0	57.8
L532P-homo	1.238	236.0	123.3	0.792	79.1	48.9

Steady-state open probability was highest for V_m=–4/0/2/4 mV for control, N588K, N588K-3:1, and N588K-homo, respectively (Figure 5.3C).
For L532P, a shift of the half-maximal activation potential $V_{1/2}$ by 23.84 mV towards positive V_m values was yielded by the optimization approach (Figure 5.3B). For inactivation, $V_{1/2}$ was shifted by 30.72 mV in the same direction. The corresponding slope factors k were identified as 22.3 mV and 24.4 mV, respectively. The voltage dependency of the time constant τ showed an almost linear and markedly flattened course for transmembrane voltages within the physiological range: 53.3 ms at –85 mV, 57.7 ms at +20 mV (Figure 5.3F). The behavior of the heterozygous models was intermediate between the control model and the homozygous mutant. The voltage for which the steady-state open probability was highest was –4 mV for control, 0 mV for L532P, 5 mV for L532P-3:1, and 15 mV for L532P-homo (Figure 5.3D).

5.1.4.2 Single Cell Simulations

The adapted Courtemanche models with the reparametrized I_{Kr} formulations were clamped to the AP course of the control model in a first step (Figure 5.4C).

Table 5.3: Resulting AP parameters for the control model and the mutant models. AP amplitude, MDP, APD at 90% and 50% repolarization, and TI were determined from single cell simulations.

	Amplitude (mV)	**MDP** (mV)	**APD$_{90}$**(ms)	**APD$_{50}$** (ms)	**TI** (%)
Control	105.64	-81.05	298.44	172.43	26.10
N588K	105.82	-81.31	255.03	129.64	46.94
N588K-3:1	105.86	-81.41	237.39	113.74	55.65
N588K-homo	105.92	-81.48	222.10	100.74	62.90
L532P	105.92	-81.64	200.78	90.76	64.56
L532P-3:1	105.99	-81.31	169.28	71.13	73.91
L532P-homo	106.01	-81.91	146.82	58.89	78.29

Both mutations increased the I_{Kr} amplitude. N588K, N588K-3:1, and N588K-homo caused increases by 104%/159%/210%, whereas L532P, L532P-3:1, and L532P-homo yielded higher amplitudes by 201%/319%/429%, respectively. As the duration of the I_{Kr} transient was mainly determined by the APD, and thus not significantly altered, the amplitude changes translated to changes of the current integral over time, as well. The current peaked earlier by between 27 and 41 ms (see Table 5.2).

In a second step, V_m of the cell models was set free and APs were elicited by recurrent stimuli with a BCL of 1000 ms (Figure 5.4A). In these AP experiments, the time of the I_{Kr} peak was earlier compared with the clamp protocol by up to 74 ms (see Table 5.2). The peak currents were reduced compared to the clamp experiments on the other hand due to the faster repolarization. Compared to the control model, they were still enhanced, though. N588K, N588K-3:1, and N588K-homo showed higher amplitudes by 58%/82%/103%, whereas L532P, L532P-3:1, and L532P-homo yielded higher amplitudes by 129%/187%/238%, respectively. The current integrals were thus also higher by +27% for N588K-homo and +55% for L532P-homo (see Table 5.2).

The APs showed a shorter duration and a less pronounced plateau, hence a more linear repolarization. Regarding the quantitative AP markers, only slight effects were observed for MDP and the AP amplitude (Table 5.3). APD and the TI differed significantly, however. MDP was hyperpolarized by less than 1 mV, the AP amplitude was increased by less than 1 mV.

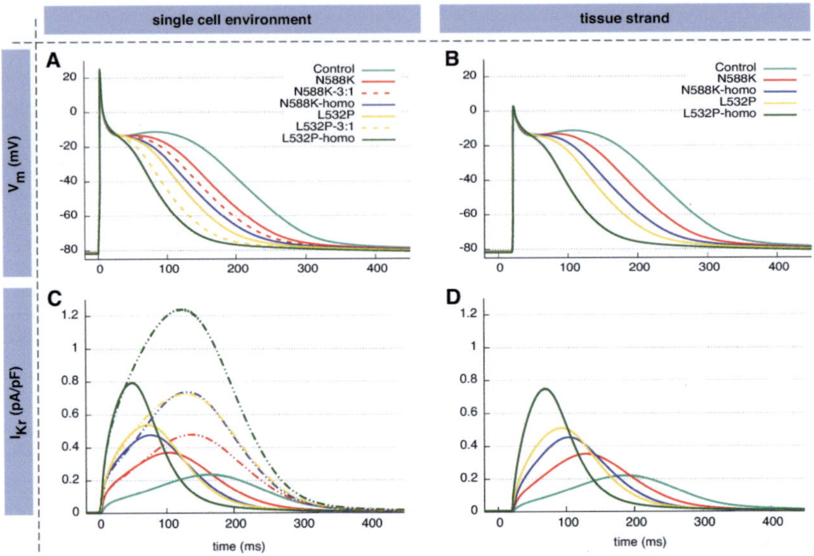

Figure 5.4: APs simulated in the single cell environment (A) and the one-dimensional tissue strand of coupled cells (B) and the corresponding I_{Kr} courses (C) and (D). Dashed lines in (A) represent heterozygous models with 75% mutant channel share. Dash-dotted lines in (C) represent I_{Kr} during AP clamp experiments using the AP of the control model as voltage protocol. The BCL was 1000 ms for all simulation.

APD_{90} was reduced by between 43 ms and 76 ms for N588K and by between 97 ms and 152 ms for L532P. APD_{90} was reduced by between 43 ms and 72 ms for N588K and by between 82 ms and 114 ms for L532P, respectively. Effects were more pronounced for the setups comprising a higher share of mutant I_{Kr}. Compared to control (26%), the TI was elevated for all mutant models (N588K: 47% to 63%, L532P: 65% to 78%).

5.1.4.3 Tissue Restitution Properties

Only the 1:1 heterozygous mutant models were investigated on the tissue level because of the low probability of myocytes being homozygous to L532P and N588K in humans.

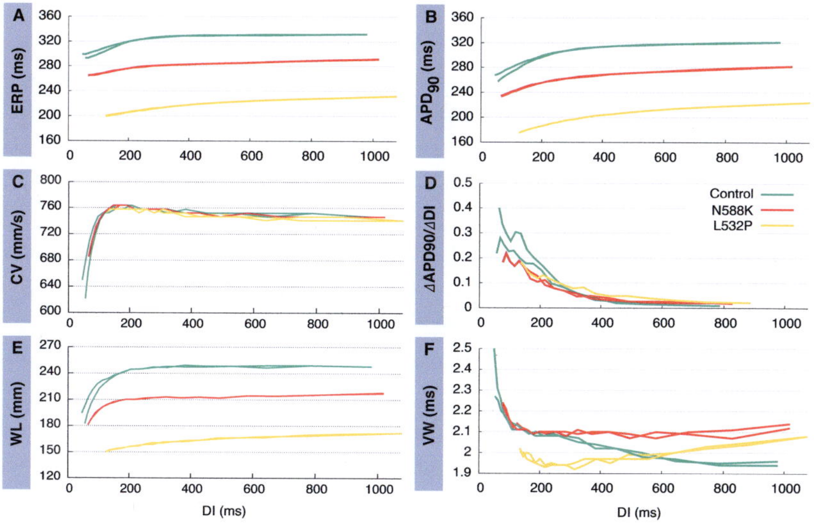

Figure 5.5: *In silico* restitution of human atrial myocardium representing healthy and hERG-mutated cells. ERP restitution (A), CV restitution (B), WL restitution as the product of ERP and CV (C), APD_{90} restitution (D) and its slope (E), as well as VW restitution (F) are shown for the fifth and the sixth beat in tissue (thus two lines per substrate) to cover beat-to-beat alternans.

When coupled to other myocytes in a tissue strand, myocytes showed a less pronounced overshoot and shorter APD (compare Figure 5.4A+B). AP amplitude was reduced by between 21.4 mV and 21.8 mV. In order to compensate for the different amplitudes, APD was compared at the time when V_m fell below –73 mV during repolarization. For the control model in tissue, APD_{-73mV} coincided with APD_{90}. Compared to the single cell simulations, APD_{-73mV} was higher by 8 to 9 ms in tissue.

Effects observed for the restitution of ERP, APD_{90}, the slope of the APD_{90} with respect to the DI ($\Delta APD_{90}/\Delta DI$), CV, WL, and the VW were more pronounced for L532P than for N588K (Figure 5.5). As was the case for the single cell simulations, effects were also more pronounced for the model variants comprising higher shares of mutant I_{Kr} than for the homozygous variant. Both mutations caused shorter ERP (Figure 5.5A) and APD_{90} (Figure 5.5B). For an intermediate BCL of 504 ms, the reduction of APD_{90} was 50 ms for N588K and 103 ms for L532P. The effect on CV (Figure 5.5C) was equivocal with conduction slowing by up to 129 mm/s and faster conduction by up to 6 mm/s for N588K and changes between –196 and +11 mm/s for L532P. Due to the higher relative amplitude of the ERP changes, the effect of the mutations on the WL (Figure 5.5E) correlated with the effect on the ERP. The restitution of the APD slope (Figure 5.5D) was flattened by introducing mutant I_{Kr}. $\Delta APD_{90}/\Delta DI$ curves for N588K and L532P intersected the control curve at DIs of 350 and 270 ms, respectively. Regarding the VW (Figure 5.5F), the restitution was unaffected by the mutations for DIs shorter than 300 ms. For longer DIs, the VW was longer by up to 9%. The VW for L532P was shorter by 0.1 ms than that for N588K consistent across most of the DI range with a slightly higher slope of the linear part causing a reduced difference for longer DIs. Beat-to-beat alternans was observed less frequently and with lower amplitude for the mutation models compared to the control model.

5.1.4.4 Dynamic Behavior of Rotors

Spiral waves could not be initiated by the S1-S2 cross-field protocol using the control model (Figure 5.6). Using the heterozygous L532P model on the other hand, rotors were sustained for the whole simulation time of 5 s with a stimulus width of 20 ms being the only exception. The N588K model failed to initiate rotors for stimuli smaller than 40 mm or later than 20 ms after the end of the ERP. For the setups that did not initiate reentry, the wavelength condition was not fulfilled for the combination of cell model and substrate geometry. If rotors were initiated, they ceased after a maximum lifetime of 2.47 s using the N588K model because the excitable substrate was consumed and the spiral wave cut itself off at an edge of the patch. Wave break was not observed using the control model and the heterozygous mutant models.
The rotor trajectories were star-shaped indicating a meandering core (Figure 5.6). The dynamic behavior of the spiral waves on the L532P substrate was more stable than on the N588K substrate as can be seen by the more regularly shaped trajectories and the smaller amount of space occupied.

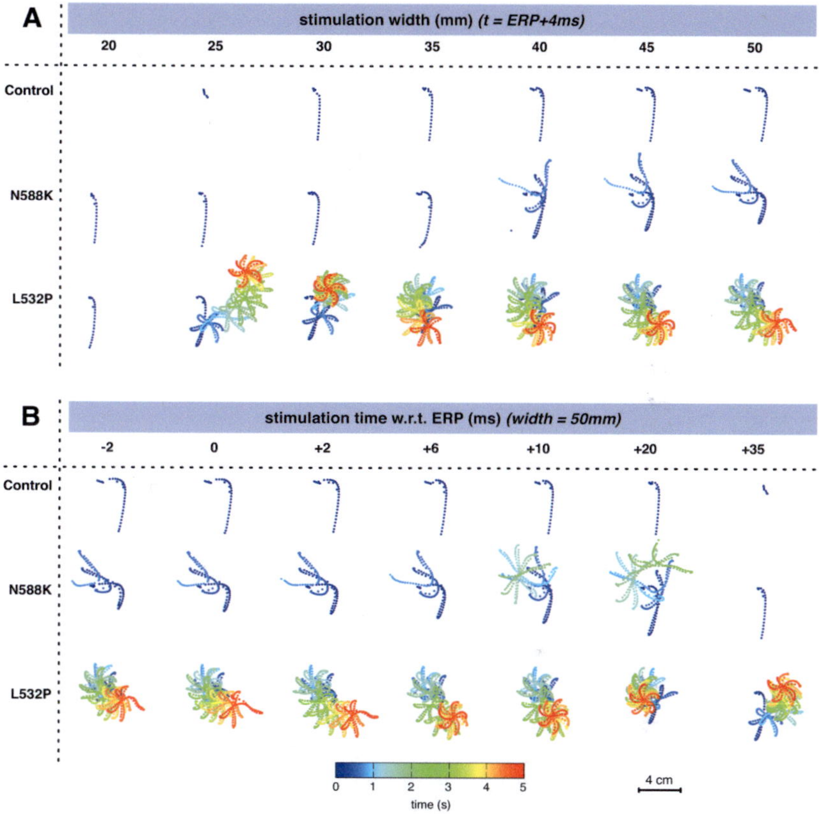

Figure 5.6: Trajectories of the phase singularities representing the rotor core in the two-dimensional tissue patch for varying stimulation widths (A) and times (B). In (A), a S2 cross-field stimulus of height 50 mm and varying width was applied at t = ERP+4 ms. In (B), the premature stimulus of size 50 mm × 50 mm was applied at varying times with respect to the end of the ERP at the left side of the tissue patch (see Figure 5.2).

Fourier transformation of the pseudo ECG signals obtained from the simulations with the premature S2 stimulus being applied 10 ms after the end of the ERP yielded DFs of 4.02 Hz for N588K and 5.37 Hz for L532P, respectively (Figure 5.7). As the control substrate could not maintain reentry, no DF could be computed.

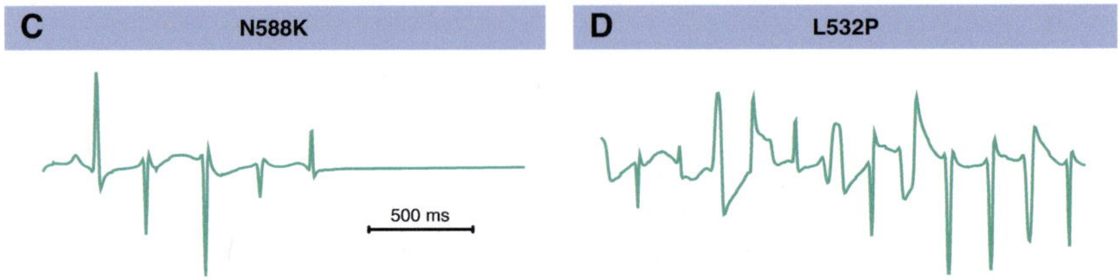

Figure 5.7: Pseudo ECGs originating from spiral waves induced by a cross-field S2 stimulus of size 50 mm × 50 mm at 10 ms after the end of the ERP (cf. Figure 5.6B). Signals for heterozygous N588K (A) and L532P (B) substrates start 0.7 s after the S2 stimulus induced reentry. Pseudo ECG amplitude is arbitrarily scaled by σ in Equation (5.6).

5.1.5 Discussion

The study presented in this chapter investigates the effect of the two hERG missense mutations N588K and L532P on human atrial electrophysiology through a multi-scale computational modeling approach. Residue N588 plays an important role in the rapid voltage-dependent inactivation of I_{Kr} [277]. This observation fits well with the results obtained in the present study indicating that the mutation N588K leads to gain of I_{Kr} function by impeded rectification. In contrast to the control model, N588K did not inactivate within the physiological V_m range. The gain of function caused by mutation L532P in residue L532 residing within the voltage sensor region was mediated via a different mechanism on the other hand. L532P I_{Kr} was enhanced through premature activation. Compared to the control model, the inactivation gate opens at more negative V_m, thus earlier during the AP. This effect potentiates through the massive depolarization caused by the fast I_{Na} kinetics. During later phases of the AP, a similar, yet less pronounced, mechanism as described for N588K contributes as well. A reason for the similar effects on I_{Kr} could be the interface between the voltage sensor (S4) hosting residue L532 and the pore domain (S5) hosting residue N588 [278].

By integrating the effects of the mutations on the single ion channel level into a comprehensive multi-scale simulation framework ranging from the ion channel via the cellular to the tissue level, the specific effects of the two missense gain-of-function mutations on higher levels of integration could be analyzed. AP clamp simulations representing a plasma membrane with a multitude of

similar channels revealed a faster rise to higher I_{Kr} peak values. AP simulation using the Courtemanche et al. model of human atrial myocytes showed that during a dynamic AP governed by the delicate balance of depolarizing and repolarizing currents, I_{Kr} was increased by 21% to 42% for the heterozygous models while the peak amplitude showed a 1.6 to 2.3-fold increase. The less pronounced effect of the mutations on the rapid delayed rectifier current I_{Kr} using the AP clamp protocol compared to the dynamic AP simulations can be explained by the mutation-induced faster repolarization causing an earlier return to lower V_m values, which in turn reduce I_{Kr} again. The shorter APD was accompanied by a more triangular AP shape in contrast to the spike-and-dome morphology of the control AP. Effects were more pronounced for L532P than for N588K on both the cellular and the tissue level. Not surprisingly, the amplitude of mutation-induced changes correlated with the share of mutant I_{Kr}, i.e. was higher for the homozygous than the heterozygous model variants. ERP and APD_{90} were reduced by $\approx$ 14% and $\approx$ 32% for N588K and L532P, respectively. For the zebrafish mutation cERG L499P corresponding to the hERG reggae mutation L532P, Hassel et al. reported an APD reduction of 19% in ventricular myocytes of zebrafish larvae [252].
An S1-S2 cross field protocol could induce stable reentry in a L532P-substrate model in contrast to the control model and N588K for which spiral waves emerged only in rare cases. This finding together with the spatially concentrated star-shaped trajectories of the rotor cores highlight the elevated arrhythmic potential of L532P. The observation that spiral waves in the N588K substrate often ceased because of interaction with the boundary of the simulation domain suggest similar investigations using a two-dimensional spherical surface in three-dimensional space. By including holes representing the orifices of the great vessels and valves, the spherical model could be extended to a simplified representation of a human atrium [279]. Regarding the transformation of the V_m space to phase space, other approaches based on e.g. the Hilbert transform were proposed in the literature. However, the applied time-delay embedding has been shown to be well-suited for noise-free simulated V_m data [266]. The DF computed for the L532P pseudo ECG was within the clinically observed range for patients in AF [280]. The rather low values for N588K, however, are most probably dominated by rotor deflections at the boundaries of the tissue patch, which could be addressed by using a spherical simulation domain as described above. For the determination of the DF in the

Fourier spectrum, more sophisticated approaches haven been proposed [281]. The simple method based on the maximum should be appropriate for noise-free simulated signals, though. Peaks reflecting harmonics of the DF were present in the signals indicating a successful DF identification.
N588K hERG currents were simulated using the Noble et al. I_{Kr} formulation [282] clamped to ventricular, Purkinje fiber, and atrial APs by McPate et al. [259]. Regarding the atrial myocytes, APs simulated using the Courtemanche et al. [47] and the Nygren [283] cell models were used as voltage protocols. They found a less pronounced shift of the voltage which causes maximum I_{hERG} and an increase of the peak current by 130% for the Nygren et al. model compared to the Courtemanche et al. model used in this study. However, the impact of the choice of the cell model should be significantly smaller in our study for all experiments except the AP clamps. For the *in silico* experiments on the cellular and tissue level, V_m was not fixed by a voltage protocol but evolved physiologically. The second *in silico* work [260, 261] studying the effect of N588K on atrial electrophysiology adapted the cell models in another way. As discussed in Chapter 4, parameter estimation problems for cardiac ion current formulation are highly underdetermined in many cases. Thus, the global model characteristics are not necessarily preserved by the approach used in their set of studies neglecting differences between experimental setups and lacking a hybridization strategy concerning parameter estimation. Compared to [260, 261], APD and AP morphology were affected to a lower degree using the approach presented in this thesis relating the amplitudes and the time constants of the WT and mutant measurements.
Using a Markov chain I_{Kr} formulation integrated in the Luo-Rudy ventricular cell model [157], Itoh et al. reported a 6% reduction of APD_{90} at a BCL of 1000 ms [258]. Zhang and Hancox found a 16% decrease for M-cells at a BCL of 400 ms for an adapted Hodgkin-Huxley-type I_{Kr} formulation integrated in the Luo-Rudy ventricular model, as well [257]. In the presented study, APD_{90} was reduced by $\approx$25% for the homozygous N588K mutant at BCLs between 400 ms and 1000 ms indicating that the effect of the N588K hERG mutation on APD is larger in the atria than in the ventricles.
The different $V_{1/2}$ activation and inactivation values for L532P-hERG found in this study compared to [252] could be traced back to the different methods applied to estimate the parameters based on the measured current traces. In the approach presented here, the slope factor k was estimated for both WT and

L532P and the result of the parameter estimation for the activation gate was considered as a priori knowledge for the estimation of the parameters of the inactivation gate. These differences as well as the missing step regarding the transformation of the parameters to the model environment also explains the differences on the AP level (Figure 5 in [252]).

5.1.5.1 Limitations

The measurement data used in this study were acquired in hERG channels, which represent the pore-forming α-subunit of the cardiac I_{Kr} channel. The β-subunit is encoded by KCNE2, which was not coexpressed for L532P. Aiming at a comparison of both mutations, N588K data were taken from pure hERG measurements, as well. Comparing hERG-N588K data with hERG-N588K + KCNE2 data shows that the effects on currents are similar, though [284]. The reported slight shift of activation towards more positive V_m associated with KCNE2 coexpression leads to the assumption that the mutation-induced effects will be gradually more pronounced than for lone hERG expression.

Both mutations were expressed homozygously. The chosen approach to approximate heterozygous expression by combining mutant and WT channels in a 1:1 ratio (and additionally a 3:1 ratio on the cellular level) appears reasonable as long as measured data for heterozygously expressed mutants are not available.

L532P measurements were conducted at room temperature and hERG channel kinetics are known to exhibit a complex temperature dependence [285]. Thus, the recordings acquired at room temperature may not exactly represent the behavior at 37° C body temperature. However, temperature dependence of the effect of hERG mutations has been shown to be rather small [259, 286]. In particular, the data by Hassel et al. [252] used in this work are in agreement with L532P experiments performed at 37° C in human embryonic kidney cells by Zhang et al. [287]. The markedly flattened time constant vs. voltage relation found in the model presented in this chapter correlates with the finding by Zhang et al., as well as the shift of activation $V_{1/2}$ by 24 mV compared with 30 mV [287].

Maximum channel conductivity is hard to estimate from current recordings in expression systems. While single-channel patch clamp recordings allow to

measure the conductivity of one channel, the acquired value would need to be multiplied with the number of channels to obtain the macroscopic conductivity of the current in the whole cell as represented in electrophysiological cell models. Protein immunoblotting could be used to estimate the amount of channel protein, however no conclusion regarding functionality could be drawn, thus neglecting possible trafficking changes.
As discussed in Section 4.1.3, a five-state Markov model is required to represent all aspects of hERG gating [210] while the Courtemanche et al. formulation [47] used in this work comprises only one activation gate governed by an ODE and one instantaneous inactivation gate. However, the Courtemanche et al. model was chosen as a phenomenological representation of atrial electrophysiology because it convinced in a benchmark of several atrial cell models [156], is well established [9, 10], and validated regarding high levels of integration. Hence, it was considered well-suited to study the effects of the hERG mutations on the cellular and tissue level. Biophysically more detailed models, e.g. the Grandi et al. model [220], come at the expense of higher computational cost and exhibit behavior partly inconsistent with experimental findings in tissue level simulations [156].
More complex and anatomically more detailed geometrical models including myocyte orientation, thus anisotropic conduction, and heterogeneous tissue properties are available [9, 183]. While reentry can be initiated by small ectopic stimuli in contrast to the large S2 cross-field stimulus used in this work, basic underlying mechanisms of rotor genesis, perpetuation, and termination can be easier illuminated in simplified models.

5.1.5.2 Conclusion

In this chapter, the effects of the two hERG missense mutations N588K and L532P on human atrial electrophysiology were studied using multi-scale simulation ranging from the ion channel level via integrated cellular models to the one-dimensional and two-dimensional tissue level. The consequences of the mutations on these higher levels of integration in terms of AP morphology changes, refractory behavior, as well as rotor initiation and sustainment capacity allow to identify individuals harboring a genetic substrate predisposing to AF. By aiding risk stratification and paving the way for genotype-guided therapeutic strategies, the findings presented here help to bridge the gap from bench to bedside. While both mutations affect the same gene, they cause qualitatively different effects suggesting more offensive approaches for subjects carrying the L532P mutation compared to N588K. In Section 6.1, geno-type specific effects of the two existing pharmacological agents amiodarone and dronedarone are evaluated regarding the two mutations. A preventive approach rendering the genetically modified substrate less vulnerable to AF by administering existing agents with a specific dose or applying a hypothetic, optimized multi-channel blocker is proposed in Section 6.3.

5.2 Chronic AF Induced Remodeling

Atria that are exposed to fibrillation for a longer time undergo remodeling processes as introduced in Section 2.3.1. In order to leverage *in silico* methods to gain mechanistic insight into AF patho-physiology and to evaluate therapeutic strategies, the results of these remodeling processes need to be represented in the models.

Established cell models have been adapted to represent AF-induced remodeling by other groups. Table 5.4 gives an overview of the existing models. Most models did not consider all existing experimental data (cf. Table 2.1) or lack reasoning for the choice of parameters. This motivated the definition of a new remodeling setup based on a rigorous literature research within the scope of this thesis. Model *AF4* by Colman et al. and the model by Koivumäki et al. consider the available literature comprehensively. However, these models were published after the model presented here was submitted as a conference contribution [294].

Parts of this work have been published as a conference paper [294] and are based on earlier work [127].

5.2.1 Methods

In the model, I_{to} was reduced by 65%, I_{K1} was increased by 100%, I_{Ks} was increased by 100%, I_{Kur} was reduced by 50%, $I_{Ca,L}$ was reduced by 55%, $I_{Na,Ca}$ was increased by 60%, and the leak current from the sarcoplasmic reticulum to the cytosol I_{leak} was increased by 50%. The cell capacitance was increased by 20%.

Table 5.4: Adaptation of cell models to represent AF induced remodeling from literature. The last row presents the proposed new remodeling setup based on a rigorous literature research of experimental data (cf. Table 2.1 and Section 2.3.1).

Model	Ref.	g_{K1}	$g_{Ca,L}$	g_{to}	g_{Kr}	g_{Kur}	g_{Ks}	g_{Na}	I_{NaCa}	I_{leak}	I_{up}	RyR	Remarks
Colman AF1	[288]	+100%	-70%	-70%									$\tau_{Ca,L}$ +60%, I_{to} activation +16 mV shift
Colman AF2	[288]	+75%	-65%	-65%									
Colman AF3	[288]	+106%	-63%	-66%		-49%							
Colman AF4	[288]	+100%	-70%	-65%		-50%	+100%		+55%	+25%	+50%	+300%	
Grandi	[220]	+ 100%	-50%	-70%		-50%	+ 100%	-10%	+ 40%	+ 25%		+100%	added late I_{Na} component, SERCA↓
Koivumäki	[289]	+62%	-59%	-62%		-38%			+50%	-15%	-16%	+100%	cell volume +58%, phospholamban to SERCA↑ sarcolipin to SERCA↓
Matene AF1	[290]	+ 73%	-63%	-65%									
Matene AF2	[290]	+ 200%	+ 50%										
Matene AF3	[290]		-63%										
Seemann	[291]	+ 110%	-65%	-65%									
Uldry	[292]		-30%	-80%	+ 50%	-90%							
Zhang AF1a	[293]	+ 102%	-74%	-85%									I_{to} activation +16 mV shift
Zhang AF1b	[293]	+ 250%											I_{to} activation +16 mV shift, I_{Na} activation shift +1.6 mV, $\tau_{Ca,L}$ +62%
Zhang AF2	[293]	+ 90%	-64%	-65%									
Loewe	[294]	+ 100%	-55%	-65%		-50%	+ 100%		+ 60%	+ 50%			

As the data on connexin expression is equivocal as reviewed in [126, 295], the initial monodomain conductance $\sigma = 76 mS/m$ of the monodomain equation was reduced by 30% for the setup *RemodCV* and left unchanged for the setup *Remod*.
The effect of the cAF induced changes on electrophysiology through remodeling were evaluated on multiple scales. On the single cell level, APs were elicited by applying a stimulus current of 1.3 nA for 3 ms at a BCL of 1000 ms. MDP, AP amplitude, as well as APD at 90% and 50% repolarization were analyzed after pacing for 50 cycles. Restitution curves were obtained through simulations in a one-dimensional tissue strand as introduced in Section 5.1.2.3. Restitution of APD_{90} and its slope, CV, ERP, and WL was determined for BCLs ranging from 180 ms to 1300 ms for the fifth and the sixth beat in tissue to cover beat-to-beat alternans.
Besides the original Courtemanche et al. model [47] representing healthy tissue (*Control*), the setup presented by Seemann et al. in 2010 [291] was used for comparison. In the Seemann et al. setup, a 30% reduction of the monodomain conductivity σ was assumed as for the *RemodCV* setup.

5.2.2 Results

The APs yielded by the remodeling variants of the Courtemanche et al. model are shown in Figure 5.8. Compared to control, the MDP was hyperpolarized by 3.2 mV for the new setup as compared to 3.7 mV for the setup by Seemann et al. [291]. AP amplitude was higher by 1.5 mV and 2.4 mV, respectively. APD was shortened due to remodeling: compared to control, APD_{50} was reduced by 55% for *Remod*, thus less drastically than for the Seemann et al. setup (69%). APD_{90} was reduced by 56% and 64%, respectively.
Compared to the Seemann et al. setup, the repolarization of the AP yielded by the new setup was less linear. However, the AP plateau was not as pronounced as for the control model and the initial notch after the overshoot was missing. Thus, the spike-and-dome morphology of the control model was not present in the new remodeling setup. The setup considering changes of the intercellular coupling (*RemodCV*) did not exhibit any differences compare to *Remod* on the single cell level as a matter of course.

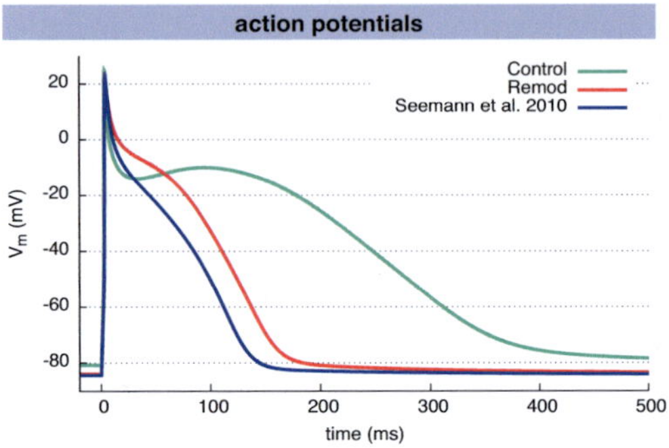

Figure 5.8: AP of an atrial myocyte under cAF remodeling conditions (red) in comparison to control (green). The blue curve represents the setup by Seemann et al. [291].

Restitution was analyzed in a one-dimensional tissue strand for the three remodeling setups. Compared to the control model, the ERP was shortened in the *Remod* setup by between 142 ms for a BCL of 341 ms and 160 ms for a BCL of 764 ms (Figure 5.9A). The difference in ERP between *Remod* and *RemodCV* was smaller than 2 ms for all BCLs. In comparison, the Seemann et al. setup shortened the ERP by between 160 ms (BCL: 326 ms) and 188 ms (BCL: 852 ms).

APD_{90} restitution exhibited a qualitatively similar course as the ERP curves (Figure 5.9B). The slope of the APD_{90} with respect to the DI did not differ significantly between the three remodeling setups and was lower by up to 0.3 compared to control for short BCLs. The Seemann et al. setup exhibited marked oscillations by up to 0.2 for BCLs shorter than 400 ms. For BCLs longer than 700 ms, no differences to control were observed (Figure 5.9D).

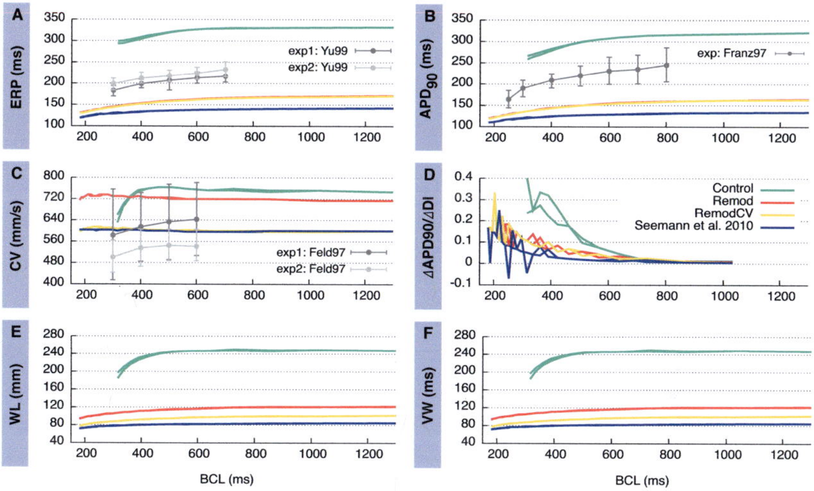

Figure 5.9: Restitutions curves of atrial myocardium with cAF induced remodeling. ERP restitution (A), CV restitution (B), WL restitution as the product of ERP and CV (C), APD_{90} restitution (D) and its slope (E), as well as VW restitution (F) are shown for the fifth and the sixth beat in tissue (thus two lines per substrate) to cover beat-to-beat alternans. The gray lines with error bars represent experimental data of chronic AF remodeled myocytes from Franz et al. [296], Yu et al. [297], and Feld et al. [298].

Remodeling caused conduction slowing by up to 39 mm/s (BCL: 504 ms) for the *Remod* setup and by up to 165 mm/s (BCL: 504 ms) for the Seemann et al. setup. *RemodCV* exhibited similar properties as the Seemann et al. setup regarding the CV with a maximum difference of 8 mm/s. The restitution was markedly flattened for all remodeling setups compared to control (Figure 5.9C).

The different remodeling setups yielded the most distinct results for the WL measure defined as the product of the ERP and the CV (Figure 5.9E). The WL was shortened by between 81 mm and 128 mm for *Remod*, by between 100 mm and 150 mm for *RemodCV*, and by between 110 mm and 166 mm for the Seemann et al. setup. The reduction was lowest for a BCL of 313 ms being the lowest BCL for which the control model yielded stable APs.

While the general progression of the VW with respect to the BCL was similar for all setups, *Remod* showed the shortest VW with values between 0.31 ms and 0.53 ms. The Seemann et al. setup showed a relatively constant VW of

about 1.25 ms. *RemodCV* and control exhibited similar VW restitution for BCLs above 800 ms. For lower BCLs, *RemodCV* showed a shortening of the VW by up to 0.2 ms for a BCL of 300 ms (Figure 5.9F).
Beat-to-beat alternans, particularly with respect to APD_{90}, was reduced by all models of cAF induced remodeling.

5.2.3 Discussion

In this section, the Courtemanche et al. model representing healthy human atrial myocytes was adapted to reflect changes induced by cAF remodeling. Maximum conductivities of the ion currents were altered based on a rigorous literature research. Since the publication of this setup as a conference contribution in 2014 [294], the data base regarding experimental data of ion channel remodeling has not changed significantly [299]. Compared to an earlier remodeling setup developed at IBT by Seemann et al. [291], the AP plateau is not completely degenerated. This observation can be attributed to the 50% reduction of I_{Kur} and secondary to the slightly less reduced $I_{Ca,L}$ (55% vs. 65%). In comparison to the control model, the repolarization of the new setup is still more linear, though.
A number of biomarkers were evaluated to assess the arrhythmogenic potential of the remodeled substrate. ERP, APD, and WL indicated a tendency towards arrhythmogeneity considering the critical WL concept. While CV was mostly dependent on the assumed monodomain conductivity σ, conduction slowing was observed in the *Remod* setup despite unaltered σ and I_{Na} compared to the control model. This observation can be explained by the hyperpolarized resting membrane voltage as a stimulus current of a given amplitude needs more time to exceed the threshold due to the capacitive properties of the membrane. Moreover, increased I_{K1} counteracts depolarizing stimuli. The slope of the APD_{90} with respect to the DI was higher, thus presumably more arrhythmogenic, for control than for any remodeling setup. Also beat-to-beat alternans as a potential pro-arrhythmic mechanism was only observed in the control substrate.
The comparison to the sparse available experimental data regarding restitution in cAF remodeled substrates shows fair agreement regarding APD_{90} [296] and ERP [297]. However, the absolute values of both markers in the cAF

remodeling setups were larger in the model than in the experimental data. The absolute values of the model CV were in the range reported by Feld et al. [298]. The slope of the CV with respect to the BCL does not match the mean values of the experiments. However, the error bars of the experimental data span a wider interval than the dynamic restitution interval (Figure 5.9C).
The model presented here is limited in the sense that only changes of the maximum ion current conductivities were considered. However, the remodeling of gating kinetics is reported very equivocally as described in detail in [127]. Structural remodeling effects such as the influence of e.g. fibrosis are beyond the scope of this work focussing on the electrophysiological effects on the single cell and one-dimensional tissue level. Future work could address inter-subject variability as suggested by Sanchez et al. [300].
In conclusion, the modification of the Courtemanche et al. model of human atrial myocytes presented in this section represents cAF induced electrophysiological remodeling and is able to reproduce the main characteristics observed experimentally. It provides mechanistic descriptions how remodeling increases susceptibility to reentry through shortened WL facilitating the initiation and maintenance of atrial arrhythmias according to the *AF begets AF* paradigm. The adapted model provides the means to evaluate tailored therapeutic strategies for cAF patients *in silico* and was used as a substrate model in Chapter 6 regarding pharmacotherapy and in Chapter 8 regarding ablation.

CHAPTER 6

Pharmacological Agents

Pharmacological treatment of atrial fibrillation (AF) with various antiarrhythmic drugs is an alternative, less invasive approach to radio-frequency or cryo-ablation of atrial tissue for cardioversion and prevention of AF recurrence. While antiarrhythmic agents are classically developed and tested using *in vitro* and *in vivo* approaches in both animals and humans, *in silico* methods can complement a thorough analysis. In this way, critical compounds can be identified and rejected at earlier stages of drug development and the number of animal studies can be reduced in the long run [9, 301, 302]. Moreover, novel ion channel targets can be characterized [303, 304] and therapies can be tailored for subgroups of the general population as a further step towards personalized medicine [305].

Computational models were employed to evaluate the effect of hypothetic and existing antiarrhythmic agents on ventricular electrophysiology in previous studies [205, 306–308]. The focus of most ventricular studies was drug safety in terms of prevention of torsades de pointes tachycardia that can cause sudden cardiac death. Mirams et al. performed a virtual thorough QT study aiming at a prediction of the drug induced proarrhythmic risk of up to 34 compounds by *in silico* modeling [309] superior to using IC_{50} values only [310]. The use of *in silico* methods for drug safety evaluation has recently been reviewed in [301].

Regarding atrial electrophysiology, Morotti et al. presented a computational study aiming at a prevention of phase-3 early afterdepolarizations as a poten-

tial mechanism of AF initiation by blocking peak I_{Na} [311]. Tsujimae et al. investigated voltage and time dependent I_{Kr} inhibition caused by the pharmacological agents dofetilide, vesnarinone, and quinidine [312]. I_{Kur} inhibitor kinetic properties were studied regarding their effect on rotor termination by Scholz et al. [303] and regarding AP prolongation by Tsujimae et al. [313]. Wilhelms et al. [205, 314] presented first work on the effects of amiodarone and dronedarone on atrial electrophysiology. While the study presented here is based on this study, the dynamic effects caused by the interplay of the circadian changes of both drug concentration and heart rate were not considered in the work of Wilhelms, thus neglecting pharmacokinetic considerations. Moreover, the drug model was advanced. Aslanidi et al. [315] studied the effect of dronedarone of APD_{90} restitution and spiral wave dynamics. Heijman et al. used a computational model to study the determinants of beat-to-beat alternans of action potential duration (APD) [316], which can translate to beat-to-beat variability of T-wave morphology [317]. Zemzemi et al. studied how inhibition of I_{Kr}, I_{Na}, and $I_{Ca,L}$ in ventricular myocytes translate to changes up to the body surface potential level [306].
The study presented in Section 6.1 is the first comprehensive study of the dynamic effects of amiodarone and dronedarone on human atrial pathoelectrophysiology considering the properties of distinct atrial substrates. Vernakalant investigated in Section 6.2 has never been studied *in silico* before to the best of my knowledge highlighted by the lack of a comprehensive understanding of its effects on different levels of integration. The study presented in Section 6.3 is the first to optimize hypothetic and existing compounds for the treatment and prevention of familial AF comprehensively.

6.1 Amiodarone & Dronedarone

Amiodarone and dronedarone are two antiarrhythmic agents that have been proposed as an effective treatment of AF [1]. As both drugs inhibit cardiac potassium currents, they are classified as class III agents according to the Singh Vaughan Williams system [318]. However, both agents exert effects on multiple channels and have to be considered multi-channel blockers, indeed. Besides differences in their pharmacodynamic properties in terms of inhibition of ion channels, amiodarone and dronedarone also differ markedly in their

pharmacokinetic properties. Amiodarone accumulates in a third compartment because of its lipophilic properties leading to a biological half-life of several weeks. Dronedarone on the other hand is less lipophilic translating to a significantly shorter half-life of less than 24 h [136].
Even though dronedarone was designed as a less thyrotoxic alternative to amiodarone with similar effects on cardiac electrophysiology, the efficacy in terms of AF recurrence prevention is much better for amiodarone than for dronedarone [72, 130, 136]. Therefore, three hypotheses are tested in this study using a multi-scale *in silico* approach: It is hypothesized that the effects of the two drugs differ because of i) the different pharmacokinetic properties causing distinct temporal variations in drug concentration, ii) different restitution properties leading to distinct effects in different heart rate regimes, and iii) distinct effects for different atrial substrates.
Parts of this work have been published as a journal article [129] and are based on a supervised student's project [319].

6.1.1 Methods

The original Courtemanche et al. model of human atrial myocytes [47] was used as the control substrate representing healthy atrial myocardium. Besides, the effect of amiodarone and dronedarone was assessed in the chronic atrial fibrillation (cAF) substrate introduced in Section 5.2 and for the two hERG mutations L532P and N588K introduced in Section 5.1 as models of familial AF. Regarding the hERG mutations, heterozygous expression was assumed and approximated by mixing mutant and wild-type (WT) I_{Kr} at a 1:1 ratio.

6.1.1.1 Modeling the Effect of Amiodarone and Dronedarone

Binding of the agents to the channel proteins and the consequent conductivity reduction were modeled using Hill's equation [320]:

$$\Theta = \frac{1}{1 + \left(\frac{IC_{50}}{D}\right)^{nH}}, \tag{6.1}$$

with Θ being the degree of channel block $\in [0,1]$ ranging from no block to complete block, IC_{50} being the half-maximal inhibitory concentration, D being the

free plasma drug concentration, and nH being the Hill coefficient quantifying cooperative binding. The IC_{50} and nH values describing the effect of amiodarone and dronedarone on cardiac ion currents were extracted from literature (Table 6.1). Amidarone affected the currents I_{Kr} [321], I_{Ks} [322], I_{Na} [323], $I_{Ca,L}$ [324], the sodium calcium exchanger I_{NaCa} [325], and the sodium potassium pump I_{NaK} [326]. Dronedarone affected I_{Kr} [327], I_{Kur} [328], I_{Ks} [329], I_{Na} [323], and $I_{Ca,L}$ [137]. Figure 6.1 shows the resulting Hill curves.
The amiodarone plasma concentration in steady-state is reported to range between 1 μg/ml and 2 μg/ml [330]. Given the molar mass of 643.31 g/mol, this corresponds to 1.55 to 3.11 μM. For dronedarone, the reported plasma concentration of 84 ng/ml to 147 ng/ml corresponds to 0.15 μM to 0.25 μM considering the molar mass of 556.76 g/mol. For a thorough exploration of the concentration space, the effect of both agents was modeled for free drug concentrations ranging from approximately 10% of the respective mean standard concentration to 10$\times$ the mean standard concentration. Within those ranges, 15 logarithmically spaced concentrations were assessed.

Table 6.1: Inhibition of cardiac ion channels by the pharmacological agents amiodarone and dronedarone. Half-maximal inhibitory concentrations IC_{50} and Hill coefficients nH were extracted from literature.

	Amiodarone			**Dronedarone**		
	IC_{50} (μM)	nH	Reference	IC_{50} (μM)	nH	Reference
I_{Kr}	2.80	0.91	[321]	0.0591	0.80	[327]
I_{Kur}	–	–		1.00	1.00	[328]
I_{Ks}	3.84	0.63	[322]	5.60	0.51	[329]
I_{Na}	4.84	0.76	[323]	0.54	2.03	[323]
$I_{Ca,L}$	5.80	1.00	[324]	0.83	2.75	[137]
I_{NaCa}	3.30	1.00	[325]	–	–	
I_{NaK}	15.60	1.00	[326]	–	–	

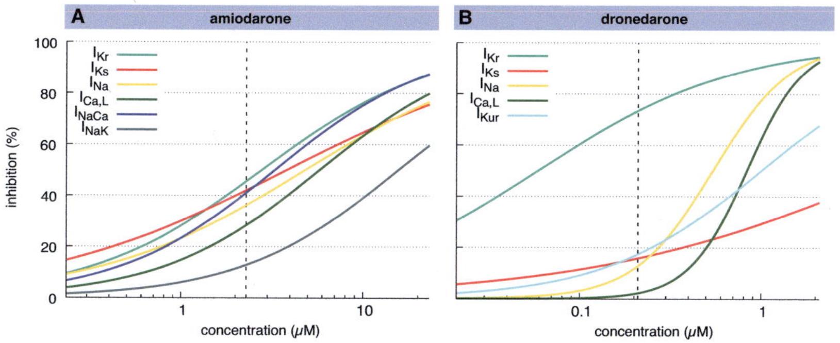

Figure 6.1: Degree of inhibition resulting from Hill-type channel block due to amiodarone (A) and dronedarone (B) based on the half-maximal inhibitory concentrations and Hill coefficients given in Table 6.1. The vertical dashed line corresponds to the standard concentration. Note the different scales on the x-axes.

6.1.1.2 Scoring

Similar to the method introduced in Section 5.1.2.3, the effect of amiodarone and dronedarone on cardiac electrophysiology was studied in a one-dimensional tissue strand with the same numerical methods as in the previous chapter (see Section 5.1.3). In order to obtain information on the frequency dependence, the system was paced at 20 different basic cycle lengths (BCLs) being distributed equidistantly in the frequency domain between 200 ms and 1300 ms. Restitution curves were computed for APD_{50}, APD_{90}, the slope of the APD with respect to the diastolic interval (DI) ($\Delta APD_{90}/\Delta DI$), action potential (AP) amplitude, maximum diastolic potential (MDP), conduction velocity (CV), effective refractory period (ERP), wavelength (WL), triangulation index (TI), and vulnerable window (VW) as introduced in Section 5.1.2. Moreover, the resulting APs for each combination of drug concentration and BCL were classified into categories. APs were considered valid if V_m exceeded –45 mV and the upstroke velocity exceeded 10 V/s. Besides normal APs and total block, consistent 2:1 block, block of a single AP, and APs with decrescent amplitude formed categories. The decrease was considered significant if the amplitude was reduced by at least 3% from beat to beat. Moreover, sequences of valid APs with more than 3% variation in APD_{90} were classified as *alternans*.

Table 6.2: Bounds for the continuous scoring of the biomarkers. ERP, APD_{50}, and VW were related to the respective values without drug influence (subscript 0).

	Value for score 1	**Value for score 6**
CV (mm/s)	800	300
$\Delta APD_{90}/\Delta DI$	-0.3	1.5
TI (%)	15	95
ERP/ERP_0 (%)	130	60
$APD_{50}/APD_{50,0}$ (%)	130	60
VW/VW_0 (%)	60	130

All acquired biomarkers were scored on a continuous scale and combined in a single score to represent the results in a compact way allowing for assessment of the interdependency between BCL and concentration. The scores ranged from 1 representing the best value to 6 being the worst score regarding arrhythmogeneity. The upper and lower bounds for the continuous, linear score of the six biomarkers considered are given in Table 6.2. AP categories were scored from 1 to 6 as follow: normal, alternans, decreasing, single block, 2:1 block, complete block. The score values for combinations of BCL and concentration not being on the grid points formed by the 20 BCL values and the 15 concentration values, for which tissue level simulations were performed were interpolated bilinearly. The overall score was computed as the mean of the six scores of the single biomarkers in Table 6.2. If one score yielded 5.5 or worse or two markers were 5.0 or worse, the overall score 6 was assigned, however.

6.1.1.3 Pharmacokinetic Scenarios

To identify the most relevant areas in the BCL-concentration space spanned by the 20 BCLs and the 15 concentrations, for which the biomarkers were evaluated, typical trajectories were defined by combining pharmacokinetic scenarios with dynamic heart rate variations (Figure 6.2). A 200 mg daily dose of amiodarone was assumed to be administered at 8 a.m. causing a 20% increase in concentration [331] with respect to the mean value. The standard concentration of 2.3 μM was used as a reference for the mean value. Thus, a reduction of 20% with respect to the standard concentration was modeled at the time of administration.

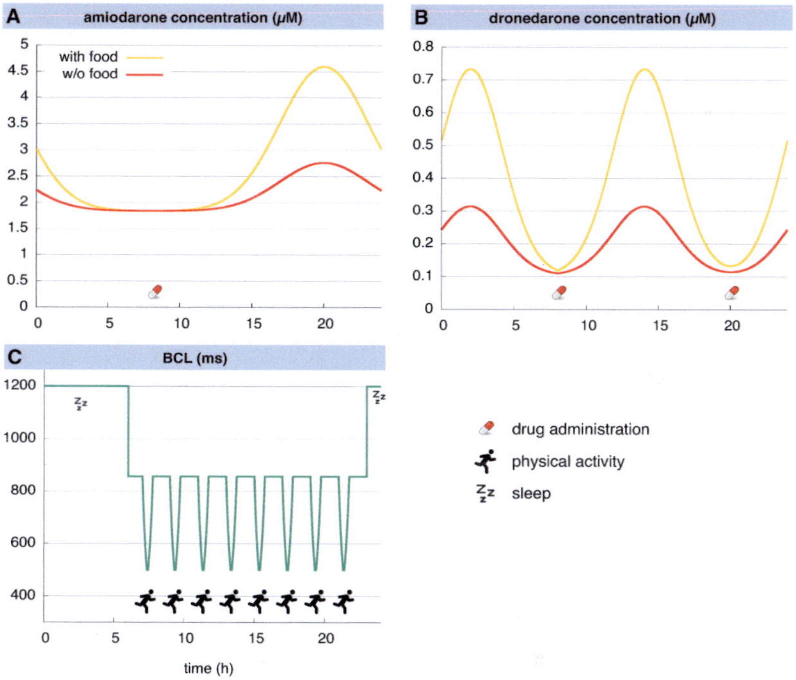

Figure 6.2: Course of the drug concentrations over a typical day modeled in the pharmacokinetic scenarios for amiodarone (A) and dronedarone (B) with and without concomitant food intake, as well as the circadian BCL course including sleep, rest, and phases of physical activity (C).

The time course between these extrema was modeled using Gaussians (Figure 6.2A). For dronedarone, in contrast, two doses of 400 mg each were administered at 8 a.m. and 8 p.m. causing an increase of 50% [332] with respect to the mean value of 0.21 μM (Figure 6.2B). In a second set of scenarios, concomitant food intake was assumed resulting in a three-fold increase of the bioavailability of both agents [136] (Figure 6.2A+B).

Regarding the circadian variation of the heart rate (Figure 6.2C), a baseline of 70 beats per minute (bpm) corresponding to a BCL of 857 ms was assumed during daytime (6 a.m. to 11 p.m.).

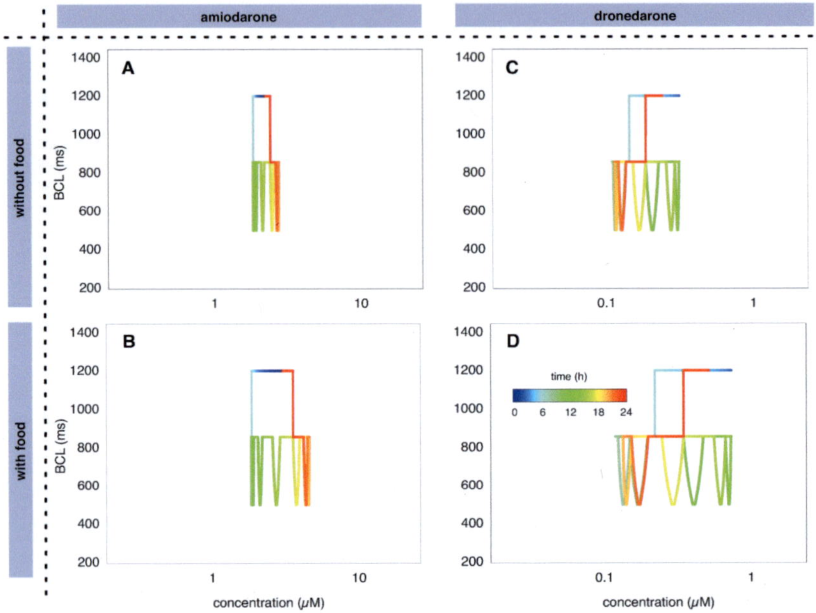

Figure 6.3: Dynamic trajectories in the BCL-concentration space for amiodarone (A)+(B) and dronedarone (C)+(D). The time of the day is color-coded. The lower panel represents drug administration with concomitant food intake resulting in a higher bioavailabilty. The axes correspond to the axes in Figure 6.6.

Episodes of physical stress were modeled by a 20 min linear increase of the heart rate to 120 bpm (BCL: 500 ms), followed by 5 min at 120 bpm and a 20 min linear decrease to the resting value of 70 bpm. Eight such episodes were distributed equidistantly during daytime. The heart rate during sleep (11 p.m. to 6 a.m.) was assumed to be 50 bpm (BCL: 1200 ms). The heart rate course was the same for all substrates (including the cAF substrate) for the sake of comparability.

6.1.2 Results

6.1.2.1 Dose and Frequency Response

The effect of variations in the drug dose and the pacing frequency (inversely correlated with BCL) were studied in the one-dimensional tissue strand. Drug-induced conduction block occurred for dronedarone concentrations above 1.09 μM in all substrates. For amiodarone, block was only observed in the cAF substrate for concentrations above 23 μM (see Figure 6.4). The concentration at which block occurred coincided with the drug concentration causing I_{Na} block of $\approx$80%. As the baseline sodium current in the drug-free scenario was reduced in the cAF substrate due to the remodeling, block occurred already at lower drug concentrations. Fast pacing, thus low BCLs, induced block in all substrates but cAF. The cutoff BCL increased with increasing drug concentration resulting in a step-like pattern and was higher for dronedarone than for amiodarone.

For valid APs which were not blocked but conducted along the strand, the frequency and dose response of the biomarkers was evaluated. The interested reader is referred to Figures S6 and S7 in the online supplementary material of [129] for the 160 graphs detailing the dose and frequency response with a fixed value of the respective other parameter for both drugs in all four substrates. Here, the results are presented in a condensed form and quantified for representative BCLs and drug concentrations.

AP amplitude decreased for higher concentrations. In the control model, it decreased from 83.9 mV without any compound applied to 54.3 mV for 23 μM amiodarone and to 62.1 mV for 1.09 μM dronedarone at a BCL of 1008 ms. For dronedarone concentrations below 0.1 μM and amiodarone concentrations below 0.32 μM, AP amplitude was almost unaffected. AP amplitude increased again when raising the dronedarone concentration from 0.56 μM to 0.78 μM for BCLs longer than 600 ms. Shorter BCLs were associated with smaller amplitudes, in general. The cAF substrate exhibited a markedly attenuated frequency dependence. The difference in amplitude between the shortest and the longest BCL was 3.1 mV in the cAF substrate compared to between 15.4 mV and 19.9 mV for the other substrates at an amiodarone concentration of 0.23 μM.

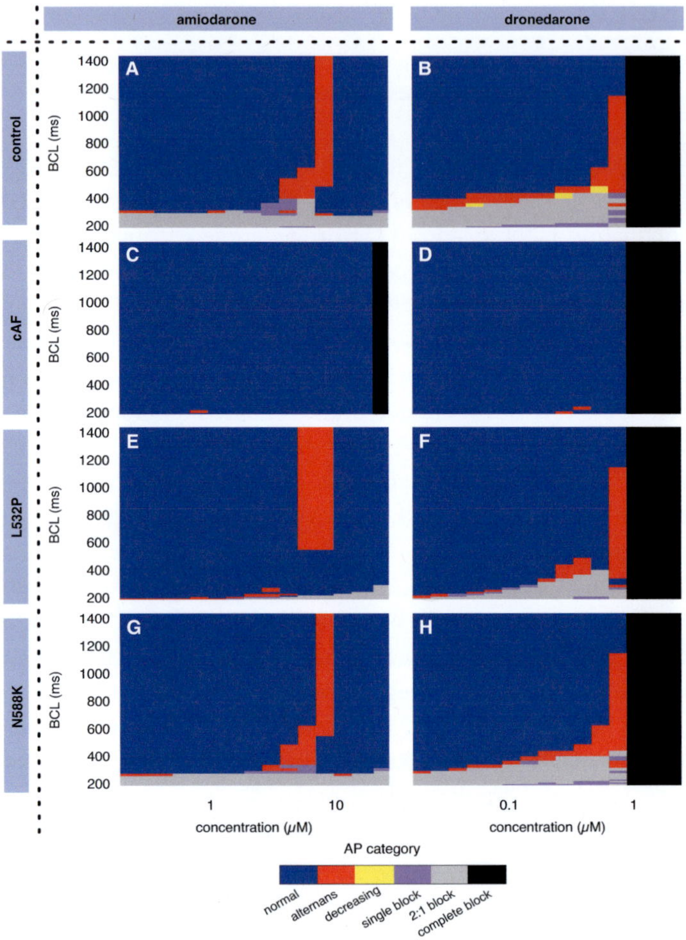

Figure 6.4: Resulting AP categories for amiodarone (A), (C), (D), and (G) and dronedarone (B), (D), (F), and (H) and the four different substrates control (A)+(B), cAF induced remodeling (C)+(D), hERG mutation L532P (E)+(F), and hERG mutation N588K (G)+(H). Alternans was defined as APD_{90} alterations of 3% or more. Sequences with a least 3% beat-to-beat decrease of AP amplitude were considered as decreasing.

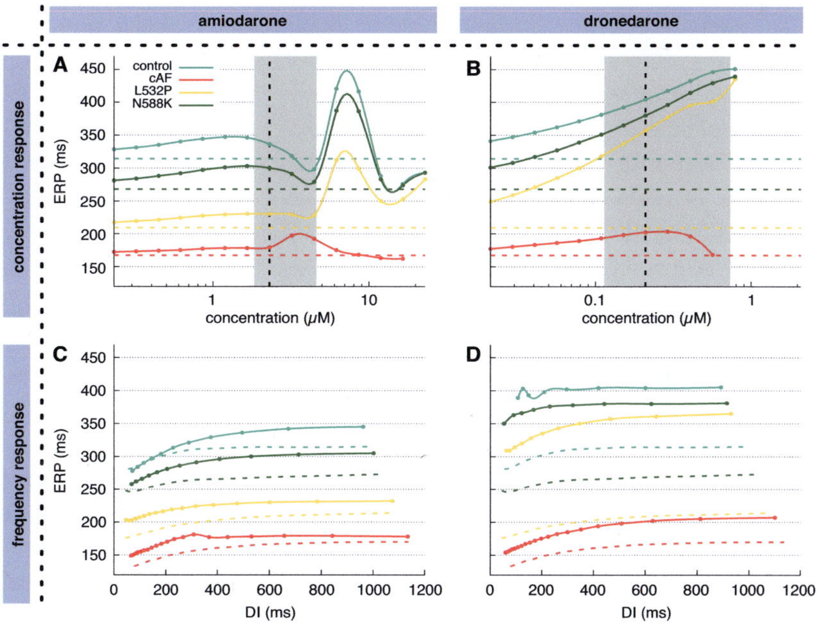

Figure 6.5: Response of ERP to different concentrations of amiodarone (A) and dronedarone (B) for a fixed BCL of 857 ms corresponding to 70 bpm. Vertical dashed lines indicate the standard concentration of the respective drug, horizontal dashed lines represent the baseline ERP for zero drug concentration. (C)+(D) show the frequency response (restitution) against the DI at the standard concentrations of amiodarone (C) (2.3 μM) and dronedarone (D) (0.21 μM). The shaded gray area in (A)+(B) represents the concentration range covered in the pharmacokinetic scenarios (Figure 6.2 and Figure 6.3). The DI range covered was different for each substrate and each concentration. Data points are indicated and were interpolated using cubic splines. Data points were neglected if no AP could be elicited due to drug-induced block.

Similar characteristics were observed for dronedarone (exemplary concentration of 0.021 μM) with a range of 3.8 mV in the cAF substrate compared to 14.1 mV to 22.9 mV in the other substrates.

Amiodarone dose-response curves for the biomarkers APD_{50}, APD_{90}, and ERP were bell-shaped in contrast to dronedarone, which caused a monotonic increase towards higher concentrations followed by a marked drop beyond a cutoff concentration. The amiodarone concentration corresponding to the peak in ERP was 3.2 μM for cAF and between 6.1 μM and 8.6 μM for control,

L532P, and N588K. The absolute value of the amiodarone induced APD_{50} increase was largest in the control substrate (+160 ms $\widehat{=}$ +86%), followed by N588K (+144 ms $\widehat{=}$ +86%), L532P (+117 ms $\widehat{=}$ +96%), and cAF (+28 ms $\widehat{=}$ +23%). In the control and N588K substrates, a less pronounced peak was observed at an amiodarone concentration of $\approx$ 1/5 of the main peak. The cutoff dronedarone concentrations were identified as between 0.56 μM and 0.78 μM in all substrates. In the cAF substrate, the cutoff was not as sharp as for the other substrates causing a decrease for dronedarone concentrations between 0.29 μM and 0.56 μM rather than an instantaneous cutoff observed for the other substrates. ERP dose response curves are shown in Figure 6.5A for amiodarone and Figure 6.5C for dronedarone at a BCL of 857 ms corresponding to 70 bpm. The dose response for APD_{90} and ERP showed similar courses.
Regarding the restitution properties, the overall course did not differ between substrates and the gross morphology of the restitutions curves was unaffected by both drugs. However, the degree of *reverse use dependence* describing the effect of less pronounced ERP prolongation for lower BCLs, thus faster heart rates, differed between substrates. It was observed for N588K and the control substrate for amiodarone. In the control case, ERP with the standard amiodarone concentration of 2.3 μM was even shorter than the baseline value for BCLs shorter than 392 ms (Figure 6.5C). Reverse use dependence was observed for dronedarone in the cAF and L532P substrates; compared to amiodarone to a lower degree, though. Restitution curves are shown in Figure 6.5C for amiodarone and Figure 6.5D for dronedarone at the respective standard concentrations.
The APD_{90} slope $\Delta APD_{90}/\Delta DI$ oscillated for short BCLs close to cutoff and high concentrations of both drugs close to cutoff. In general, the slope was steeper towards lower BCLs (most pronounced for the L532P substrate followed by control and N588K).
Increasing drug concentrations caused conduction slowing correlating with the degree of I_{Na} block. This effect on CV was observed for dronedarone concentrations above 0.1 μM as was the case for AP amplitude. Marginal intersubstrate differences were reflected in minimal CV values under amiodarone administration of 268 mm/s, 324 mm/s, 267 mm/s, and 268 mm/s for control, cAF, L532P, and N588. Values for dronedarone were 417 mm/s, 505 mm/s, 414 mm/s, and 416 mm/s, respectively. CV frequency dependence was only

observed for BCLs shorter than 500 ms with a tendency towards slower conduction. In the cAF substrate, CV was unaffected by a BCL decrease down to 200 ms. The WL was calculated as the product of ERP and CV resulting in a general tendency towards shorter WLs for higher amiodarone concentrations. The peaks observed in the ERP dose response translated to the WL course, though. These peaks counterbalanced the amiodarone induced ERP decrease and almost restored the baseline WL without any drug. For dronedarone, a WL increase was observed for concentrations up to 0.15 μM in the cAF substrate and up to 0.29 μM in all other substrates. For higher concentrations, WL dropped. WL prolongation compared to baseline was up to 52 mm (+22%) for control, 19 mm (+16%) for cAF, 101 mm (+64%) for L532P, and 70 mm (+34%) for N588K.
Regarding the MDP, amiodarone caused a hyperpolarization whereas dronedarone depolarized the MDP. The amplitude of this effect was smaller than 2.5 mV for all drug concentrations at a BCL of 1008 ms. Faster pacing did prevent full repolarization of V_m yielding higher MDPs by up to 4.8 mV, 2.1 mV, 6.1 mV, and 6.2 mV for control, cAF, L532P, and N588K, respectively. The TI as a marker quantifying the linearity of the repolarization, i.e. the absence of an AP plateau, showed a qualitatively similar course as the ones for the APD markers. For amiodarone, higher concentrations were associated with a slightly higher TI with the exception of a marked drop around 3 μM in the cAF substrate and around 6 μM in the other substrates. For dronedarone, the general tendency was towards lower TI values for higher concentrations in all substrates but cAF, which showed no significant sensitivity for concentrations up to 0.6 μM.
The baseline duration of the VW with no drug administered was between 1.5 ms and 2.0 ms for all substrates but cAF for which it was 0.3 ms. Amiodarone shortened the VW down to 0.3 ms in the former substrates and 0.1 ms in the cAF substrate. The VW was unaffected by dronedarone concentrations far from the cutoff concentration. Frequency dependence was marginal for BCLs significantly above the cutoff value.

6.1.2.2 Scores

The biomarkers were scored according to Table 6.2. The interested reader is referred to Figure S8 in the online supplementary material of [129] for details of the resulting scores for all markers under both drugs in all four substrates. Here, selected results are presented in a condensed form. Figure 6.6 shows the resulting total score. The baseline value without any drug administered was 2.33, 2.57, 2.75, and 2.53 for the control, cAF, L532P, and N588K substrates at a BCL of 1008 ms.

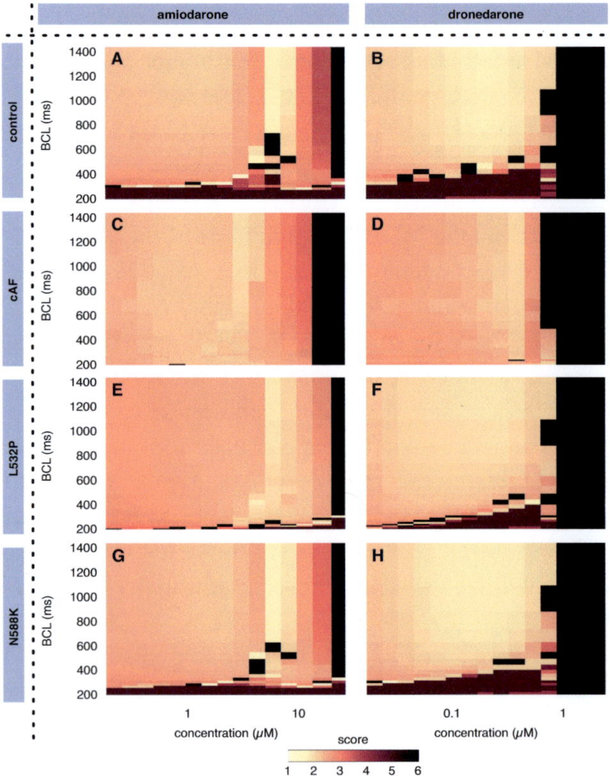

Figure 6.6: Total score resulting from amiodarone (A), (C), (E), and (G) and dronedarone (B), (D), (F), and (H) administration in the four different substrates control (A)+(B), cAF induced remodeling (C)+(D), hERG mutation L532P (E)+(F), and hERG mutation N588K (G)+(H). Scores range from 1 (best) to 6 (worst). The total score is based on the individual scores for AP category (see Figure 6.4), CV, $\Delta APD_{90}/\Delta DI$, TI, ERP/ERP_0, $APD_{50}/APD_{50,0}$, and VW/VW_0. In case one of the individual scores of the markers evaluated to 5.5 or worse, or two markers yielded 5.0 or worse, the total score 6 was assigned. Otherwise, the mean of the seven individual scores was considered.

Regarding the individual biomarkers, CV yielded higher, thus worse, score values for elevated drug concentrations with no significant frequency or substrate dependency. Only for BCLs close to cutoff, a tendency towards higher scores was observed which was more pronounced for dronedarone than for amiodarone. The worst CV scores for high drug concentrations were 6 for amiodarone in all substrates and 5 for dronedarone for all but the cAF substrate for which the maximal score was 4.

The bell-shaped ERP amiodarone dose response translated to a bathtub-shaped ERP score dose response curve. The minima occurred at amiodarone concentrations of 6.17 μM, 3.19 μM, 4.44 μM, and 6.17 μM in the control, cAF, L532P, and N588K substrates. Lower BCLs were associated with slightly higher scores at low amiodarone concentrations. At higher concentrations, the opposite behavior was observed, i.e. lower scores for lower BCLs. Regarding dronedarone, elevated concentrations caused lower ERP scores in all substrates but cAF for which a minimum was observed at 0.15 μM. In the other three substrates, peaks to high, thus bad, scores were observed for low BCLs close to cutoff for some concentrations. The $APD_{50}/APD_{50,0}$ score showed a qualitatively similar course as the ERP/ERP_0 score.

The APD_{90} slope scores were dominated by peaks to critical values close to the concentrations yielding APD_{90} (and ERP) minima for amiodarone and close to cutoff BCLs for dronedarone. In general, shorter BCLs yielded slightly higher $\Delta APD_{90}/\Delta DI$ scores.

Regarding TI, minima were observed at amiodarone concentrations yielding APD_{90} (and ERP) minima. In vicinity to these concentrations, shorter BCLs and higher concentrations were associated with higher scores resulting in a step-like pattern. For lower concentrations in the control substrate, also longer BCLs yielded lower scores. The course of the TI score for dronedarone was consistent with the ERP score. The frequency dependence causing higher scores for shorter BCLs was more pronounced for TI than for ERP, though. In the L532P substrate, low concentrations ($<3\,\mu$M amiodarone, $<0.1\,\mu$M dronedarone) yielded TI scores as high as 4.9.

Regarding the VW, higher amiodarone concentrations caused lower scores in general. This tendency was less pronounced for dronedarone. Hot spots with peaks to critical values were observed for short BCLs close to cutoff for several concentrations of both compounds. Dronedarone applied to the cAF substrate caused such hot spots also for longer BCLs.

6.1.2.3 Circadian Variation

The total score was evaluated along the trajectories in the BCL-concentration space representing the circadian variation of the drug concentration and the heart rate (Figure 6.3). The amiodarone score in the *food* scenario considering concomitant drug and food intake varied between 1.6 and 2.5 in the control substrate (Figure 6.7A), between 1.8 and 2.5 for cAF (Figure 6.7C), between 2.1 and 2.4 for L532P (Figure 6.7E), and between 1.7 and 2.4 for N588K (Figure 6.7G). The same scenario applied to dronedarone caused total score values between 1.6 and 5.1 in the control substrate (Figure 6.7B), between 1.9 and 6.0 for cAF (Figure 6.7D), between 1.7 and 5.1 for L532P (Figure 6.7F), and between 1.6 and 5.1 for N588K (Figure 6.7H).

Compared to the baseline score trace with zero drug concentration, the score under amiodarone was improved. The only exception was observed for the control substrate during phases of high concentration and low heart rate in the *food* scenario (Figure 6.7A). Dronedarone improved the score compared to baseline in most cases. Worse scores under dronedarone were observed during peaks to critical values (Figure 6.7B,D,F,H). These peaks occurred in all substrates during phases of high concentration and low heart rate considering the *food* scenario and during phases of low concentration and intermediate heart rate in the cAF substrate (Figure 6.7D) considering the *non-food* pharmacokinetic scenario.

Phases of elevated heart rate, thus shorter BCL, reflecting physical stress lead to elevated scores during phases of low amiodarone concentration. During phases of high concentration, the score was reduced during stress with the exception of the cAF substrate in which a stress induced increase was observed for all concentration phases.

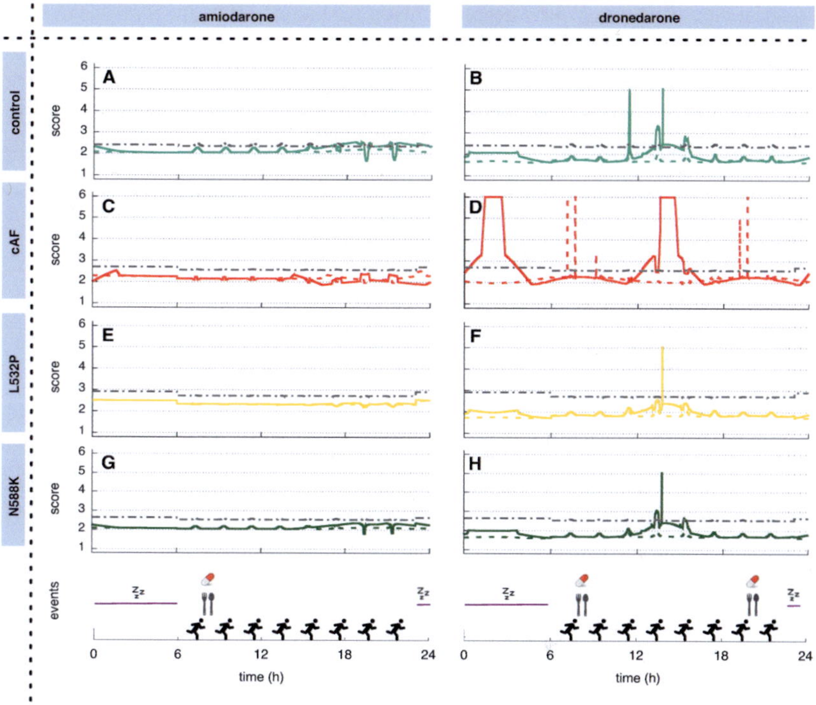

Figure 6.7: Circadian variation of the total score (Figure 6.6) along the trajectories through the BCL-concentration space representing a typical day (Figure 6.2 and Figure 6.3). The antiarrhythmic drugs amiodarone (A), (C), (E), and (G) and dronedarone (B), (D), (F), and (H) were assumed to be administered together with food (solid lines) or without (dashed lines) resulting in different bioavailability of the agents. The gray, dash-dotted lines indicate the baseline score at zero drug concentration. Resulting scores are shown in four different substrates: control (A)+(B), cAF induced remodeling (C)+(D), hERG mutation L532P (E)+(F), and hERG mutation N588K (G)+(H). The lower panels indicate times of sleep, drug (and possible food) intake, as well as phases of elevated heart rate representing physical activity.

The circadian variation of the drug concentration lead to higher scores during phases of high amiodarone concentration with the exception of the cAF and the L532P substrates, which showed no consistent trend.

The dronedarone scores peaked to critical values of 5.0 or above during phases of high concentration and short BCL in all substrates in the *food* scenario. In the scenario without concomitant food intake, peaks above 2.5 were only observed in the cAF substrate. Moreover, the peaks occurred under different circumstances: low concentration and short BCL in contrast to high concentration and short BCL. In the *food* scenario, elevated dronedarone levels caused higher scores, in general. In the cAF substrate however, the score was lowest during the transition from high to low concentration and the other way around. In the *non-food* scenario, the circadian variation of the dronedarone concentration was reflected in significant score changes only in the cAF substrate. Shorter BCLs representing physical stress yielded higher scores in all substrates.

6.1.3 Discussion

The dynamic effect of amiodarone and dronedarone on human cardiac electrophysiology was investigated in this study under consideration of physiological circadian variation of drug concentration and heart rate using a computational model. Moreover, the influence of the substrate was assessed comprising cAF induced remodeling and two hERG mutations associated with familial AF. Under high drug concentrations, AP could no longer be elicited due to the degree of sodium channel block. For short BCLs, the tissue could not fully repolarize between two consecutive wavefronts leading to depolarized MDP. This may favor ectopic beats as any stimulus of given amplitude is more likely to reach the V_m threshold and trigger an AP. Alternans on the AP level under amiodarone occurred only for high concentrations corresponding to the concentration peaks in the pharmacokinetic scenario assuming concomitant food and drug intake. For dronedarone however, APs exhibited alternans for the whole concentration range at short BCLs close to cutoff, particularly in the control substrate. This proarrhythmic mechanism [333, 334] is potentially one of the factors contributing to the inferior efficacy of dronedarone compared with amiodarone in terms of the prevention of AF recurrence [72, 130, 136]. A further factor contributing to the inferior efficacy can be found in the fact that the total score peaked to critical values in all substrates in the dronedarone *food* scenario. In the cAF substrate, these peaks could even be observed in the *non-food* scenario during phases of low dronedarone concentration right before the next drug intake. Under amiodarone, the circadian variation of BCL and drug concentration caused only minor score oscillations, though.

Acceleration of the heart rate reflecting phases of physical activity caused peaks to critical scores in all dronedarone concentration phases. For amiodarone on the other hand, shorter BCLs improved the score during phases of high concentration in all but the cAF substrate. Reverse use dependence was also substrate dependent and occurred in the control and N588K substrates under amiodarone and the other two substrates under dronedarone.
The finding that the amiodarone concentration yielding the best, thus lowest, score was lower by 50% in the cAF substrate compared to the control substrate and the two hERG mutations implies and highlights that the responder rate of pharmacological AF therapy and preventive approaches could be raised by tailoring the drug regimen in a group-specific way considering the atrial substrate. For dronedarone, a less pronounced tendency in the other direction was observed proposing elevated doses for cAF patients. Generally speaking, the effects in the cAF substrate differed markedly from the others. The drop of the biomarkers APD, ERP, and VW at the cutoff concentrations was not as abrupt but showed a rather smooth transition starting at lower concentrations compared to the other substrates. The VW was significantly shorter by a factor of $\approx$5 and the ERP score did not decrease for higher dronedarone concentrations. All these differences lead to peaks to critical score values under dronedarone in the cAF substrate even in the pharmacokinetic scenario assuming smaller variations of the drug concentration.
Wilhelms proposed I_{Na} block as the predominant mechanism by which amiodarone terminates spiral wave reentry [205]. Such two-dimensional tissue level effects were beyond the scope of the study presented here and should be addressed by future research. Preferably, investigations regarding the effects of drugs on rotor inducability and perpetuation should be performed on closed two-dimensional surfaces in three-dimensional space (cf. Section 5.1.5). The results presented here regarding the effect of amiodarone on ERP and CV are in line with experimental findings by Shinagawa et al. [335]. They report prolonged ERP in atrially tachypaced dogs under chronic amiodarone administration. The restoration of ERP absolute values and ERP rate adaptation to control values observed in the tachypaced dogs could not be reproduced, though. A reason for this might be the slightly different pharmacodynamic effects of amiodarone regarding acute and chronic administration further discussed in the next section. The CV reduction of $\approx$200 mm/s with flat restitution reported by Shinagawa et al. were reproduced here for an amiodarone concen-

tration of 4.4 μM. In their study, regional variations of the effect of amiodarone were described. This spatial heterogeneity could be integrated in a heterogeneous anatomical model (cf. Section 9.1) in future work once appropriate pharmacodynamics data on the ion channel level become available.
Sun et al. superfused rabbit muscle preparations acutely with either 10 μM dronedarone or 10 μM amiodarone [336]. They reported a similar degree of APD_{90} reduction for both compounds. Their observation cannot be explained by any IC_{50} and nH values found in the literature, however. In guinea pig experiments [329], MDP was not significantly affected by dronedarone as was the case for the *in silico* experiments presented here.
Scoring systems are widely used to quantify the complex effects of drugs in a condensed way. However, they are often based solely on IC_{50} values [337], neglect frequency dependence, thus restitution, of the dynamic system [309], neglect substrate dependence [338, 339], or require experiments using large animal models [340]. Besides markers derived from simulations using biophysically detailed models facilitating mechanistic insight, data-driven approaches using machine learning methods resulting in black box descriptions have been proposed. Kramer et al. used logistic regression on IC_{50} values of I_{Kr} (hERG), $I_{Ca,L}$ (Cav1.2), and I_{Na} (Nav1.5) obtained through automatic patch clamping [337]. Mistry et al. proposed to combine the degree of block of these channels in a single scalar measure [341]. Babcock et al. proposed to use gene expression levels instead of measured currents [342]. Pharmacokinetic properties were mostly neglected in prior work with few exceptions using basic representations as used in this study [301].

6.1.4 Limitations

The Hill-based drug models employed in this study are based on drug receptor interaction data from the literature, which are sometimes reported equivocally [321, 323, 324, 326, 327, 329, 343–361]. As pointed out before [362], dose response curves obtained under comparable experimental conditions from the same species for all cardiac ion current would be desirable. Recent developments aim to build methods allowing to incorporate measures considering and quantifying the uncertainty caused by the variability in the data [363] as well as the intrinsic variability across the population [300, 338, 364] based on e.g. Bayesian inference [365].

While the Hill-based conduction block model used in this study does not allow to consider voltage- or state-dependent block which has been described for some currents [312, 366, 367], these effects should not play a significant role considering the timescale at which binding and unbinding of the compound to the channel occurs, which is much longer than the timescale of channel state transitions and voltage changes. Therefore, simple conductance block models should be suitable except for agents affecting the probability of state transitions (allosteric block) [339]. The mode of action of amiodarone and dronedarone is mainly mediated via non-voltage-dependent effects and the available data describing voltage-dependent block were too sparse to model this effect reliably. Moreover, the non-competitive anti-β-adrenergic effect of both drugs [366, 367] was neglected and could be included in a future extension of the model in a similar way as in the work by Keller et al. [368].

It has to be stressed that the models of the drugs are based on data representing their acute effects rather than chronic administration. Differences between chronic and acute effects have been reported particularly for amiodarone with a possible mechanism being a modulation of gene expression [133, 369]. The available data on the ion current level were not sufficient to identify a complete set of Hill curve parameters representing the effects of chronic amiodarone administration.

The *in silico* modeling approach chosen in this study does not necessarily allow to translate the results to *in vivo* settings in terms of absolute concentrations as in the latter, the free drug concentration can hardly be assessed reliably [370]. Binding to plasma proteins has been reported for both drugs in vitro reducing the bioavailability as only the free drug concentration is pharmacologically active [371]. Even though the levels of plasma protein binding are not known precisely (e.g. 96.3±0.6% [372] vs. 99.97–99.99% [371] for amiodarone), this uncertainty does not affect the validity of the results in terms of relative concentration levels. The calibration of the biomarkers taken into account in the scoring process was based on the dynamic range observed in the simulation results and not on a robust and extensive empirical data set. Thus, validation and probably also refinement of the calibration is needed to draw clinically relevant conclusions from the score in a quantitative way rather than qualitatively as done in this study.

The circadian variation of the drug concentrations was based on a very simplistic model and does not claim to represent the exact course observed *in vivo*. Moreover, the course of the heart rate can only be a stereotypical showcase and does not claim to cover the whole range of possible scenarios in the real world population as a matter of course. The pharmacokinetic properties of both drugs are reported equivocally in the literature. As dronedarone kinetics are hard to assess in vivo, no data from humans were available and the amplitude of the circadian variation was assumed to be 50% due to the shorter elimination half time compared with amiodarone [136]. Considering the above mentioned aspects, a detailed pharmacokinetic model appears questionable to date and a variation within a certain range served the purpose of this study.

6.1.5 Conclusion

The results presented in this study show how atrial electrophysiology is differentially affected by the antiarrhythmic compounds amiodarone and dronedarone in a concentration-dependent and heart rate-dependent manner. The insights gained from *in silico* modeling regarding AP alternans as a proarrhythmic mechanism provide possible explanations for the superior efficacy of amiodarone over dronedarone in the treatment of AF. The newly proposed arrhythmia score aggregating several biomarkers from the cellular and tissue level peaked to critical values for dronedarone but not for amiodarone. The elucidated effects may aid in the design and optimization of patient group-specific pharmacotherapy. The drug effects differed significantly in a cAF remodeled substrate. By considering the atrial substrate in tailored therapies, the responder rate can be improved.

6.2 Vernakalant

Vernakalant is a recent compound, which has proven to be effective for the acute cardioversion of AF in a large share of patients in clinical studies. In this respect, vernakalant is superior to both placebo and the agent amiodarone, which was investigated in Section 6.1 [72, 140–144, 373, 374]. However, it was ineffective in patient with AF lasting for more than seven days and patients with atrial flutter (AFlut) [145]. The underlying mode of action and the reasons for the strong time dependence are not understood in their entirety. The experimental data ranges from one study on isolated ion channels [375], to a study in isolated tissue preparations [376] up to an *in vivo* study assessing the effect of vernakalant on atrial and ventricular ERP in humans [377]. The results on these different levels of integration have never been consolidated in a coherent framework and could not be linked until now. In this study, a multi-scale computational modeling approach is employed to elucidate the complex non-linear effects of vernakalant on cellular electrophysiology by linking the experimental data from the single channel level up to tissue level data.

Parts of this work have been published as a conference contribution [378] and are based on a supervised student's project [379].

6.2.1 Methods

The effect of vernakalant was studied using the Courtemanche et al. model of human atrial myocytes [47] representing a healthy substrate as well as in a variant representing cAF induced remodeling as introduced in Section 5.2. The cellular models were integrated in a one-dimensional tissue strand as detailed in Section 6.1. The effect of vernakalant was modeled based on Hill's equation (Equation (6.1)) using the following pairs of half-maximal inhibitory concentrations IC_{50} and Hill coefficients nH for the cardiac ion currents: 21.0 μM / 0.92 for I_{Kr} [375], 13.0 μM / 0.92 for I_{Kur} [375], 30.0 μM / 0.82 for I_{to} [375], and 84.0 μM / 1.0 for $I_{Ca,L}$ [376]. This model based on literature values is referred to as *M1* (Figure 6.8C). A second model *M2* was formulated with only $I_{Ca,L}$ being affected (42.0 μM / 1.0) (Figure 6.8D) besides sodium channel block as a hypothesis based on the experimentally observed behavior [376].

I_{Na} block was considered in both models. Due to the pronounced frequency dependence of vernakalant induced I_{Na} block, it could not be well represented by a single pair of IC_{50} and nH values. Therefore, the degree of I_{Na} block was determined by fitting g_{Na} aiming at the reproduction of experimentally observed changes of the AP upstroke velocity dV_m/dt_{max} [376] for each frequency and drug concentration individually.

dV_m/dt_{max} at zero drug concentration and the desired frequency was taken as a reference value to determine the relative reduction for a specific vernakalant concentration. The degree of I_{Na} block was optimized in the tissue strand environment. The resulting degree of block at concentrations of 10 μM and 30 μM were used to determine frequency-specific IC_{50} and nH values.
Besides the AP upstroke velocity dV_m/dt_{max}, further markers were evaluated. ERP, APD_{90}, AP amplitude, and MDP were introduced above. APD_{20} was determined at 20% repolarization and PLT_{20} was defined as the mean potential in the time window between 20% and 30% repolarization [376].

Table 6.3: Frequency-dependent estimates of half-maximal inhibitory concentrations IC_{50} and Hill coefficients nH for I_{Na} based on dV_m/dt_{max} reduction data [376] for the two models of vernakalant (M1 and M2).

		M1		M2	
		IC_{50} (μM)	nH	IC_{50} (μM)	nH
control	**0.5 Hz**	36.15	2.67	35.79	2.67
	1.0 Hz	36.25	1.16	35.27	1.07
	3.0 Hz	15.07	0.95	17.34	1.25
cAF	**0.5 Hz**	76.89	1.26	39.45	1.87
	1.0 Hz	61.32	1.10	61.88	1.18
	3.0 Hz	36.99	1.27	37.32	1.10

6.2.2 Results

The optimization of I_{Na} block using a bisection method converged for all substrates, frequencies, and concentrations and reproduced the experimentally observed relative reduction of AP upstroke velocity dV_m/dt_{max} with a residual of 0.4±1.8%. Table 6.3 lists the resulting IC_{50} and nH values for all three frequencies in both substrates. For faster pacing, lower IC_{50} values and smaller Hill coefficients were identified. This translated to a higher degree of block for vernakalant concentrations between 1 μM and 35 μM (Figure 6.8A+B). The frequency dependence was attenuated in the cAF substrate compared to control.

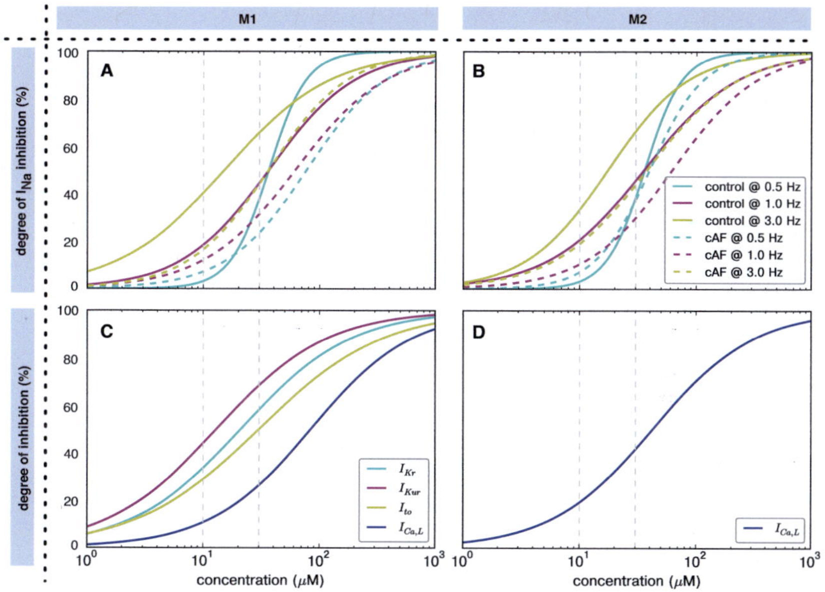

Figure 6.8: Dose response of veranakalant induced I_{Na} block depending on the pacing frequency and the substrate in *M1* (A) and *M2* (B) (cf. Table 6.3). The vertical lines indicate the concentration span covered in the study by Wetter et al. [376]. The frequency and substrate independent degree of block of other cardiac ion currents is shown in (C) for *M1* and (D) for *M2*.

By pacing the coupled cell models in the one-dimensional tissue strand under the influence of vernakalant, APs were elicited (Figure 6.9). 2:1 block occurred in the control substrate for 3 Hz pacing frequency and the drug model *M1*. All others combinations conducted APs robustly. AP alternans was observed, though. The resulting AP markers and their correspondence to the experimental findings in [376] are presented in Table 6.4. While *M1* reproduced the ERP prolongation reported in [376], the drug induced increase of divergence between ERP and APD_{90} was not reproduced. This divergence caused by concomitant ERP prolongation and APD_{90} shortening was described particularly for the control substrate [376]. *M2* on the other hand reproduced the APD_{90} shortening and the elevation of PLT_{20} but did not exhibit ERP prolongation. The other investigated AP markers were sufficiently reproduced by both drug models.

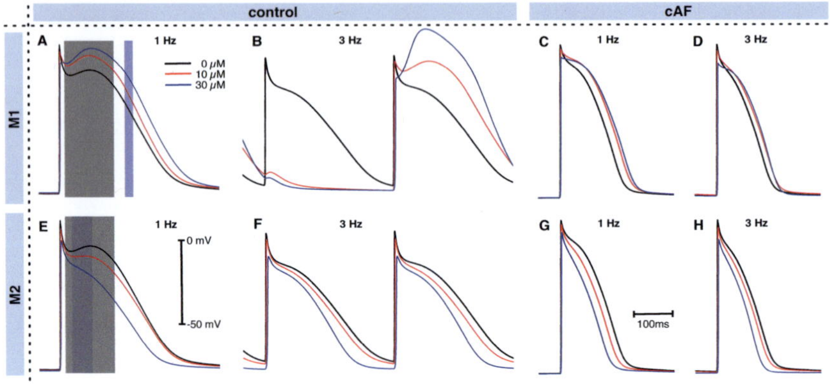

Figure 6.9: Vernakalant-induced change of the AP and its frequency dependence for the two drug models *M1* (A)–(D) and *M2* (E)–(H) in the control (A), (B), (E), and (F) and cAF substrates (C), (D), (G), and (H). AP curves are shown for the 5th beat in the tissue strand for 1 Hz and 3 Hz pacing frequency corresponding to BCLs of 1000 ms and 333 ms, respectively. For 3 Hz in the control substrate, the 6th beat is shown as well because of 2:1 block observed using *M1*. The time between APD_{20} and APD_{30} used to calculate PLT_{20} is highlighted by the shaded areas in (A) and (E) for zero drug concentration (gray) and 30 μM veranakalant (blue).

6.2.3 Discussion

In this study, it was shown that inhibition of the potassium currents I_{Kr}, I_{Kur}, and I_{to} together with the L-type calcium current $I_{Ca,L}$ by vernakalant prolongs the atrial ERP dose-dependently. The frequency-dependent and dose-dependent block of I_{Na} causes AP upstroke slowing and attenuated AP amplitudes. The model *M1*, which is based on pharmacodynamics data from literature, explains ERP prolongation, which can be considered vernakalant's major antiarrhythmic mode of action. The results presented here are in line with *in vivo* data from human by Dorian et al. reporting ERP prolongation to be dose-dependent but not significantly frequency-dependent between 1.6 Hz and 3.3 Hz [377]. In their study, atrial ERP was prolonged by between 12% and 14% for the higher investigated dose of 4.6 mg/kg applied intravenously.

Table 6.4: Resulting g_{Na} reduction based on dV_m/dt_{max} tuning and AP markers obtained using the two *in silico* models *M1* and *M2* in comparison to experimentally observed data [376].

				g_{Na}	dV_m/dt_{max}	ERP	APD_{90}	APD_{20}	PLT_{20}	APA	MDP
control	0.5 Hz	10 μM	M1	-3.1%	-8.3%	+4.1%	+3.8%	+31.0%	-0.0%	-1.4%	-0.2%
			M2	-3.1%	-6.4%	-0.6%	-0.7%	-86.1%	+8.4%	-1.4%	+0.1%
			[376]		-6.4%		-6.5%	+129.3%	+28.3%	-4.5%	-1.6%
		30 μM	M1	-37.8%	-37.8%	+16.0%	+11.2%	+50.0%	-6.9%	-0.7%	-0.3%
			M2	-38.3%	-38.0%	-8.2%	-10.1%	-79.5%	+49.0%	-10.4%	+0.3%
			[376]		-38.0%		-18.7%	+475.6%	+53.3%	-21.0%	-6.3%
	1.0 Hz	10 μM	M1	-18.2%	-15.6%	+6.4%	+5.4%	+692.0%	+29.5%	-4.7%	-0.3%
			M2	-20.7%	-19.5%	-0.3%	-1.5%	+295.2%	+43.1%	-5.1%	+0.3%
			[376]		-17.9%	+7.2%	+1.2%	+135.8%	+36.1%	-5.4%	+0.7%
		30 μM	M1	-44.5%	-43.9%	+18.8%	+12.7%	+787.1%	+17.0%	-3.0%	-0.5%
			M2	-45.7%	-46.0%	-12.4%	-15.8%	+87.9%	+83.6%	-12.9%	+0.7%
			[376]		-45.6%	+11.0%	-4.1%	+430.2%	+63.3%	-18.6%	-2.9%
	3.0 Hz	10 μM	M1	-40.4%	-19.1%			+844.1%	+3.0%	-0.4%	+3.7%
			M2	-33.5%	-22.5%	-5.3%	-6.9%	+49.6%	+14.3%	-4.1%	+1.7%
			[376]		-22.1%	+10.7%	+11.2%	+90.1%	+4.6%	-8.2%	-3.2%
		30 μM	M1	-65.7%	-60.8%		+19.4%	+710.7%	-90.1%	+24.0%	+3.6%
			M2	-66.5%	-63.1%	-8.9%	-19.4%	+265.5%	+46.8%	-13.6%	+5.5%
			[376]		-62.7%	+31.3%	+15.0%	+100.8%	+52.5%	-36.1%	-10.4%
cAF	0.5 Hz	10 μM	M1	-7.1%	-7.2%	+11.6%	+11.9%	+52.3%	+3.2%	-1.7%	-0.1%
			M2	-7.2%	-7.3%	-8.7%	-9.3%	-29.3%	+6.3%	-1.7%	+0.0%
			[376]		-7.3%		+7.3%	+42.9%	+16.1%	-4.3%	-2.7%
		30 μM	M1	-23.4%	-23.2%	+18.0%	+16.6%	+75.7%	+17.5%	-5.9%	-0.1%
			M2	-37.5%	-24.2%	-17.4%	-20.8%	-45.6%	+20.5%	-6.5%	+0.0%
			[376]		-24.3%		+16.4%	+109.9%	-6.9%	-10.4%	-5.3%
	1.0 Hz	10 μM	M1	-11.9%	-13.2%	+12.4%	+12.7%	+47.5%	+7.2%	-2.9%	-0.1%
			M2	-10.3%	-10.9%	-9.5%	-10.5%	-27.7%	+10.0%	-2.5%	+0.1%
			[376]		-10.1%	+8.5%	+5.9%	+36.6%	+38.0%	-3.5%	-2.6%
		30 μM	M1	-31.2%	-31.0%	+18.9%	+17.3%	+67.1%	+25.7%	-8.2%	-0.1%
			M2	-29.8%	-30.9%	-19.5%	-23.1%	-46.6%	+26.7%	-7.9%	+0.1%
			[376]		-30.3%	+30.3%	+15.9%	+76.4%	+52.0%	-9.9%	-3.9%
	3.0 Hz	10 μM	M1	-16.0%	-15.3%	+11.6%	+10.5%	+56.5%	+13.2%	-4.2%	-0.3%
			M2	-19.1%	-18.5%	-5.4%	-7.4%	-7.1%	+16.8%	-4.6%	+0.4%
			[376]		-16.2%	+16.3%	+11.2%	+36.7%	+800.0%	-16.6%	-3.9%
		30 μM	M1	-43.4%	-44.2%	+15.6%	+10.6%	+107.8%	+41.0%	-12.1%	+0.4%
			M2	-44.0%	-45.3%	-15.0%	-21.4%	-11.9%	+42.8%	-11.8%	+1.2%
			[376]		-43.9%	+23.7%	+14.1%	+40.1%	+1070.0%	-16.6%	-14.3%

Frommeyer et al. recently reported an increase of APD by 9 ms and ERP by 16 ms in whole-heart Langendorff-perfused rabbit models [380]. Burashnikov et al. reported a rate-dependent prolongation of post repolarization refractoriness in LA canine preparations which was accounted to block of the sodium channel [381].

The second model *M2* comprised only $I_{Ca,L}$ block besides I_{Na} inhibition with the model parameters for $I_{Ca,L}$ block not being based on literature data from the subcellular level but chosen to match experimentally observed AP properties. This model affected the delicate balance of depolarizing and repolarizing currents during the AP plateau and repolarization in a way possibly explaining the effects of vernakalant on APD_{90} and PLT_{20}. PLT_{20} suggested as a marker in [376] has to be considered with caution, however, as APD_{20} strongly depends on the AP morphology. If the AP exhibits a pronounced spike-and-dome morphology (30 μM in Figure 6.9A), APD_{20} is shifted to later phases in the AP compared to early values for a more linear repolarization (30 μM in Figure 6.9E). The cell model by Maleckar et al. [218] yielded qualitatively similar results (data not shown). Thus, the results of this study are unlikely to be sensitive to the choice of a particular cell model.

Both investigated drug models provide hypotheses for part of the experimentally observed effects of vernakalant. However, none of the drug models is capable of reproducing the effects in their entirety and providing comprehensive mechanistic insight. This finding highlights a missing piece in the puzzle regarding our understanding of vernakalant's mode of action and brings up new questions. Besides potential effects on the MDP mediated by I_{K1} or $I_{K,ACh}$ and affecting ERP via the availability of the h gate of the sodium channel, the frequency-dependence, and possibly state-dependence, of I_{Na} block is not understood. This puts the ball in the experimentalists court as appropriate wet-lab data is required to formulate a more complex model representing the effects of vernakalant. In particular, a Markov model directly describing the frequency dependence appears better suited than a set of models comprised of one Hill formulation per frequency. State-dependency of block might as well need to be covered in order to reproduce the different effects on ERP and APD_{90}. Models of the discrete kinetics of drug interaction can e.g. be parametrized using the methods recently proposed by Moreno et al. [382].

In conclusion, this study fosters our understanding of the cellular mode of action of vernakalant on the one hand. On the other hand, it points out relevant gaps in our current knowledge and will thus hopefully fuel and direct future wet-lab and computational research on this aspiring antiarrhythmic agent. As such, it serves as an example how the interplay between experimentalists and modelers can lead to mutual benefit and cross-fertilize and speed up research.

6.3 Optimization of Drug Therapy for Familial Atrial Fibrillation

Early onset AF has a significant familial component [383]. Individuals carrying certain gene mutations, as e.g. the two hERG mutations N588K and L532P introduced in Section 5.1, are more susceptible to AF. In this study, multi-channel blockers are evaluated regarding their potential to revert the AP of atrial myocytes affected by these mutations to the control AP of non-mutated, WT myocytes. Towards this end, a hypothetic multi-channel blocker is designed and optimized for each mutation. Moreover, the potential of the two existing compounds amiodarone and dronedarone (cf. Section 6.1) is assessed by tuning the concentration levels. The optimization aims at a minimization of the root mean square difference (RMSD) between the control and the mutant AP. The properties of the myocytes under the influence of the tailored pharmacological agent is then assessed in a dynamic way considering APD_{90} restitution and calcium transients.
Parts of this work have been published as conference contributions [384, 385] and are based on a supervised student's project [319].

6.3.1 Methods

The Courtemanche et al. model of human atrial myocytes [47] served as a reference for the healthy, WT myocytes. The hERG mutations N588K and L532P were modeled by altering the I_{Kr} formulation as introduced in Section 5.1. For the design of the hypothetic multi-channel blocker, the maximum conductances g_x of the nine atrial ion currents I_{Kr}, I_{Kur}, I_{Ks}, I_{to}, I_{K1}, I_{Na}, $I_{Ca,L}$, $I_{b,Na}$, and $I_{b,Ca}$ were scaled individually by a factor $\Theta_x \in [0,1]$:

$$I_x = g_x \cdot \Theta_x \cdot (V_m - E_x) \ , \tag{6.2}$$

with E_x being the equilibrium potential of the ion type carrying the respective current. The existing compounds amiodarone and dronedarone were modeled by the Hill equation-based approach introduced in Section 6.1.

The cost function for the minimization was the RMSD ΔAP between the mutant and the control AP over a fixed time span of 500 ms:

$$\Delta AP := \sqrt{\frac{1}{500}\sum_{i=1}^{500}\left(V_{m,mut}\left(t_i,\Theta\right) - V_{m,ctl}\left(t_i\right)\right)^2} \ , \tag{6.3}$$

with $\Theta \in \mathbb{R}^9$ altering the mutant AP. In order to minimize ΔAP, Θ was optimized in the nine-dimensional space for the hypothetic multi-channel blocker. For the existing compounds amiodarone and dronedarone, the scalar concentration D translating to a specific degree of block Θ_x for each channel according to Equation (6.1) and Table 6.1 was subject to optimization. APs were elicited with a BCL of 1000 ms and analyzed in steady-state conditions.

The cell model was implemented in *Matlab* and solved by *ode15s* with a variable time increment for simulations on the single cell level. Tissue level simulations were conducted in the one-dimensional tissue strand introduced in Section 5.1 with a fixed time step of 10 μs. Optimization on the single cell level was performed using the TRR algorithm introduced in Section 4.1.1.3, which is well-suited for multi-dimensional, non-linear minimization problems. The start vectors were drawn randomly using a uniform distribution. On the tissue level, the constrained Broyden-Fletcher-Goldfarb-Shanno algorithm belonging to the class of quasi-Newton hill-climbing methods provided by the *Python* library *SciPy* [386] was utilized. The parameters yielded by the optimization on the single cell levels were used as the initial guess on the tissue level.

To evaluate the optimization result, APD_{90} was analyzed in the tissue strand for 30 BCLs ranging from 200 ms to 1300 ms distributed linearly in the frequency domain to obtain its restitution with respect to the DI.

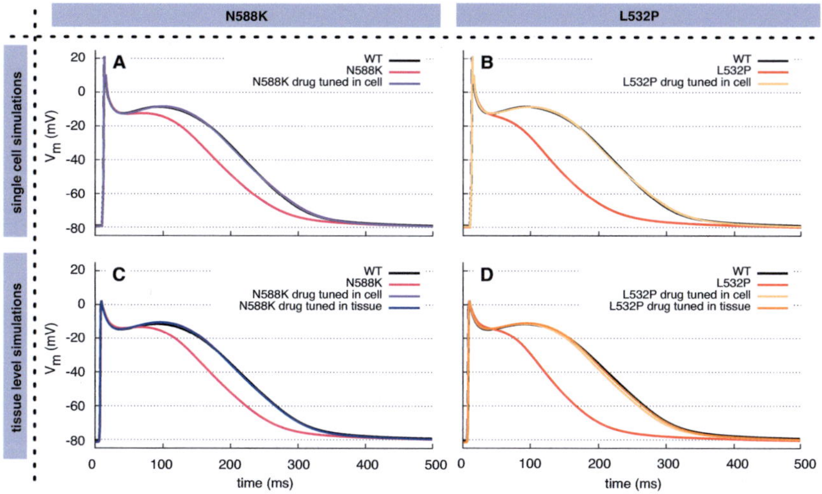

Figure 6.10: AP curves from single cell (A)+(B) and tissue level (C)+(D) simulations obtained using WT and hERG mutation cell models. The optimized multi-channel blockers given in Table 6.5 were applied to mutant myocytes to restore the WT AP. In (A) and (B), the WT APs are partly covered by those of the mutant models under drug influence. In (C) and (D), the APs obtained by tissue level optimization partly cover the single cell optimization result, additionally.

6.3.2 Results

By optimizing the degree of inhibition for each channel individually, the deviation between the WT and the mutant APs could be reduced. The RMSD was lowered from 8.3 mV to 0.5 mV for N588K (Figure 6.10A) and from 18.2 mV to 0.5 mV for L532P (Figure 6.10B) in the single cell environment. The maximum deviation observed for a single time step was reduced from 36.2 mV to 3.1 mV and from 17.1 mV to 2.5 mV, respectively. The corresponding optimal scale factors Θ_x are listed in Table 6.5. Transitioning to the tissue level, the factors Θ_x defining the optimized hypothetic compound remained unchanged for N588K. In the tissue strand simulation, the RMSD was 0.63 mV (Figure 6.10C). Concerning, the L532P substrate the single cell result yielded an RMSD of 1.8 mV that could be reduced to 0.6 mV by optimization on the tissue level. Compared to the optimal compound on the single cell level, I_{Kr} was reduced by additional 3% and $I_{b,Na}$ by additional 1% (Figure 6.10D).

Table 6.5: Scaling factors Θ of the hypothetic multi-channel blocker for atrial ion currents ranging from 1 (no effect) to 0 (complete blockage). The given combinations yielded the lowest RMSD between mutant and WT APs in single cell and tissue simulations.

	L532P		N588K	
	Cell	**Tissue**	**Cell**	**Tissue**
Θ_{Kr}	0.42	0.39	0.56	0.56
Θ_{Kur}	0.59	0.59	0.61	0.61
Θ_{Ks}	0.95	0.95	0.88	0.88
Θ_{to}	1.00	1.00	0.99	0.99
Θ_{K1}	1.00	1.00	1.00	1.00
Θ_{Na}	1.00	1.00	0.99	0.99
$\Theta_{Ca,L}$	0.86	0.86	0.83	0.83
$\Theta_{b,Na}$	0.97	0.98	0.96	0.96
$\Theta_{b,Ca}$	0.92	0.92	0.96	0.96

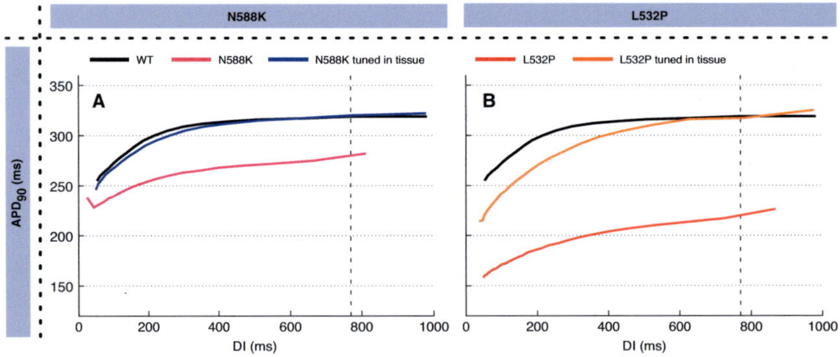

Figure 6.11: Restitution of the APD_{90} for WT and mutant atrial myocytes. The multi-channel blockers (see Table 6.5) were optimized at a BCL of 1000 ms corresponding to the vertical dashed line and applied to the hERG mutant cells at BCLs between 200 ms and 1300 ms.

The compounds that performed optimal for the fixed BCL of 1000 ms were analyzed regarding their dynamic APD_{90} restitution properties (Figure 6.11). For higher pacing rates, thus lower DIs, the APD of the mutant cells under the influence of the tuned compounds was shorter compared to WT. This effect was more pronounced for L532P (maximum deviation of 34.2 ms at a DI of 62 ms, Figure 6.11B) than for N588K (maximum deviation of 6.2 ms at a DI of 178 ms, Figure 6.11A).

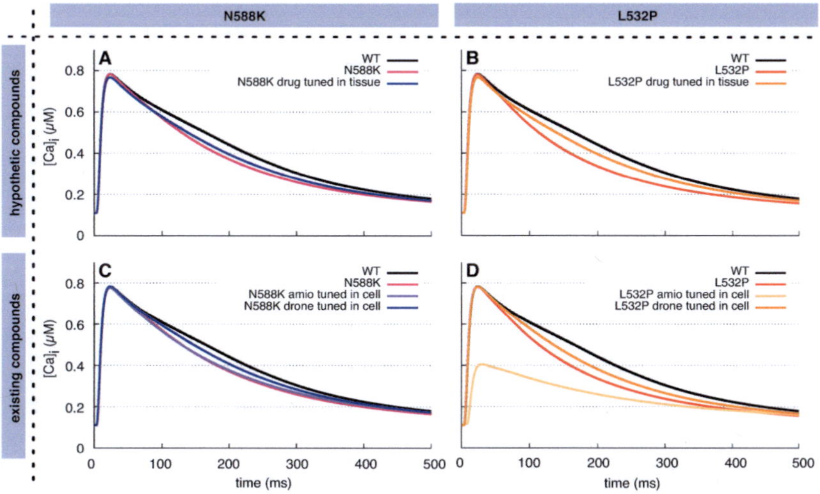

Figure 6.12: Calcium transients observed during APs in the N588K (A)+(C) and L532P (B)+(D) hERG mutant cells. In (A) and (B), the optimized hypothetic multi-channel blockers were administered, whereas amiodarone and dronedarone were administered at optimized concentrations in (C)+(D).

A second property that was not considered during the optimization but determines the cell's electrophysiological characteristics are calcium transients that were ameliorated by the optimized compounds but not fully restored (Figure 6.12A+B).

Besides the design of hypothetic multi-channel blockers with arbitrary ratios of channel inhibition, the concentration of the existing compounds amiodarone and dronedarone was optimized on the cellular level. The objective function was Equation (6.3) as above. The N588K mutant AP could be reverted up to 1.3 mV by 0.04 μM of dronedarone, thus almost as good as using the hypothetic compound (0.5 mV). Amiodarone, however failed to restore the WT AP yielding a residual RMSD of 6.3 mV at the optimal concentration of 0.76 μM not much lower than the initial value of 8.3 mV (Figure 6.13A).

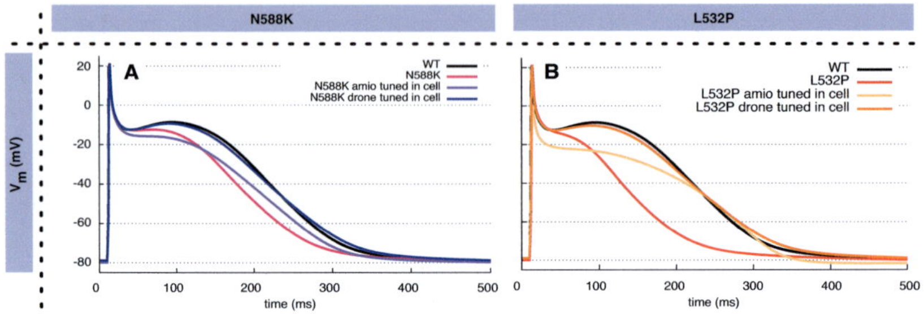

Figure 6.13: APs obtained by applying the optimized concentrations of amiodarone and dronedarone to restore the WT AP in cells affected by hERG mutations L532P (A) and N588K (B).

The results for L532P were comparable with a residual RMSD of 1.76 mV for the optimal dronedarone concentration of 0.088 μM and 17.21 mV for the optimal amiodarone concentration of 10.72 μM. The optimal dronedarone concentration and the optimized hypothetic compound regarding ΔAP differed in the resulting Ca^{2+} transients (Figure 6.12C+D). For N588K, dronedarone restored the WT transient slightly better whereas the result was opposite for L532P.

6.3.3 Discussion

In this study, the electrophysiology of hERG mutant atrial myocytes was restored to the healthy state in terms of AP morphology and APD. The WT AP could be restored by significant block of I_{Kr} and I_{Kur} ($\geq$39%) and less pronounced block of I_{Ks}, $I_{Ca,L}$, $I_{b,Na}$, and $I_{b,Ca}$ ($\leq$17%). On the tissue level, I_{Kr} inhibition had to be slightly reduced for L532P to obtain optimal AP restoration. The presented results show that on the AP level, changes in I_{Kr} conductance and kinetics can be counterbalanced by combined reduction of ionic current conductances without altering their kinetics. APD_{90} restitution and calcium transients were used as independent quality metrics to assess the restoration of the electrophysiological properties using measures that were not considered in the optimization cost function. For N588K, APD_{90} restitution was almost restored by the hypothetic multi-channel blocker, whereas deviation of up to 15% were observed for fast pacing in the L532P substrate.

The existing antiarrhythmic agents amiodarone and dronedarone exhibited markedly different potential with respect to the restoration of the WT AP. Dronedarone performed very well and achieved levels of restoration close to the hypothetic multi-channel blocker with just one degree of freedom (the concentration) instead of nine (the levels of block). Amiodarone on the other hand could not reduce the RMSD between the mutant and the WT AP significantly. This observation underlines the importance of the complex, non-linear interaction between the different atrial ion currents and prevent solely considering the main effect (in this case inhibition of potassium channels) when characterizing the mode of action.

This is the first work using computational methods or experimental approaches to restore mutant APs to the state of healthy control myocytes by hypothetic or existing pharmaceutical compounds to the best of my knowledge. The limitations regarding the models of amiodarone and dronedarone with respect to acute vs. chronic administration and the Hill equation-based formulation discussed in Section 6.1.4 apply to this study as well. Future work could include the metrics that were used for validation in this study (restitution properties and calcium transients) into the cost function. However, validation has to be performed in other ways, then.

In conclusion, the study presented in this section provides insight into the pharmacodynamic response of hERG mutant myocytes rendering patients vulnerable to AF and may aid in the design and advancement of tailored therapeutic and preventive approaches considering the atrial substrate as recently outlined in a roadmap for personalized drug development [305].

PART III

IDENTIFYING ATRIAL FLUTTER PATHS

CHAPTER 7

Augmenting Anatomical Models with a Priori Knowledge

Today's medical imaging technologies provide the means to obtain the anatomy of individual patients in unprecedented detail. However, some properties cannot be image *in vivo*. One important aspect is the orientation of myocytes which influences excitation propagation significantly. Moreover, the contrast in most imaging modalities does not allow to identify the presence of interatrial connections (IACs) or at least their conductive properties. Their presence and intactness determines the LA activation pattern, though. The same holds for scar tissue introduced by ablation or fibrosis induced by remodeling processes, which can only be imaged by late Gadolinium-enhanced magnetic resonance imaging (MRI) with a limited resolution [178–181]. Another challenge is the estimation of the long-term extent of the scar as late gadolinium enhanced MRI of acute ablation lesions significantly overestimate the chronic scar volume [387]. Moreover, it is necessary to introduce standard ablation patterns in the *in silico* models in an automated manner in order to assess their effect before applying them in the patient.
Therefore, data acquired in animal models, human *ex vivo* studies, or invasive electroanatomic mapping studies is used to learn about these features. These general patterns can then be applied to augment anatomical models of an individual with a priori knowledge in a rule-based manner. Section 7.1 describes a method to annotate myocyte orientation which is mesh-type-agnostic,

i.e. can be applied to meshes with arbitrary elements (triangles, tetrahedra, hexahedra etc.). Section 7.2 introduces an extension allowing to connect the right atrium (RA) and the left atrium (LA) via well-defined IACs in order to control interatrial conduction.
Part of this work is based on earlier work [23] and a supervised student's project [388] and has been published as a conference contribution [389].

7.1 Myocyte Orientation

As introduced in Section 2.1.1.2, myocytes tend to align along pronounced muscular bundles and finer, non-transmural structures. This fact gives rise to anisotropic conductive properties, which in turn influence excitation propagation significantly [55, 390, 391] with consequences for the development and perpetuation of atrial arrhythmias [33, 392].
Diffusion tensor imaging (DTI) is an MRI-based imaging technique that can provide information on myocyte orientation. However, acquisition in the atria is difficult due to the very thin wall compared to the ventricles and the motion due to the beating of the heart. This requires the atria to be fixated and an acquisition time of several hours in contrast to first *in vivo* data for the ventricles [393]. Other techniques such as histographs [394] or extended volume surface imaging [395, 396] were used to map the myocyte orientation of a specific specimen to an anatomical model of the same specimen. After early studies with manually placed myocyte orientation [57, 58, 397–399] and simple interpolation methods [400, 401], the first comprehensive approach to augment models with transmurally varying myocyte orientation in a rule-based manner semiautomatically was presented within the scope of the dissertation of Dr.-Ing. Martin Krüger [23].
The method presented by Krüger et al. is based on several anatomical studies [19, 20, 22] and was evaluated and validated in [23, 183, 402]. However, it was designed and implemented for models represented in structured grids with a fixed resolution of 0.33 mm.

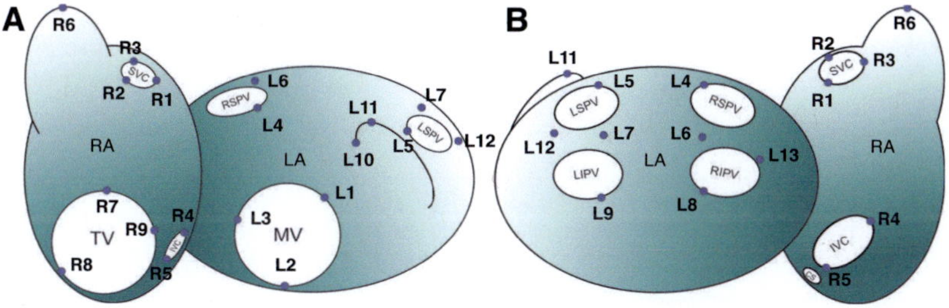

Figure 7.1: Schematic representation of the 22 landmark points (blue) given in Table 7.1. R1 to R9 are located in the RA, L1 to L13 are located in the LA. (A) shows the anterior aspect, (B) the posterior aspect. Figure based on supervised student's work [388].

Structured grids built of uniformly-sized hexahedra carry the disadvantage of requiring a high resolution in order to represent the curved atrial surface without pronounced jagged boundaries causing spurious currents [403]. Moreover, the whole domain has to be modeled using elements of the same size. Particularly for bidomain simulations including passive regions (e.g. blood) this represents a major restriction and a computational bottleneck. Therefore, tetrahedral meshes are often better suited for finite element simulation of cardiac electrophysiology. Another type of grids are triangular surface meshes that are commonly used in fast, simplified excitation propagation simulation using e.g. the fast marching algorithm (Chapter 8). Therefore, the existing method to annotate myocyte orientation was extended and improved aiming at a mesh-type-agnostic approach, thus being suited for structured and unstructured grid with arbitrary building blocks.

7.1.1 Methods

In order to get an abstract representation of the elements of the mesh (cells), each cell was represented by a single point located at its centroid. This transformation provided the means to design the algorithm in a mesh-type-agnostic way while maintaining the distance between elements.

Table 7.1: Definition of the 22 landmark points used in the annotation that are required as an input to the algorithm. Points R1 to R9 are located in the RA, L1 to L13 are located in the LA.

Point	Location
R1	boundary of the superior vena cava (SVC), septal, close to R4
R2	boundary of the SVC, anterior towards the tricuspid valve (TV)
R3	boundary of the SVC, junction with the right atrial appendage (RAA)
R4	boundary of the inferior vena cava (IVC), superior
R5	boundary of the IVC, inferior
R6	tip of the RAA
R7	boundary of the TV, anterior/superior
R8	boundary of the TV, posterior/inferior
R9	boundary of the TV, septal
L1	boundary of the mitral valve (MV), close to the left atrial appendage (LAA)
L2	boundary of the MV, posterior/inferior
L3	boundary of the MV, septal
L4	right superior pulmonary vein (RSPV), superior/medial, in line with L6 and L8
L5	left superior pulmonary vein (LSPV), superior/medial, in line with L7 and L9
L6	between RSPV and right inferior pulmonary vein (RIPV)
L7	between LSPV and left inferior pulmonary vein (LIPV)
L8	RIPV, inferior/medial
L9	LIPV, inferior/medial
L10	end of Bachmann's bundle (BB) in the LA
L11	tip of the LAA
L12	left lateral of the LPVs, between the LPVs and the LAA
L13	right lateral (septal) of the RPVs

The proposed method can be applied without user interaction once the position of 22 anatomical landmarks (Figure 7.1) are defined [23]. These nine points in the RA and 13 points in the LA can either be marked manually or provided by the tool performing the preprocessing including the segmentation of the atria. Table 7.1 and Figure 7.1 give a detailed description of the location of these initial points. The two atria need to be separated, i.e. right and LA elements may not share common nodes. If such nodes are present in the model, they are resolved by node duplication: a common node is split into two nodes (one for the LA, one for the RA) with the same coordinates.

For the annotation of the myocyte orientation and the definition of additional, derived points, connections between points had to be found. Paths $\mathbf{p}$ from a starting point $\mathbf{a_0}$ to an end point $\mathbf{a_{N-1}}$ via potential intermediate points were computed using a modification of the Dijsktra algorithm [171, 172] which penalizes deviance from the direct connection between the points:

$$\|\mathbf{p}(\mathbf{a_0},\mathbf{a_{N-1}})\|_2 = \min\left(\sum_{i=1}^{N-1}\left(\|\mathbf{a_i}-\mathbf{a_{i-1}}\|_2 + \frac{\|(\mathbf{a_n}-\mathbf{a_0})\times(\mathbf{a_i}-\mathbf{a_0})\|_2}{\|\mathbf{a_n}-\mathbf{a_0}\|_2}\right)\right), \tag{7.1}$$

with N being the number of points along the path and $\mathbf{a_i}$ being the location of point i. If the starting point a_0 and the end point a_{N-1} are the same, the path is circular and referred to by $\mathbf{p_c}$ in the following. Some paths were restricted to a plane, e.g. the crista terminalis (CT) and the pectinate muscles. Therefore, the penalty term was changed to the distance between the point on the path and the plane defined by the normal vector $\mathbf{n}$ for paths $\mathbf{p_p}$ restricted to a plane:

$$\|\mathbf{p_p}(\mathbf{a_0},\mathbf{a_{N-1}})\|_2 = \min\left(\sum_{i=1}^{N-1}\left(\|\mathbf{a_i}-\mathbf{a_{i-1}}\|_2 + \frac{\|(\mathbf{a_i}-\mathbf{a_0})\cdot\mathbf{n}\|_2}{\|\mathbf{n}\|_2}\right)\right). \tag{7.2}$$

The paths along which myocyte orientation was annotated as well as the rules to derive auxiliary points used to define these paths are given in Table 7.2 and Table 7.3. In the LA, separate sets of rules were applied to the endocardial (Table 7.5) and epicardial layer (Table 7.6) using the the auxiliary points defined in Table 7.4. A schematic representation of the paths is shown in Figure 7.2. Once the sequence of points defining a path was found, the myocyte orientation was annotated as the normalized difference vector between the current element and the preceding one. Depending on the course of the path and the structure of the underlying mesh, this approach can lead to local discontinuities in myocyte orientation which are not modeled deliberately based on anatomical observation but have to be considered artifacts. Therefore, the orientation along the paths was smoothed by a moving average filter implemented as a symmetric sliding window of size eleven.

As the annotation of myocyte orientation was motivated by the observation of bundles with a finite thickness, the orientation of the elements along the path was copied to adjacent elements using a spherical shape element with a defined radius (see Tables 7.3, 7.5, and 7.6). This interpolation and dilation step resulted in a tubular structure with coherent myocyte orientation.

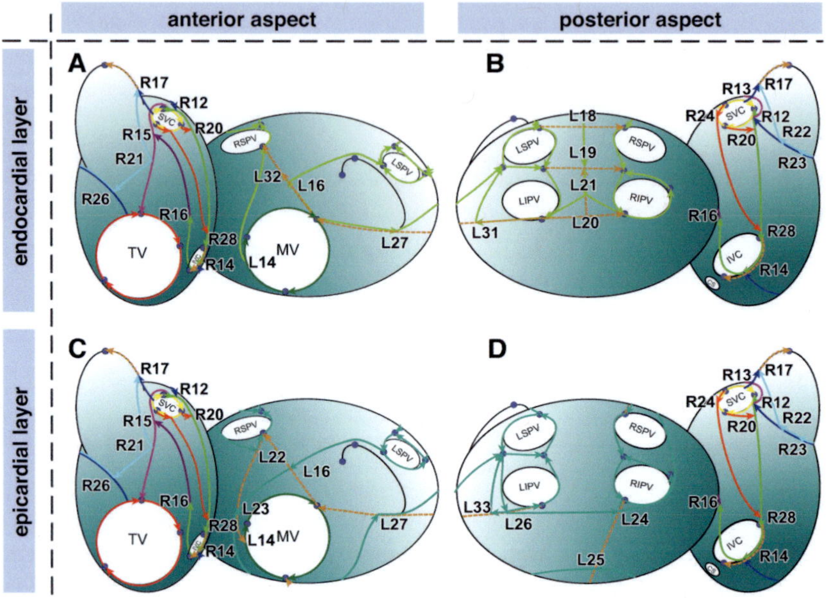

Figure 7.2: Schematic course of the paths along which myocyte orientation was annotated. In the LA, the paths in the endocardial layer ((A) and (B)) and the epicardial layer ((C) and (D)) were annotated using two distinct set of rules, whereas the paths did not differ between layers in the RA. Different colors represent distinct tissue classes. Blue points represent the 22 initial landmarks. Dashed lines were only used to compute the location of auxiliary points and not used to align myocyte orientation. (A) and (C) show the anterior aspect, (B) and (D) the posterior aspect. Figure based on supervised student's work [388].

For atrial wall segments that are thicker than twice the radius of the dilation shape element, the annotation of fibers and tissue classes was thus not necessarily transmural. However, particularly complete separation of adjacent regions by a dilated path is crucial for some steps. Therefore, the spherical shape element can optionally be replaced by two semi-spheres connected by a cylinder with the same radius and a variable height yielding a precisely transmural annotation in each element. This extended approach guarantees transmurality even for pathological wall thicknesses (see e.g. Chapter 11) on the expense of computation time.

Table 7.2: Definition of additional points in the RA used during the annotation procedure. Missing points in the sequential numbering were identified as non-necessary during the development of the algorithm.

Point	Location	Point	Location
R10	10% along pR7R8	R22	59% along PM_1
R11	3% along pR12R4	R23	43% along PM_1
R12	3% along pR3R1	R24	50% along R1R2
R13	85% along pR2R3	R26	22% along PM_1
R14	60% along pR4R5	R28	90% along pR12R4
R15	20% along pR12R7	R29	80% along pR12R4
R16	25% along pR14R15	R31	65% along pR12R4
R17	6.6 mm along pR13R6	R38	40% along pR2R7
R18	50% along pR14R15	R39	50% along R2R24R28
R20	29% along pR12R4	R40	25% along pR7R8
R21	22% along pR12R7		

The interpolation and dilation steps can cause myocyte orientations to deviate slightly from the tangential direction with respect to the surface which is not physiological. Therefore, the orientation was projected onto the plane defined by the closest surface element and normalized. For hexahedral meshes, the surface mesh considered in this step was smoothed in order to avoid artifacts due to mesh structure-induced jagged edges.

Besides the annotation of a vector defining the myocyte orientation, a scalar value representing the tissue class was added for points along the paths and dilated similarly. Initially, the entire RA was set to the class RA while the LA was divided into two layers (LA_{endo} and LA_{epi}) for volumetric models.

The CT tapers from 3.96 mm at the SVC to 2.64 mm at the IVC [20]. Therefore, the radius was linearly decreased from 3.96 mm at R3 via R12 to 2.64 mm at R4. The number of pectinate muscles (PMs) differs between individuals and was thus implemented as a variable M with a default value of 15. The PMs depart from the CT (pR10R8) towards the TVR (pR11R4R14) with the junctions being distributed equidistantly. Each PM was defined as a path along a plane ($\mathbf{p_p}$) being defined by the start and the end point and R18.

Table 7.3: Paths defining atrial myocyte orientation in the RA. A path is defined by the start point, the end point, and potential intermediate points.

Name	Material restriction	Material label	Radius (mm)	Additional remarks
p_cR1R2R3	RA	SVC	4.29	
p_cR6R7R8	RA	TVR	6.27	
pR12R7	RA, SVC, TVR	TL	3.96	
pR3R12	RA, SVC	CT	3.96 - 2.64	
p_pR12R4	RA, SVC	CT	3.96 - 2.64	plane defined by R12, R4, R14
pR4R14R16	RA	CT	2.64	
pR16R15	RA, TL	CT	4.62	
PM_1	RA	PM	1.32	extended width of 2.64 mm for the first 4.95 mm
PM_2-PM_M	RA	PM	0.66	
pR13R17	RA	PM	1.98	
p_cR17R22R23R26R21	RA	RAA	2.64	
pR2R24R28	RA, CT, SVC	ICB	4.80	
pR1R20	RA, CT, SVC	ICB	2.64	
pR2R7	RA	BB	2.00	

For the annotation of the LA elements, two distinct sets of rules (see Tables 7.5 and 7.6) were applied for the endocardial and the epicardial elements. Volumetric models have to be separated into endocardial and epicardial layers by preprocessing steps as e.g. described in [404]. Before annotating the respective layers, the seed points were moved normal to the atrial wall such that they were located within the right layer. For surface models, endocardial and epicardial data arrays are created allowing to choose the appropriate set for the desired application in a flexible way.

7.1.1.1 Pulmonary Veins & Atrial Appendages

The anatomy of the atrial appendages and the pulmonary vein ostia exhibits pronounced interindividual variability. As this variability also affects wall thickness and incidence angle, a standard path dilation with a spherical shape element does not guarantee transmural separation of these structures.

Table 7.4: Definition of additional points in the LA used during the annotation procedure. $\mathbf{c}_{\mathbf{BoBo}}$ represents the center of the bounding box around a path.

Point	Location	Point	Location
L14	80% along pL2L3	L54	$\mathbf{c}_{\mathbf{BoBo}}$ pL7L9L26L12
L16	50% along pL1L4	L55	45% along pL13L22
L18	50% along pL5L4	L56	50% along pL1L2
L19	50% along pL7L6	L57	60% along pL13L22
L20	50% along pL9L8	L58	30% along pL6L7
L21	50% along pL19L20	L59	70% along pL7L7
L22	10% along pL4L14	L60	20% along pL12L26
L23	50% along pL4L14	L61	20% along pL4L6
L24	10% along pL8L2	L62	50% along pL7L5
L25	80% along pL8L2	L63	20% along pL9L7
L26	20% along pL9L1	L64	80% along pL6L8
L27	75% along pL9L1	L65	70% along pL9L7
L31	30% along pL9L1	L66	60% along pL4L6
L32	70% along pL9L1	L67	20% along pL7L5
L33	5% along pL26L1	L68	closest LA point to R16
L34	6.93 mm along pL1L11	L69	70% along pL13L2
L35	10% along pL13L22	L70	30% along pL6L7
L36	25% along pL3L2	L72	80% along pL13L58
L39	$\mathbf{c}_{\mathbf{BoBo}}$ pL6L8L13	L73	20% along pL13L58
L44	$\mathbf{c}_{\mathbf{BoBo}}$ pL4L6L13L22	L74	50% along pL60L7
L49	$\mathbf{c}_{\mathbf{BoBo}}$ pL5L7L12		

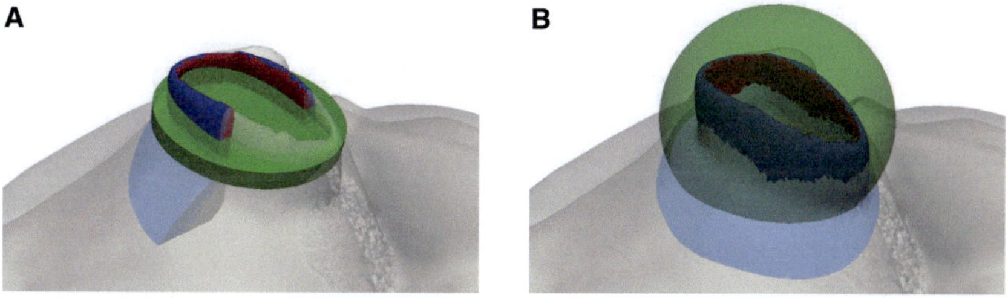

Figure 7.3: Annotation of the PVs. If non-labeled tissue (blue) was found within the green cylinder in (A), an outwards-oriented PV was assumed to be present. The PV was cut open for visualization reasons within the semi-transparent LA wall in (A) but not in (B). All elements within the green sphere in (B) were labeled as PV tissue. Figure based on supervised student's work [388].

Table 7.5: Paths defining atrial myocyte orientation in the endocardial layer of the LA. A path is defined by the start point, the end point, and potential intermediate points. The paths were restricted to the material LA_{endo}. Abbreviations: mitral valve ring (MVR).

Name	**Radius** (mm)	**Additional remarks**
p_cL1L2L3	5.50	marked as material MVR
pL4L6L8L13L6	2.64	
p_cL5L7L9L31L12	2.64	
pL21L9	2.64	temporary path to separate PV and MVR regions
pL21L8	2.64	temporary path to separate PV and MVR regions
pL5L4	3.00	temporary path to separate PV and MVR regions
pL18L19L21L9	2.64	
pL1L32L12L7	2.64	
pL1L16L5	3.30	
pL14L4	2.64	
p_cL34L5L10L12R21	2.60	marked as material LAA
p_cL6L8L13	-	marked as material RIPV
p_cL4L6L13L22	6.30	marked as material RSPV
p_cL7L9L26L12	-	marked as material LIPV
p_cL5L7L12	-	marked as material LSPV

Not all anatomical models present during the development of this approach contained outwards-oriented PV ostia. In order to check if an annotatable PV is present, the normal vector of the plane defined by the three seed points around the PV and the center of the bounding box of the path defined by these three points ($\mathbf{c}_{\mathbf{BoBo}}$) was computed. $\mathbf{c}_{\mathbf{BoBo}}$ was then translated along the normal vector of the plane by half the maximum distance between $\mathbf{c}_{\mathbf{BoBo}}$ and the points along the path. An outwards-oriented PV was defined as present if non-annotated tissue was found within a cylinder of height 2 mm centered around the translated $\mathbf{c}_{\mathbf{BoBo}}$ and aligned with the normal vector of the plane (see Figure 7.3A). If PV was found, a sphere was defined to identify the elements belonging to it. The sphere was centered at the average location of all points along the PV path and the radius was set equal to the maximum distance between that point and the points along the path (see Figure 7.3B). For the annotation, $\mathbf{c}_{\mathbf{BoBo}}$ was translated from its initial position by 15 mm along the outwards-pointing normal vector of the plane. This served as a distant reference point in order to sort the PV points by descending distance to it. Then, the same averaging approach as used for the appendages was applied.

Table 7.6: Paths defining atrial myocyte orientation in the epicardial layer of the LA. A path is defined by the start point, the end point, and potential intermediate points. The paths were restricted to the material LA_{epi}.

Name	**Radius** (mm)	**Additional remarks**
p_cL1L2L3	5.50	marked as material MVR
p_cL6L8L13	3.30	marked as material RIPV
pL26L24L13L22L4L6	3.30	
p_cL5L12L26L9L7	3.30	
pL5L16L23L25L27	3.30	
pL26L33L12L7	3.30	
pL8L24	3.30	
pL5L4	3.63	temporary path to separate inter-pulmonary vein region
pL22L4L6L8L24	3.30	
pL26L9L5L16	3.30	
pL7L5L16L23L25L27L12	3.30	
pL26L24L13L22L4L6	3.30	
p_cL34L5L10L12R21	2.60	marked as material LAA
p_cL4L6L13L22	5.30	marked as material RSPV
p_cL7L9L26L12	-	marked as material LIPV
p_cL5L7L12	-	marked as material LSPV
pL5L10L1	2.00	marked as BB

Regarding the atrial appendages, the points defining the circular paths around the base of the appendages (p_cR17R22R23R26R21 and p_cL34L5L10L12R21) were translated towards their tips (R6 and L11). R17, R22, and R23 were moved until they were at least 0.66 mm away from previously annotated points. The threshold for R21 and R26 was 1.32 mm, and 1.65 mm for all LA points. Circular paths were then computed and smoothed using the translated points. Moreover, the center of the bounding box of each path ($\mathbf{c_{BoBo}}$) was calculated. The path was dilated using a cylindrical shape element determined specifically for each point along the path. The cylinder was confined by four planes defined by: i) $\mathbf{c_{BoBo}}$, the tip of the appendage and the preceding point on the path, ii) the two aforementioned points and the subsequent point on the path, iii) $\mathbf{c_{BoBo}}$, the current point on the path, and the preceding point on the path translated normally in that node of the current element being closest to the tip of the appendage, and iv) $\mathbf{c_{BoBo}}$, the current point on the path, and the subsequent point on the path translated normally in that node of the current element being most remote to the tip of the appendage. Planes i and ii confined the cylinder

radially while planes iii and iv defined the height. The isolating paths obtained through this method were then additionally dilated radially to a minimum width (see Tables 7.3, 7.5, and 7.6). All elements connected to the tip of the appendage via elements not being on the isolating paths were annotated as belonging to the appendage in a final step. For this purpose, all these elements were sorted by their distance to the tip in descending order and successively assigned the average orientation of the adjacent elements.
In conclusion, the myocyte orientation in the RA was annotated first. Afterwards, the endocardial layer of the LA and the epicardial layer of the LA followed. Finally, the PVs and the atrial appendages were annotated.

7.1.1.2 Interpolation and Region Growing

Besides distinct bundles, there are areas in the atria that show coherent preferential myocyte orientation, e.g. the posterior LA wall in the endocardial layer. The paths described above define the orientation along the boundaries of these regions. Tissue areas which were isolated from other non-annotated tissued by two boundary paths $p1$ and $p2$ were annotated by subsequent interpolation. Each element within the region was assigned the weighted average of the closest elements in the boundary paths. The weight was the inverse distance to the respective elements, thus assigning a higher weight to the orientation of the closer path. The interpolated orientation of node i ($\mathbf{f_i}$) was defined as:

$$\mathbf{f_i'} = \left(1 - \frac{d(\mathbf{i},\mathbf{p})}{d(\mathbf{i},\mathbf{p}) + d(\mathbf{i},\mathbf{q})}\right) \cdot \mathbf{f_p} + \left(1 - \frac{d(\mathbf{i},\mathbf{q})}{d(\mathbf{i},\mathbf{p}) + d(\mathbf{i},\mathbf{q})}\right) \cdot \mathbf{f_q} \,, \tag{7.3}$$

$$\mathbf{f_i} = \frac{\mathbf{f_i'}}{||\mathbf{f_i'}||_2} \,, \tag{7.4}$$

with $\mathbf{p}$ being the closest node on the first path $p1$, $\mathbf{q}$ being the closest node on the second path $p2$, $\mathbf{f_p}$ and $\mathbf{f_q}$ the respective orientations, and $d(\mathbf{x},\mathbf{y})$ the euclidean distance between nodes $\mathbf{x}$ and $\mathbf{y}$. As the conductive properties are orientation-dependent but direction-independent, thus the same for $0°$ and $180°$, the myocyte orientation is only defined for $-90° \leq x < 90°$ which was considered during the interpolation. If the scalar product of $\mathbf{f_p}$ and $\mathbf{f_q}$ yielded values <0, $\mathbf{f_q}$ was flipped by $180°$. This method was applied for the

region between the RAA and the first PM, the intercaval region, and the region between pR12R7R8R9 and pR14R16R15 in the RA. For the latter region, the plane defined by the points R14, R17, and R4 divided the domain into two half spaces. Only points in the half space including R8 were considered during the interpolation. Moreover, points in the half space defined by the plane R14, R7, and R18 and oriented towards R4 were neglected. The tissue class inferior isthmus was annotated for the points that lie in the half space not including R8 spanned by R14, R17, and R4 and also lie in the half space not including R20 spanned by R28, R2, and R39.
In the endocardial layer of the LA, interpolation was performed using the paths around the PVs and the temporary paths defined in Table 7.5, which were required to isolate the region and removed after the interpolation. Moreover, the area between pL14L4 and pL1L16L5 was interpolated. In the epicardial layer, the area between the pulmonary veins in the posterior wall confined by pL5L4 and the four paths pL22L4L6L8L24, pL26L9L5L16, pL7L5L16L23L25L27L12, and pL26L24L13L22L4L6, respectively.
Besides paths, also planes can serve as boundaries for the interpolation. This method was used for the interpolation of the PMs since the paths were deliberately not dilated transmurally. While the myocyte orientation in the interpectinate regions was interpolated based on the adjacent PMs, the tissue class was labeled as RA.
Remaining tissue elements that were not annotated during path dilation and interpolation were handled during a final outside-in region growing step. The elements in a non-annotated region were assigned the orientation of the closest connected annotated element if the region is surrounded by elements of only one tissue class. If more than one tissue class was present, the principal orientation of the adjacent regions was determined as a weighted average with the weight being the inverse distance to the boundary. Each node $\mathbf{i}$ inside the non-annotated region was then assigned a weighted average of the principal orientations of the N adjacent regions with the weight λ_j of region j defined as:

$$\lambda_i = \frac{d(\mathbf{r_j},\mathbf{i})^{-1}}{\sum_{l=0}^{N-1} d(\mathbf{r_l},\mathbf{i})}, \tag{7.5}$$

with $\mathbf{r_j}$ being the node in region j, which is closest to node $\mathbf{i}$.

The last tissue class being labeled was the sinus node. It was modeled as an ellipsoid with semi-principal axes of length 2 mm, 2 mm, and 4 mm plus the average distance between points across the mesh. The ellipsoid was centered at R3 and the longest axis was aligned along pR3R20. The myocyte orientation was not altered during this step.

7.1.2 Results

The algorithm annotating myocyte orientation in biatrial meshes was evaluated in a cohort of eight anatomically personalized models derived from MRI data. The characteristics of the patients and volunteers in which the data were acquired, as well as the anatomical properties of the subject's hearts are introduced in more detail in Chapter 9 (Section 9.1.1, see also Table 9.1). For each subject, a volumetric hexahedral mesh composed of cubic voxels, a triangular surface mesh, and a volumetric tetrahedral mesh was generated in order to thoroughly evaluate the methods regarding mesh type independency. The presented method applied to an isotropic voxel grid width a fixed element side length of 0.33 mm was already validated in [23]. Therefore, the focus here is laid on differences between mesh types.

The overall pattern of resulting myocyte orientation and the annotated tissue labels are shown in Figure 7.4. A comparison of the results obtained for different underlying mesh types shows gross correspondence. In contrast to the volumetric voxel meshes (left column in Figure 7.4) and tetrahedral meshes (middle column in Figure 7.4), no fiber crossing in different layer occurred in the surface meshes (right column in Figure 7.4) as a matter of course. In Figure 7.4, the epicardial rule set was applied to the surface mesh. In principle, endocardial and epicardial rule sets could be applied to the respective surface meshes which could subsequently be merged. Figure 7.5 shows a close up of the LA in the region where the BB joins the LAA. In this region, the endocardial layer is aligned almost perpendicular to the myocytes within the BB, thus causing transmurally crossing myocyte orientation.

The resulting circular myocyte orientation within the LAA is shown in Figure 7.6. The circumferential alignment and the smooth transition between the LA wall and the LAA indicate that the method introduced in Section 7.1.1.1 performed well in both types of volumetric meshes.

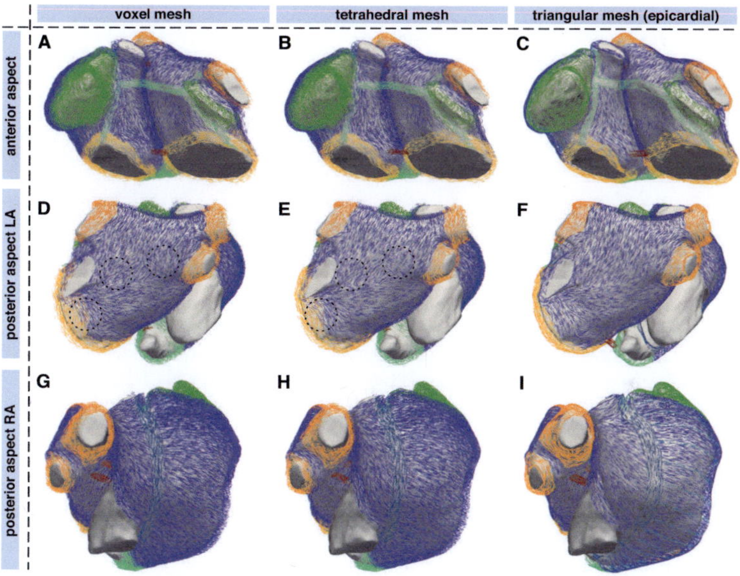

Figure 7.4: Annotated myocyte orientation in a volumetric voxel mesh ((A), (D), and (G)), a tetrahedral mesh ((B), (E), and (H)), as well as a triangular mesh of the epicardial surface ((C), (F), and (I)) of model #5. The color of the lines aligned with myocyte orientation encodes the annotated tissue class. The smoothed endocardial surface is shown in grey. The distinct endocardial and epicardial two layer architecture can e.g. be seen in the posterior wall region and at the junction with the inferior PVs in (D) and (E) (dashed circles). In (F), no crossing fibers are present as only the epicardial layer is present. The orientation along the IACs introduced in Section 7.2 are already annotated in green (BB) and red (remaining IACs).

Model #4 deviated from the norm of anatomical properties in terms of the number of PVs and the shape of the LAA. The subject had two RIPVs (Figure 7.7A) and an L-shaped LAA (Figure 7.7B) instead of the standard cone shape. The algorithm coped with this challenge even though no explicit rules to handle additional PVs were implemented.

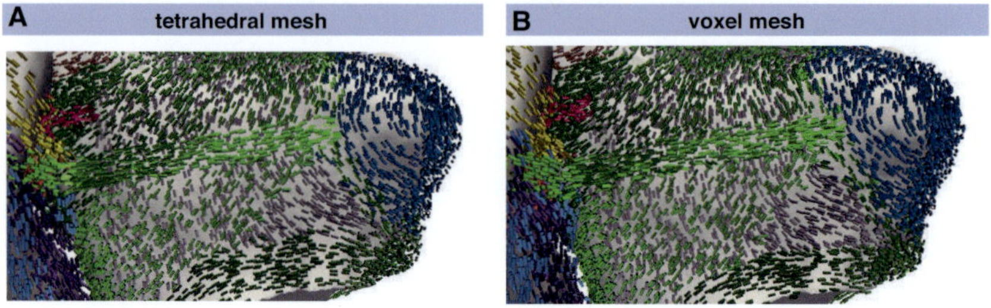

Figure 7.5: Close up of the annotated myocyte orientation in the BB region in model #4 represented by cylinders superimposed on the smoothed blood pool shown in grey. The two-layer architecture is clearly visible. Endocardial orientation cylinders are shown in grey while the epicardial ones are colored in green. The tissue class labels in both the tetrahedral mesh (A) and the structured voxel grid (B) are encoded by color. Figure based on supervised student's work [388].

7.2 Interatrial Connections

The RA and the LA are electrically isolated by the septum and interatrial conduction is only possible via distinct IACs. The presence, location, and conductive properties, which all express tremendous variability, affect excitation propagation and the activation pattern significantly, particularly in the LA [27, 55, 405–408]. However, these IACs are delicate structures, which makes them hard to identify in imaging data. Moreover, their sole presence gives no information about their conductive properties. The gold-standard to assess the intactness of IACs is to perform pacing during invasive electroanatomic mapping studies.
Because of their crucial relevance for atrial activation and arrhythmogenesis [405] on the one hand and the difficulties to image the IACs on the other hand, it is desirable to augment models with initially separated atria with IACs in a rule-based, flexible manner. An algorithm providing these means is presented in this chapter.

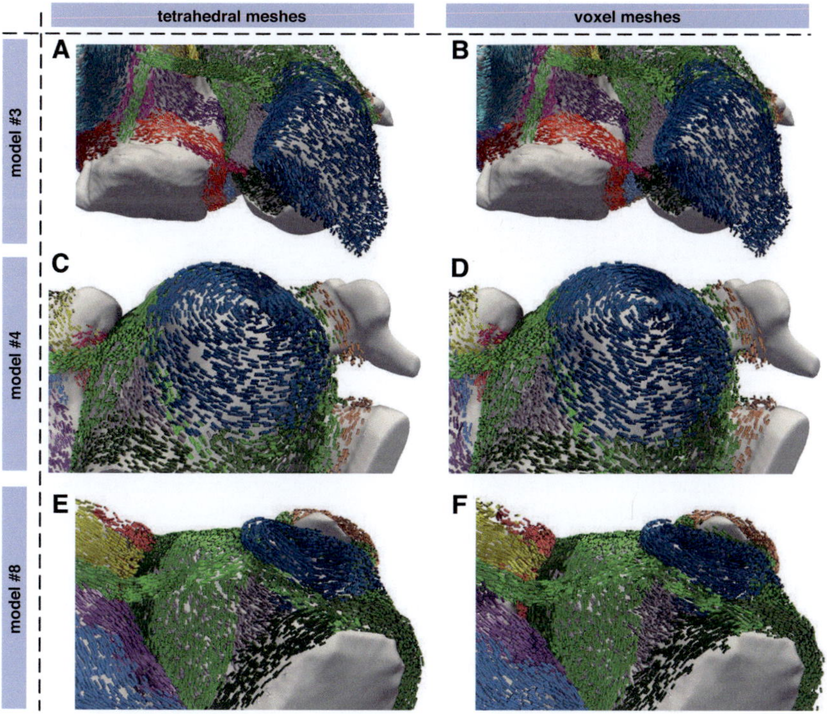

Figure 7.6: Close up of the annotated myocyte orientation of the LAA region in model #3 ((A) and (B)), model #4 ((C) and (D)), and model #8 ((E) and (F)) represented by cylinders superimposed on the smoothed blood pool shown in grey. The tissue class labels in both tetrahedral meshes ((A), (C), and (E)) and structured voxel grids ((B), (D), and (F)) are encoded by color. The orientation along the IACs introduced in Section 7.2 are already annotated. Figure based on supervised student's work [388].

7.2.1 Methods

IACs are defined by a start point $\mathbf{r_0}$ in the RA and an end point $\mathbf{l_0}$ in the LA. A cylinder with a predefined radius r was aligned along the connecting line between $\mathbf{r_0}$ and $\mathbf{l_0}$ to restrict the search space for the points derived to actually set the connection. In a first step, the points $\mathbf{r_1}$ and $\mathbf{l_1}$ were defined as the nodes within the search space being located closest to $\mathbf{l_0}$ and $\mathbf{r_0}$, respectively.

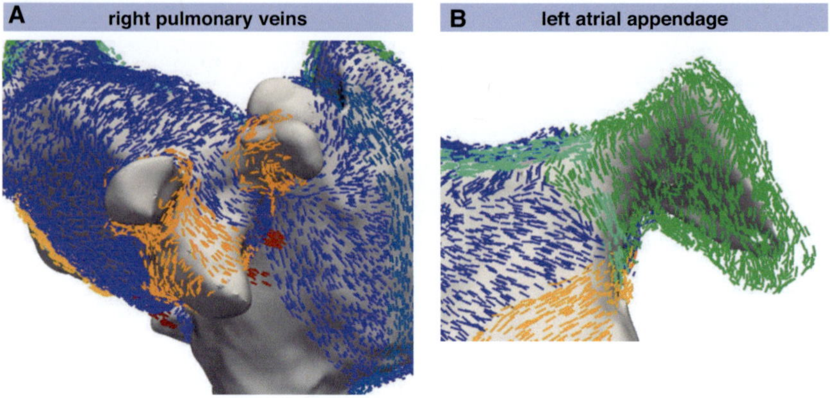

Figure 7.7: Close up of the annotated myocyte orientation in the RPV (A) and LAA (B) region of model #3. The color of the lines aligned with myocyte orientation encodes the annotated tissue class. The smoothed endocardial surface is shown in grey. The two RIPVs were annotated together (A). The L-shaped LAA was completely labeled with the right tissue class and myocyte orientation was modeled approximately circumferential.

The midpoint of the line segment defined by $\mathbf{r_1}$ and $\mathbf{l_1}$ was named $\mathbf{m}$ and used to identify the actual start and end points of the IAC: $\mathbf{r_2}$ defined as the RA point being closest to $\mathbf{m}$ within the search cylinder, and $\mathbf{l_2}$ being the closest LA point to $\mathbf{m}$.
Paths between $\mathbf{r_0}$ and $\mathbf{r_2}$, as well as between $\mathbf{l_0}$ and $\mathbf{l_2}$ were computed using Equation (7.1). These paths were dilated with a radius of 0.83 mm and used to annotate myocyte orientation and tissue labels. The actual bridge was inserted into the model as a pill-shaped object built of a cylinder running from $\mathbf{r_2}$ to $\mathbf{l_2}$ with the predefined bridge radius and a hemisphere with the same radius attached to each end of the cylinder. The hemispheres formed connections to the atrial walls providing a smooth transition without jagged edges.
For voxel-based meshes, the elements within the IAC could just be labeled. For unstructured grids, the surface of the IAC was generated of triangles using the fundamental forms provided by the *VTK* library [409]. For volumetric tetrahedral grids, the surface was then filled with tetrahedra using Delaunay triangulation provided by the *TetGen* library [410].

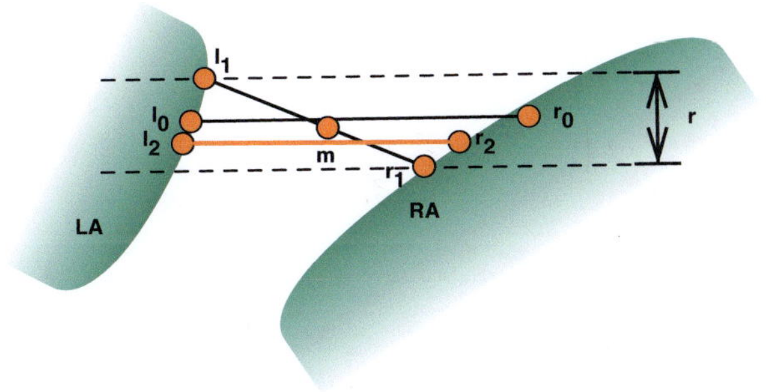

Figure 7.8: Sketch of how the final IAC start point in the RA $\mathbf{r_2}$ and the end point in the LA $\mathbf{l_2}$ are determined starting from the initial points $\mathbf{r_0}$ and $\mathbf{l_0}$. A search cylinder with radius r is defined around the direction connection between $\mathbf{r_0}$ and $\mathbf{l_0}$. The point $\mathbf{l_1}$ is the closest LA point to $\mathbf{r_0}$ within this cylinder. $\mathbf{r_1}$ is defined analogously. $\mathbf{r_2}$ and $\mathbf{l_2}$ are determined as the points within the respective atrium being closest to $\mathbf{m}$ which splits the direct connection between $\mathbf{r_1}$ and $\mathbf{l_1}$ in half.

The interface between the surface of the IAC and the atrial walls was treated in an automated post-processing step guaranteeing proper connectivity of the elements. Myocyte orientation was aligned with the path running from $\mathbf{r_2}$ to $\mathbf{l_2}$ within the cylinder. The dilation step with a spherical element and the radius of the cylinder did also cover the hemispheres.
The implemented algorithm can augment biatrial models with freely defined IACs as well as several standard IACs (Figure 7.9) based on the seed points introduced in Section 7.1.1 (see Table 7.2 and Table 7.4): BB, two connections on the posterior side (middle posterior connection (MPC), lower posterior connection (LPC)), a connection via the coronary sinus (CS), as well as two connections on the anterior side (upper anterior connection, lower anterior connection). The standard search radius for IACs was set to the maximum of $2\times$ the average mesh resolution and 1 mm. The radius of the connections was 1.65 mm. The MPC ran from point R31 in the RA to point L55 in the LA, the LPC from R29 to L35. The lower anterior connection linked the points R40 and L36. The upper anterior IAC connected the points R1 and L22. The connection at the CS was established via R14 and L1 with a search radius of the maximum of $3\times$ the average mesh resolution and 1 mm.

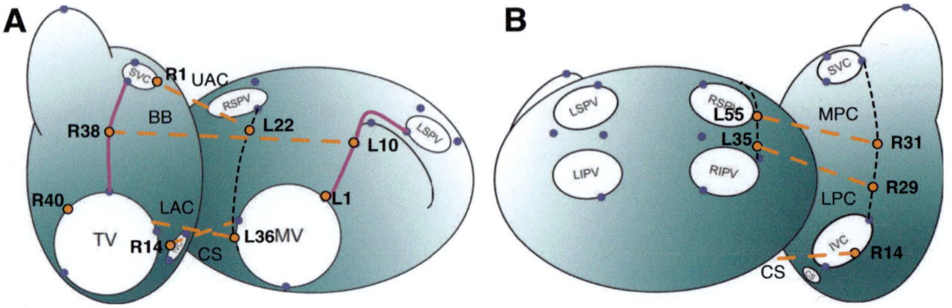

Figure 7.9: Schematic course of the IACs (dashed orange lines) connecting the start points in the RA and the end points in the LA directly. The RA and LA extension of BB is indicated by the magenta line. The dashed black lines represent auxiliary paths used to locate start and end points (orange) of the IACs. Blue points represent the 22 landmarks points. (A) shows the anterior aspect, (B) the posterior aspect.

The BB differs from the other IACs in terms of spatial extent. The search radius for the start and end points $\mathbf{r_2}$ to $\mathbf{l_2}$ was 8 mm (cf. Figure 7.8). Besides the actual IAC bridging the septum from R38 to L10, the BB reaches out to the bases of the RAA and the LAA (see Table 7.3 and Table 7.6). This extension can either be restricted to existing elements, thus only affecting tissue labels and myocyte orientation or modeled as a tube-like structure protruding from the atrial walls. For the latter option, a radius of 2.31 mm was used.

7.2.2 Results

The algorithm to introduce IACs in a rule-based manner was tested using the models of all eight subjects in all three mesh variants resulting in 24 models as was the case for the myocyte orientation. Elements were successfully introduced in the meshes as exemplary shown for the voxel-based model (Figure 7.10A) and the tetrahedral model (Figure 7.10B) of subject #4. In (Figure 7.10B), the coalescence of the BB tube and the LA tetrahedra in the fused mesh can be appreciated. Moreover, the default connections BB, posterior IACs, and CS are included in Figures 7.4, 7.5, and 7.6.

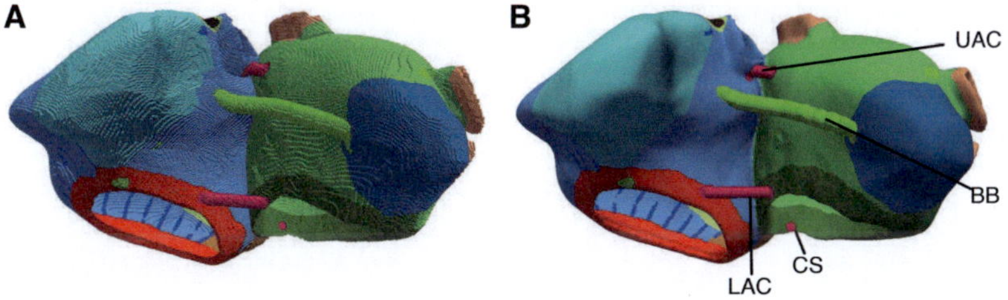

Figure 7.10: Voxel-based model (A) and tetrahedral model (B) of subject #4 with inserted IACs. The presented anterior aspect shows BB, the two additional upper (UAC) and lower (LAC) anterior connections, as well as the RA landing point of the IAC via the CS. Tissue class labels are color-coded. Figure based on supervised student's work [388].

7.3 Atrial Ablation Patterns

Besides the anatomy, the myocyte orientation, and the IACs, also non-excitable scar tissue plays a vital role determining the atrial activation patterns and arrhythmogenesis. Radio-frequency ablations aims at rendering tissue non-excitable. For an *in silico* evaluation of different ablation patterns in order to identify the optimal option, it is thus imperative to introduce standard ablation patterns in anatomically individualized models.
In this section, an approach to augment models with standard ablation patterns based on the methods presented in the previous sections of this chapter is presented.

7.3.1 Methods

Ablation lines are defined by a start point, and end point and optionally a number of additional intermediate points. The points were connected with a path defined by Equation (7.1) which was later on dilated with a spherical shape element of a predefined radius. The spherical shape element can be centered at the endocardial or the epicardial surface depending on the desired application.

Table 7.7: Paths defining ablation patterns A to J based on [411] and K to M based on [412]. The location of the points defining the patterns is given in Table 7.4.

Pattern	Path	Pattern	Path
A	pL8L6L4L5L7L9L56	**H**	p_cL8L13L69L4L5L12L26L9 pL26L56
B	p_cL5L12L7 p_cL60L26L9L59L74 p_cL4L58L72L57L69 p_cL70L8L13L73	**I**	all paths from pattern H plus pL8L1
C	p_cL8L13L69L4L6 p_cL9L7L5L12L26 pL6L57 pL12L65	**J**	all paths from pattern H plus pL13L68 pL5L11
D	p_cL8L13L69L4L6 p_cL9L7L5L12L26	**K**	p_cL8L13L69L4L5L12L26L9 pL20L2 pL5L10L34L12
E	all paths from pattern D plus pL61L62 pL26L56	**L**	all paths from pattern K plus pL9L7L5 pL4L5L8
F	all paths from pattern D plus pL66L67 pL26L56 pL6L57 pL12L65	**M**	all paths from pattern D plus pL5L10L34L12
G	all paths from pattern F plus pL63L64		

Moreover, transmural ablation scars can be introduced using a pill-shaped dilation element with varying height at each point depending on the wall thickness as introduced in Section 7.1.1. A border zone with a fixed width around the scar was included by applying the algorithm twice: first with a width defined as the sum of the border zone and the scar width, thus labeling the border zone. The second run considered only the width of the actual scar and overwrote the tissue label within the scar.

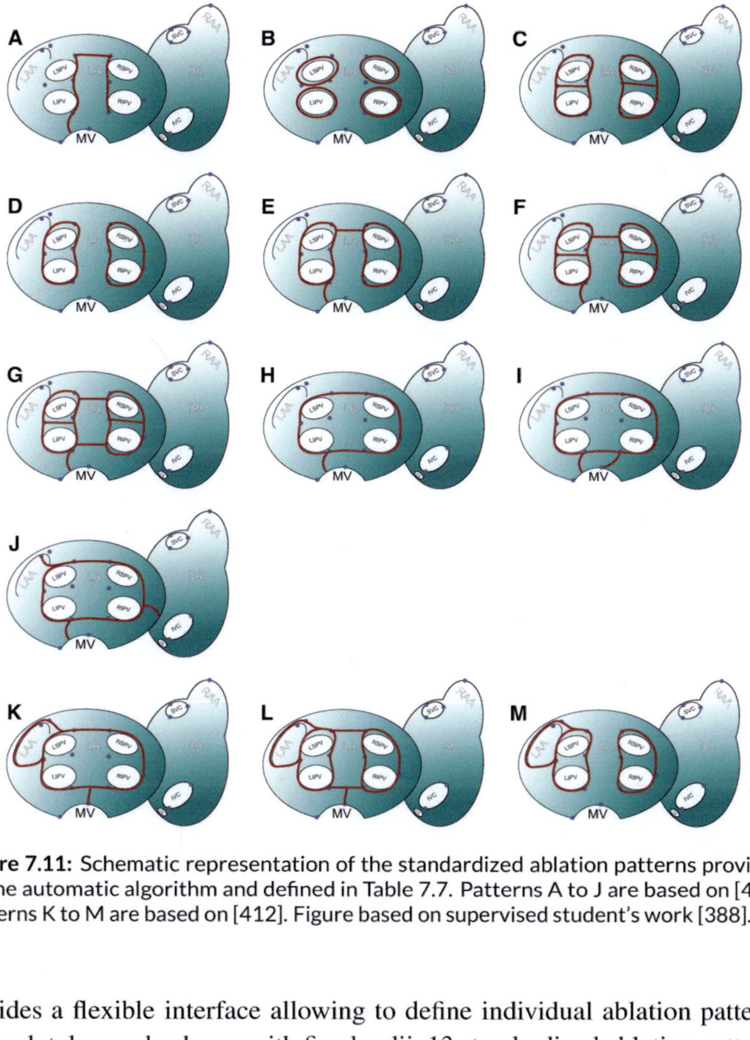

Figure 7.11: Schematic representation of the standardized ablation patterns provided by the automatic algorithm and defined in Table 7.7. Patterns A to J are based on [411], patterns K to M are based on [412]. Figure based on supervised student's work [388].

Besides a flexible interface allowing to define individual ablation patterns through tubes and spheres with fixed radii, 13 standardized ablation patterns based on the points derived from the anatomical landmarks (Table 7.4) can be automatically generated. Table 7.7 lists the paths that make up the standardized ablation patterns based on publications by Reumann et al. [411] and Deisenhofer et al. [412]. The pattern A to M are schematically visualized in Figure 7.11.

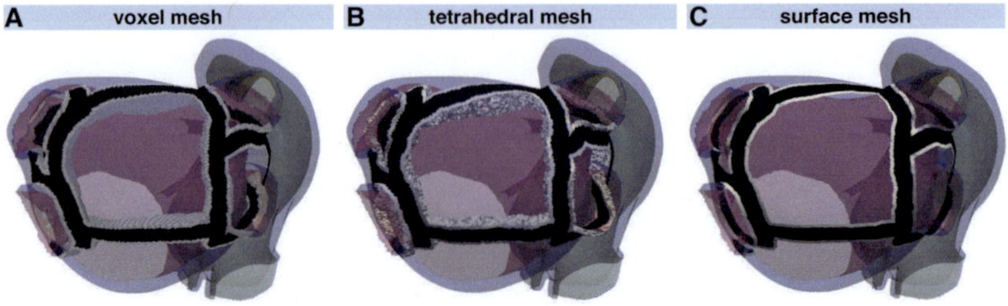

Figure 7.12: Resulting ablation by applying pattern G in model #4. The core lesion with a radius of 2 mm (black) is surrounded by a border zone with a width of 1 mm (white) in the semi-transparent biatrial model. Transmural ablation was applied in the voxel grid (A) and the volumetric tetrahedral mesh (B) revealing the different mesh structures at the interface between the border zone and LA myocardium. In the triangular surface mesh (C), ablation was applied to the epicardial side.

7.3.2 Results

The automatic placement of the nine ablation patterns introduced in Table 7.7 was assessed using models from all eight subjects in all three types of meshes: structured voxel grids, volumetric tetrahedral meshes, and triangular surface meshes. Moreover, all four variants to place the ablation (starting from the endocardium, from the epicardium, from within the wall, and transmurally) were performed successfully yielding a total of 1248 results. Figure 7.12 shows transmural ablation of pattern G including a border zone in model #4 in the three different mesh types.

7.4 Discussion

The rule-based algorithm to annotate myocyte orientation and tissue labels was originally introduced and thoroughly evaluated in [23]. The myocyte orientation pattern was compared to manual placement based on histology data [57, 401] and image data in models of the Visible Human dataset [413, 414]. Moreover, anatomical images from literature were used a qualitative reference [19, 392, 401] and a high resolution microscopic image stack of sheep atria [415] served as a quantitative reference with myocyte orientation determined by a gradient-based structure tensor approach [416]. The rule-based approach was able to reproduce the overall pattern of fiber orientation observed in the microscopy data even though the anatomy of the sheep atria differed from human atria. Comparison to previously published manually annotated datasets revealed similar major axes for most of the elements.

The main progress achieved by the work presented here is a coherent and consistent description of the set of rules used to annotate myocyte orientation, tissue classes, as well as standard ablation patterns. Moreover, the implementation provides a mesh-type-agnostic algorithm that can be applied to all common data structures used in computational modeling of cardiac electrophysiology and biomechanics. Furthermore, the implementation is flexible regarding the resolution of the underlying mesh. By replacing the few remaining absolute distance measures by normalized values, the algorithm could be used for pediatric scenarios or hearts of small animals, as well. The object-oriented design of the software using modern software engineering methods yielded an extendable software with maintainable code.

CHAPTER 8

Analysis of Atrial Flutter Vulnerability

The long-term success rate of atrial fibrillation (AF) ablation is unsatisfactory low, particularly in patients suffering from persistent AF. Besides AF recurrence, the development of post-ablational atrial flutter (AFlut) represents a major problem [8, 65–68]. In more than half of the patients, sustained AF is reinitiated within 5 years after ablation or AFlut develops [417]. More than 40% of patients in the *STAR AF II* study by Verma et al. suffered from recurrent AF within 18 months independent from the ablation approach chosen [149]. 20% of recurrences after AF ablation in elderly are due to AFlut [418]. In the general AF population, 18.5% of patients were diagnosed with AFlut during a median follow-up time of 421 day post ablation [419]. Liang et al. observed AF or organized atrial tachycardia in 53% of 300 patients within the first six weeks after pulmonary vein (PV) antral isolation [420]. AF and AFlut are often even combined endpoints in studies evaluating the success of AF ablation [417]. Waldo and Feld highlighted the inter-relationships between AF and AFlut [421]. AF precedes AFlut in most cases forming the required line of block between the vena cavae by fibrillatory conduction. Moreover, ablation of atrial tissue can lead to a substrate for AFlut. Particularly gaps in linear lesions forming isthmuses or revitalized tissue areas forming zones of slow conduction render the atria vulnerable. Also PV isolation has been associated with a substantial risk to develop AFlut [422–424]. Castréjon et al.

reviewed the occurrence of organized atrial tachycardia such as AFlut after AF ablation and discuss that more extensive left atrium (LA) ablation renders the atria more vulnerable to AFlut [425]. However, the exact origin of the pathologic substrate is not understood. Therefore, a method to assess the vulnerability to AFlut in personalized computational models is presented in this chapter. Besides an identification of possibly AFlut sustaining pathways in the observed state of the patient (*baseline*), the approach allows to assess the effect of different therapeutic strategies such as ablation patterns, pharmacological compounds, or other anatomical and electrophysiological interventions *in silico* before actually performing them.

The monodomain reaction-diffusion model presented in Section 3.2.1 and used to simulate excitation propagation in Chapters 5 and 6 is based on the diffusion of ions and reactions of the plasma membrane. As such, it considers electrotonic effects and source-sink relations resulting in e.g. convex or concave wavefronts. On the one hand, the monodomain approach provides the means to simulate complex excitation patterns as chaotic fibrillation including wave breaks. Moreover, the underlying cell models can be arbitrary complex to incorporate e.g. advanced calcium handling providing the means to study early or delayed afterdepolarizations. On the other hand, the monodomain model is computationally expensive [426]. The simulation of 1 s excitation propagation in a volumetric three-dimensional model of the atria takes several hours wall-clock time on modern machines. Hence, they are not suitable for a thorough exploration of parameters regarding effects on the three-dimensional whole organ level, as e.g. the vulnerability to arrhythmia caused by ectopic stimuli from a multitude of locations and at varying time steps.

Eikonal approximations of the continuous dynamics of the reaction-diffusion system allow to simulate excitation propagation in terms of activation times with significantly reduced computational load [161] as only one static, non-linear partial differential equation (PDE) derived from e.g. the monodomain model has to be solved, which makes it interesting for simulations of cardiac activation [427, 428]. In contrast to level set methods in general, shortest path [429] and fast marching methods assume monotonously expanding wavefronts, however. Thus, a specific approach considering multiple fronts, reentry, and anisotropic conduction was developed for cardiac electrophysiology [162, 176] based on a fast marching method on structured grids [430–433]. Several extensions provide the means to consider wavefront curvature and

the mesh structure if that is needed for the specific application [434, 435]. Ablation of ventricular tissue in order to prevent scar-related ventricular tachycardia was presented as a potential application for this method [162].
Dang et al. compared different standard ablation patterns for AF using an idealized computational model [436]. Reumann et al. evaluated different patterns regarding AF prevention in a more complex model [411]. Hwang et al. proposed a method to test AF ablation patterns *in silico* using a monodomain approach on anatomically, but not electrophysiologically personalized models [437]. Thus, no substrate information regarding fibrosis, zones of slow conduction or the degree of electrophysiological remodeling is considered. McDowell et al. presented a proof-of-concept how computational modeling can predict ablation sites terminating rotors driving AF in personalized models including fibrosis distribution [438]. Bayer et al. evaluated the potency of PV isolation, mitral and roof lines, ablation guided by rotor mapping, and lesions streamlining sinus activation regarding the termination of AF *in silico* [439]. In a very recent work, Zahid et al. employed the minimum cut algorithm to predict optimal ablation sites for AFlut in the LA [440]. The potential of clinically-derived computational models to optimize catheter ablation of AF was recently reviewed by Zhao et al. [441]. They conclude that high-resolution three-dimensional models of functionally and structurally mapped atria of the exact patient are imperative to provide clinically relevant insights on a personalized level.
Lines et al. presented a method to parametrize a monodomain simulation in a standard bi-atrial model aiming to incorporate electrograms acquired during electroanatomic mapping studies in order to replicate clinically mapped AFlut *in silico* [442]. The extracellular potentials at 32 computational nodes served as a boundary condition for the solution of the monodomain system. While the algorithm synchronized the simulation to the synthetic reference simulation, the algorithm is computationally expensive and only allows to study clinically observed cases *in silico* but cannot provide information on the vulnerability to AFlut.
The method presented here is the first allowing to comprehensively assess the vulnerability to AFlut in personalized models considering both anatomical and electrophysiological properties allowing to evaluate therapeutic approaches such as ablation *in silico*.
Part of this work is based on a supervised student's project [443].

8.1 Methods

A pipeline consisting of several methods was developed in order to assess the vulnerability to AFlut. In this section, the different steps in the workflow are presented.

8.1.1 Fast Marching Simulation of Excitation Propagation

The basic concept of the eikonal-based simulation of excitation propagation and the fast marching scheme were introduced in Section 3.2.2. The existing concepts were extended to consider restitution of conduction velocity (CV) and effective refractory period (ERP). Restitution of both parameters with respect to basic cycle length (BCL) was determined by pacing in a one-dimensional tissue strand using the Courtemanche et al. cell model [47] coupled in a monodomain approach as introduced in Chapter 5. The resulting curves for CV and ERP were approximated by exponential decays:

$$CV\,(BCL) = A - B \cdot \exp\left(-\frac{BCL}{C}\right)\,, \tag{8.1}$$

with A, B, and C being determined through standard *Matlab* curve fitting methods. The BCL was defined as the time passed since the last activation of the respective node and initialized with a user-defined value either globally or for each node individually. The restitution of the ERP was described similarly. In this study, an implementation of the fast marching approach was used to trigger excitations from a multitude of locations sequentially in order to identify potential loops along which AFlut can be sustained as described in the next section. The algorithm was implemented in a modular and extensible *C++* framework.

8.1.2 Identification of Flutter Loops

For each stimulus location, activation times were computed and stored together with information regarding the spread of excitation in terms of a vector pointing from the activating to the activated node. Wavefront collision sites are points of latest activation on circular paths composed of two paths originating from the stimulus site to opposite sides. On the one hand, these paths are the shortest in the sense of wave propagation, i.e. they are not artificially prolonged by zig-zag patterns but determined as the shortest connection by the fast marching algorithm. On the other hand, they are locally the longest as two independent waves collided on the loop. A wavefront collision for node i was identified if the following condition was fulfilled for any neighboring node j:

$$\frac{\mathbf{a_i}}{\|\mathbf{a_i}\|_2} + \frac{\mathbf{a_j}}{\|\mathbf{a_j}\|_2} < 0.99 \; , \tag{8.2}$$

with $\mathbf{a_i}$ being the vector pointing from the node that activated node i to node i itself. The condition identifies all points at which the vectors meet at an angle $\in (\pi/2, 3\pi/2)$ including π, thus pointing in opposite directions. From the sites of collisions, loops were defined by the two traces along the steepest negative activation time gradient leading back to the stimulus location. A loop was thus composed of a circular, ordered series of nodes. Along the loop, the round trip time (RTT) was calculated considering the heterogeneous and anisotropic tissue properties in terms of CV and ERP (cf. Equation (8.1)). If a loop did not fulfill the wavelength (WL) condition

$$\max_i \left(ERP_i(RTT)\right) < RTT \; , \tag{8.3}$$

it was disregarded. Here, ERP_i was the ERP of node i considering a BCL equal to the RTT according to Equation (8.1). i comprised all nodes spanning the loop candidate.

The fact that the loops were traced back all the way to the initial stimulus site introduced artifacts as a dynamic wave would cut short between the two traces from the site of collision to the stimulus site in many cases. In the easier case, both half loops shared a part of the loop. Under such circumstances, all common nodes could be neglected, thus shrinking the loop (Figure 8.1A).

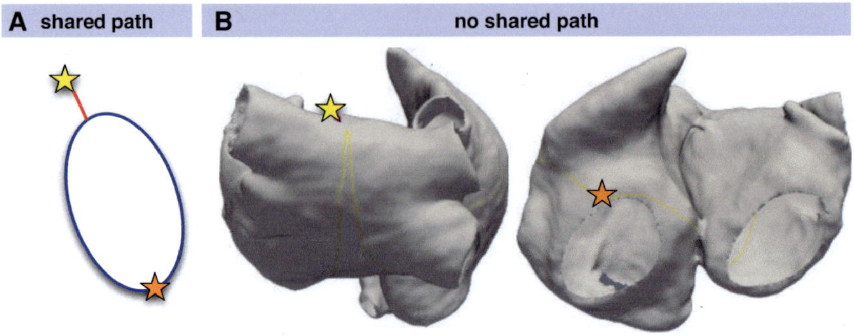

Figure 8.1: Artifacts introduced by loop tracing from sites of wavefront collision (orange star) to the stimulus location (yellow star). As in (A) both half loops share part of the loop (red segment), the loop can be constricted to the blue circle. In (B), the wavefronts collided on the anterior wall and the shared path was already disregarded (note the distance between the yellow star and the yellow loop on the LA roof). However, the loop would still be cut short by a propagating wave between the LPC and the IAC at the CS.

In most cases, however, this approach did not remove all artifacts. In Figure 8.1B, a shortcut of the two half loops running adjacent on the posterior LA wall can be anticipated between the posterior IACs and the IAC via the CS. Therefore, a geometric snake approach considering anisotropy was implemented in order to constrict the loops like a rubber band by minimizing the spline energy. Evolving snakes on triangular meshes were proposed before for mesh scissoring operations and constriction detection [444–448] and were adapted to the requirements of the specific application in this work.
The geometric snake is an active contour model that is restricted to a polygonal surface mesh. In this work, the parametrization-free implementation for triangular meshes proposed by Bischoff and Kobbelt [444, 445] was used. A snake was represented as a polygon in space (Figure 8.2). The vertices of the snake are referred to as *snaxels* and represented by lower case vectors in the following. Snaxels were constrained to lie on edges of the mesh. Furthermore, the segments of the snake (connections between snaxels) had to lie in the interior of triangles. An oriented snaxel **s** could thus be defined as:

$$\mathbf{s} = \mathbf{f_s} + p_s \cdot (\mathbf{t_s} - \mathbf{f_s}) \,, \tag{8.4}$$

with the points $\mathbf{t_s}$ and $\mathbf{f_s}$ defining the supporting edge on which the snaxel **s** lies and $p_s \in (0,1)$ defining the position on the edge.

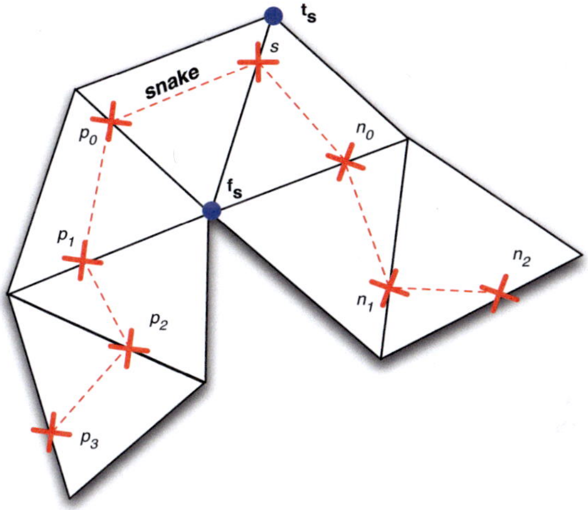

Figure 8.2: Geometric snake on a triangular mesh. The snake segments run on the surface of the triangles from snaxel to snaxel. Each snaxel is constrained to its supporting edge. Snaxel $\mathbf{s}$ is supported by the edge running from $\mathbf{f_s}$ to $\mathbf{t_s}$ and directly connected to its predecessor $\mathbf{p_0}$ and its successor $\mathbf{n_0}$.

The snake evolves by assigning a scalar speed v_s to each snaxel $\mathbf{s}$:

$$p_s \leftarrow p_s + \Delta t \cdot v_s \,, \tag{8.5}$$

with Δt being a virtual time increment. The time increment was chosen as 0.5 in this study striking a good balance between stability and convergence speed. By performing the update step, the snaxel was shifted along the supporting edge of the mesh $\mathbf{e_s}$ (Figure 8.3):

$$\mathbf{e_s} = \mathbf{t_s} - \mathbf{f_s} \,. \tag{8.6}$$

In order to avoid local oscillations, not only the direct neighbors were considered when calculating the velocity:

$$v_s = \frac{1}{\left(\frac{\sqrt{\mathbf{e_s} \cdot \mathbf{D_s} \cdot \mathbf{e_s}}}{CV_S(RTT)}\right) \cdot \sum_{i=0}^{N-1} a^i} \cdot \sum_{i=0}^{N-1} \left[a^i \left(d\left(\mathbf{p_i}, \mathbf{s}\right) + d\left(\mathbf{n_i}, \mathbf{s}\right)\right)\right] \,, \tag{8.7}$$

with N being the order of the approach, a being the order divisor $\in$ (0,1], and D_i being the anisotropy tensor according to Equation (3.20).

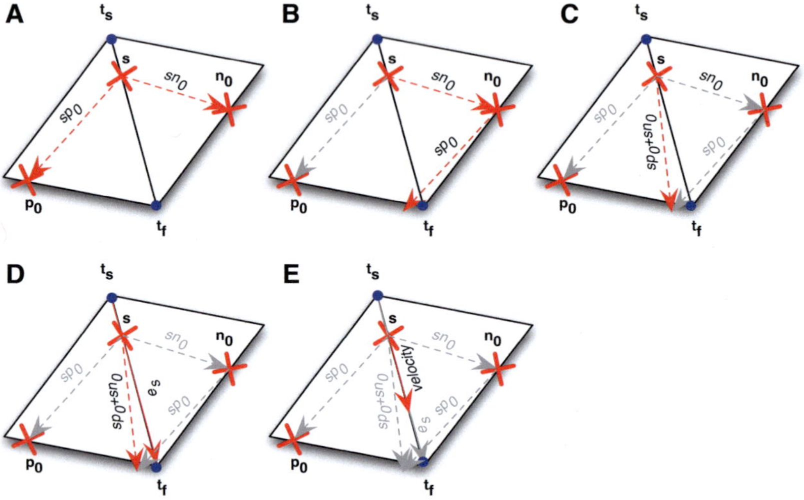

Figure 8.3: Concept of the snaxel velocity calculation for order N=1 and isotropic tissue properties. Snaxel **s** is connected to its first order neighbors $\mathbf{p_0}$ and $\mathbf{n_0}$ (A). The sum of the connecting vectors $\mathbf{sp_0}$ and $\mathbf{sn_0}$ (B)+(C) is projected onto the supporting edge $\mathbf{e_s}$ (D). The projection is scaled by the conduction velocity in order to obtain the velocity of the snaxel (E).

As snaxels were located on edges between two nodes and the material properties CV and ERP was defined for each node, the closer node was considered (referred to by upper case vectors using the same letter). Thus, $CV_{\mathbf{S}}(RTT)$ was the CV of the closest node to snaxel **s** considering the RTT of the last iteration as the BCL according to Equation (8.1). p_i is the ith predecessor of snaxel s and n_i is the ith successor. In this study, the order N was chosen as 30 and a was set to 0.91 based on experience gained in pilot studies. The anisotropic distance projected on the supporting edge and weighted by the heterogeneous CV $d(\mathbf{p_1}, \mathbf{p_2})$ was defined as:

$$d(\mathbf{p_1}, \mathbf{p_2}) = \frac{1}{CV_{P_1}(RTT)} (\mathbf{p_1} - \mathbf{p_2}) \mathbf{D_{P_1}} \cdot \frac{\mathbf{e_s}}{\|\mathbf{e_s}\|_2} . \tag{8.8}$$

If an update step shifted a snaxel on one of the supporting nodes or beyond them ($p_s \leq 0$ or $p_s \geq 1$), the snaxel was duplicated and distributed on all adjacent edges with an initial p value of 0.05. Thus, the new snaxels were located 5% away from the crossed node with respect to the length of their new supporting edge. During the evolution, one more constraint was checked and enforced. No two consecutive snake segments could lie within the same triangle. If this was the case because a snaxel was distributed after passing a supporting node, the interior snaxel was disregarded and the first and third snaxel were connected directly. Snaxel collisions caused by snaxels crossing each other on the same supporting edge were resolved by merging the respective snake segments. After each iteration, the WL condition Equation (8.3) was checked. Snakes not fulfilling it were disregarded immediately. The iterative algorithm was stopped once the absolute RTT reduction over the last 20 iterations was less than 7 ms or the relative reduction was less than 10%. This choice of parameters yielded stable convergence and is further discussed in Section 8.3.

The presented approach controls the topology, detects and resolves self-collisions at sub-element size precision, and inherently avoids error prone back projections of snaxels onto the mesh.

8.1.3 Eikonal-Diffusion Phase Interpolation

The methods introduced above allow to identify paths in an atrial model that can potentially sustain AFlut. However, the paths are not necessarily the dominant one and might thus not be expressed in dynamic scenarios. An example is shown in Figure 8.4 where several paths run from the septal side of the tricuspid valve (TV) to the right atrial appendage (RAA) and to the CS region. Each path is locally the shortest and long enough to sustain AFlut according to the WL condition. However, according to Huygen's principle only one path will dominate the excitation pattern distal to the constriction at the TV where all paths narrow. Thus, the remaining paths will be suppressed. In order to identify the dominant path, i.e. to distinguish between theoretically vulnerable paths and practically inducible paths, the initial state for a dynamic simulation had to be extrapolated from a single loop to the entire simulation domain.

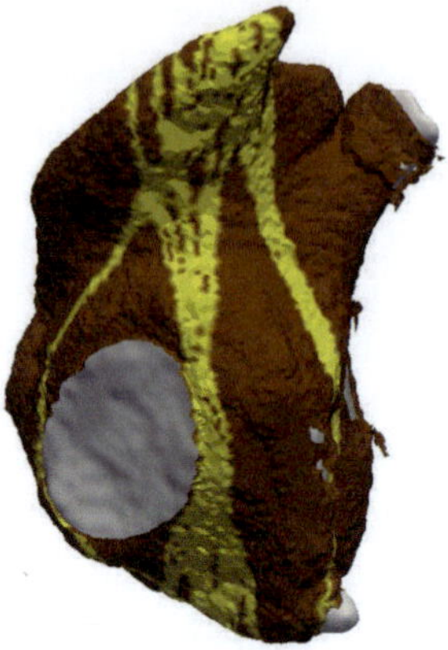

Figure 8.4: Example of an AFlut vulnerability map. The vulnerable paths are marked in yellow on the brown substrate of the RA; the blood pool is indicated in gray. Several paths run from the septal side of the TV to the RAA.

Jacquemet proposed an eikonal-diffusion approach for the initiation of reentrant cardiac propagation [449, 450]. The eikonal-diffusion equation can be derived from the monodomain equation Equation (3.12) using singular perturbation theory [449, 451, 452]:

$$\|\mathbf{c}\nabla t_a\|_2 = 1 + \nabla \cdot (\mathbf{D}\nabla t_a) \qquad x \in \Omega\,, \tag{8.9}$$

$$\mathbf{n} \cdot \mathbf{D}\nabla t_a = 0 \qquad x \in \partial\Omega\,, \tag{8.10}$$

with the symmetric positive definite tensors **c** and **D** being the link to the monodomain equation, Ω being the computation domain, and **n** being the unit vector normal to the boundary $\partial\Omega$. The scaled propagation velocity **c** in mm/rad (mm/s $\times$ T/2π) was defined as:

$$\mathbf{c} = \left(\frac{T^2\,k_m\sigma}{4\pi^2\,\beta\,C_m}\right)^{1/2}, \tag{8.11}$$

and the scaled diffusion tensor **D** in mm^2 defined as:

$$\mathbf{D} = \frac{T\,\sigma}{2\pi\,\beta\,C_m}\,, \tag{8.12}$$

with the period of the reentry T (RTT), the surface to volume ratio β, and the membrane capacitance per unit area C_m defined as introduced in Section 3.2.1. The parameter k_m depends on the cell model and results in a plane wave CV of $\sqrt{k_m \sigma / \beta C_m}$. In this study, k_m was set to $2.0833\,\mathrm{ms}^{-1}$ as suggested in [449, 450].
As we aim to simulate reentrant activity, the activation time was scaled:

$$\tau(x) = 2\pi \frac{t_a(x)}{T} \mod 2\pi\,, \tag{8.13}$$

with T being the period of the reentry, thus RTT in our case. To compensate for the 2π jumps occurring in the phase τ, a transformation to phase space was established by $\phi := \exp(j\tau)$, with j denoting the imaginary unit. This transformation yields an adapted eikonal-diffusion equation [449]:

$$\|\mathbf{c}\nabla\phi\|_2 = 1 + \mathrm{Im}(\nabla \cdot (\phi^* \mathbf{D} \nabla \phi)) \qquad x \in \Omega\,, \tag{8.14}$$

$$|\phi| = 1 \qquad x \in \Omega\,, \tag{8.15}$$

$$\mathbf{n} \cdot \mathbf{D}\nabla\phi = 0 \qquad x \in \partial\Omega\,, \tag{8.16}$$

with Im() denoting the imaginary part and * being the conjugate vector.
For $\mathbf{D} \to 0$, Equation (8.9) reduces to the classical eikonal equation Equation (3.13). If $\mathbf{D}$ is non-zero, wavefront curvature-dependent effects are included. A purely diffusive case can be considered for $\mathbf{D} = \lambda\tilde{\mathbf{D}}$ with $\lambda \to +\infty$:

$$\nabla \cdot (\mathbf{D}\nabla\tau) = 0 \qquad x \in \Omega \setminus \Gamma\,, \tag{8.17}$$

$$\mathbf{n} \cdot \mathbf{D}\nabla\tau = 0 \qquad x \in \partial\Omega \setminus \Gamma\,, \tag{8.18}$$

$$\tau(x) = \tau_0(x) \qquad x \in \Gamma\,, \tag{8.19}$$

with Γ being the subdomain posing a Dirichlet boundary condition when formulating a Laplacian interpolation problem [453] to compute an initial phase distribution ϕ_0 for the whole domain Ω.

Algorithm 8.1 Iterative eikonal solver algorithm proposed by Jacquemet [450].

Generate initial estimate for ϕ using e.g. Laplacian interpolation
while $\|\theta\|_2$ < tol **do**
  Compute $\mathbf{A}(\phi)$ and $\mathbf{f}(\phi)$
  Solve $\mathbf{A}(\phi)\,\theta = \mathbf{f}(\phi)$ for θ
  Substract mean: $\theta \leftarrow \theta -$ mean(θ)
  Under-relaxation: $\theta \leftarrow \theta \cdot \min(1, \theta_{max}/\max(|\theta|))$
  $\phi \leftarrow \phi \exp(j\theta)$
end while

The initial estimate for the solution of Equation (8.14) satisfying the constraint Equation (8.15) and the boundary condition Equation (8.16) was iteratively refined using a linearized eikonal approach [450, 454]. In each iteration, the phase of each node was shifted:

$$\phi_i \leftarrow \phi_i \cdot \exp(j\theta_i) \ , \tag{8.20}$$

with θ defined as follows:

$$\|\mathbf{c}\nabla\phi\|_2 - \mathrm{Im}(\nabla\cdot(\phi^*\mathbf{D}\nabla\phi)) - 1 = \|\mathbf{c}\nabla\phi\|_2^{-1}\,\mathrm{Im}(\phi\nabla\phi^*\mathbf{c}^*\mathbf{c}\nabla\theta) + \nabla\cdot(\mathbf{D}\nabla\theta) \ . \tag{8.21}$$

This scheme approximates Equation (8.14) up to first order in $\nabla\theta$ and is equivalent to the Newton root finding method applied to the PDE [449, 450]. The interested reader is referred to [450] regarding the details of the discretization to triangular surface meshes resulting in a linear system representing the linearized eikonal-diffusion equation:

$$\mathbf{A}(\phi)\,\theta = \mathbf{f}(\phi) \ , \tag{8.22}$$

with explicit expressions of $\mathbf{A}$ and $\mathbf{f}$ as derived in [449]. The iterative algorithm is summarized in Algorithm 8.1. The tolerance was set to 10^{-9} and the under-relaxation threshold was set to 0.1 [449]. The method was implemented in *Matlab* leveraging sparse matrix functions as proposed in [450] and spatially varying tensors $\mathbf{c}$ and $\mathbf{D}$ in order to consider heterogeneous tissue properties in terms of CV and its anisotropy.

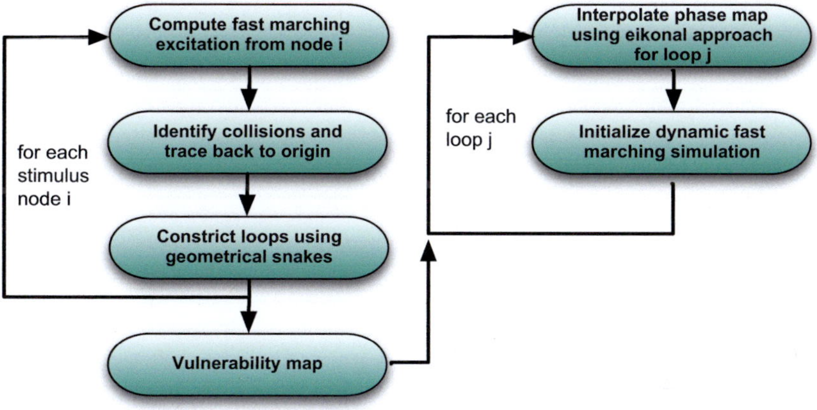

Figure 8.5: Overview of the algorithm to compute vulnerability maps (left) and optionally transfer the AFlut scenarios to dynamic simulations (right).

The resulting phase on the whole computational domain was transferred to an initial state of the dynamic fast marching simulator introduced in Section 3.2.2. The nodes in the first 50% of the cycle were included in the $REFRACTORY$ list, the next 20% in $KNOWN$, the next 20% were included in the $TRIAL$ list, and the last 10% in $UNKNOWN$. Nodes in the $KNOWN$ list have a fixed activation time influencing the activation time of the nodes in the $TRIAL$ list. The element with the smallest timestamp in the $TRIAL$ list is added to the $KNOWN$ list and all $UNKNOWN$ neighbors are added to the trial list. The BCL of all nodes was initialized with the RTT and the time of the last activation t_a of each node i was set by mapping the phase back to an activation time and starting the dynamic simulation at time $t = RTT$:

$$t_a(x) = RTT\frac{\phi(x)}{2\pi} \ . \tag{8.23}$$

Figure 8.5 summarized the pipeline used to generate AFlut vulnerability maps and transfer the results to dynamic simulations.

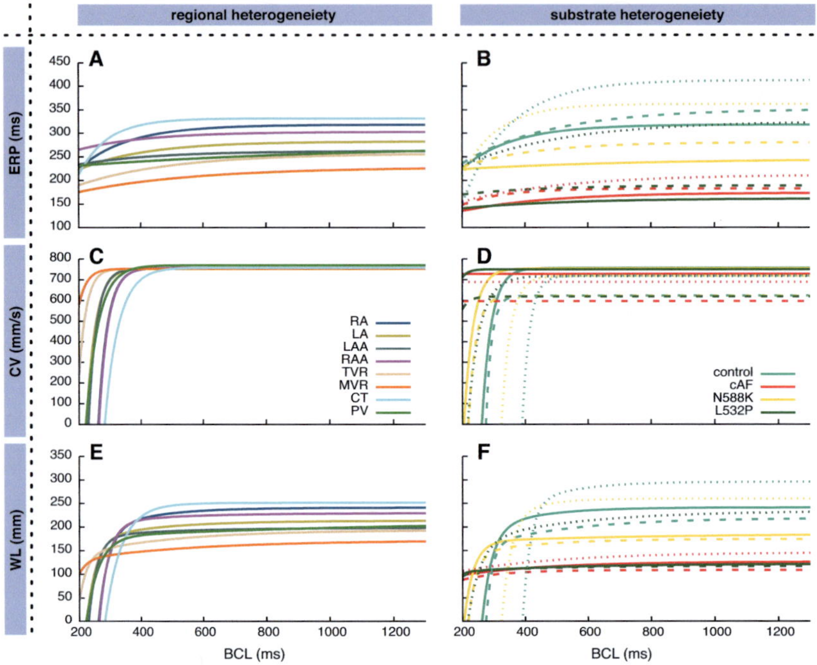

Figure 8.6: Fitted exponential restitution curves of ERP (A), (B) and CV (C), (D), as well as the WL as the product of the former measures (E), (F) for different anatomical regions in the atria (A), (C), (E) and different substrates (B), (D), (F). In (B), (D), and (F), the dashed lines represent the respective substrates under the influence of 2.3 μM amiodarone whereas the dotted lines represent the influence of 0.21 μM dronedarone. Exponential curves according to Equation (8.1) were used to fit the output of monodomain tissue strand simulations. The coefficients are listed in Table 8.1.

8.2 Results

The restitution of CV and ERP was determined through monodomain simulations in a one-dimensional tissue strand as detailed in Section 5.1.2 using variants of the Courtemanche et al. cell model [47]. CV and ERP were determined for 50 BCLs between 200 ms and 1300 ms distributed linearly in frequency domain. The monodomain conductivity σ was set to 0.076 S/m yielding a CV of 750 mm/s at a BCL of 1000 ms in the RA model.

Table 8.1: Coefficients of exponential curves representing the restitution of CV and ERP according to Equation (8.1) and the anisotropy k according to Equation (3.19) for different anatomical structures in the atria and different homogeneous substrates. Parameters were estimated based on the output of monodomain tissue strand simulations.

	CV				ERP		
	A (mm/s)	B (mm/s)	C (ms)	k	A (ms)	B (ms)	C (ms)
RA	537.4	3.02×10^6	30.3	3.75	318.4	312.9	165.0
LA	536.4	8.73×10^5	30.2	3.75	282.2	149.7	216.1
SN	1129.7	6.35×10^6	30.3	1.00	318.4	312.9	165.0
scar	0	0	1.0	1.00	318.4	312.9	165.0
CT	538.4	2.85×10^5	45.1	6.56	331.5	1000.0	94.0
PM	417.7	2.35×10^6	30.3	10.25	318.4	312.9	165.0
BB	587.5	3.30×10^6	30.3	9.00	318.4	312.9	165.0
inf. isthm.	537.4	3.02×10^6	30.3	1.00	318.4	312.9	165.0
PV	547.1	1.26×10^5	40.7	3.75	276.1	55.8	915.4
RAA	537.4	3.67×10^6	29.9	3.75	302.7	92.3	224.0
LAA	536.7	2.49×10^6	27.1	3.75	262.3	62.2	255.7
TVR	534.7	1.56×10^6	23.9	3.75	256.8	128.9	305.4
MVR	534.6	2.83×10^5	25.8	3.75	227.9	88.7	382.9
control	453.6	2.55×10^5	30.3		318.4	312.9	165.0
cAF	436.0	0	1		173.6	79.7	276.2
N588K	452.3	3.79×10^5	30.4		245.7	30.9	575.3
L532P	449.8	1.53×10^5	18.1		161.8	37.6	337.2

Different anatomical structures were investigated to account for regional heterogeneity using the data presented by Krueger et al. [158]. Furthermore, the four substrates introduced in Chapter 5 were analyzed with and without the influence of the pharmacological compounds amiodarone and dronedarone (cf. Section 6.1). Figure 8.6 shows the exponential fit of the restitution curves based on the coefficients in Table 8.1. The A and B coefficients for the CV of the different substrates were scaled with a factor of 0.6 yielding a total RA activation time of 192 ms in the control model without any drug applied.
The ERP for long BCLs ranged between 225.0 ms for the mitral valve ring (MVR) to 331.5 ms for the crista terminalis (CT). CT and the RA myocardium showed a steeper decrease towards shorter BCLs compared to the remaining regions. The CV for long BCLs differed by less than 1% for the different anatomical structures (Figure 8.6C).

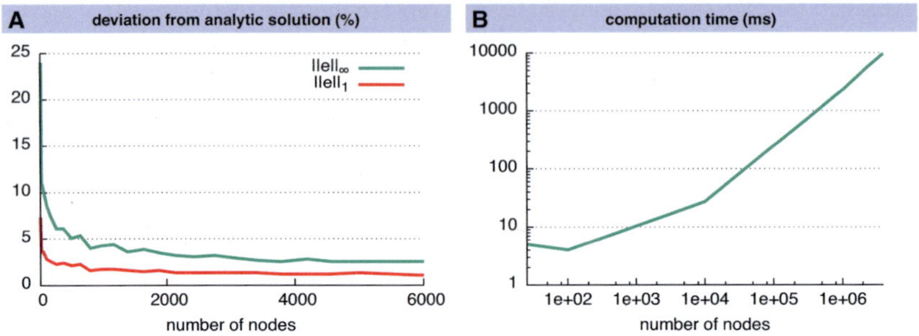

Figure 8.7: Deviation of the fast marching solution from the analytic solution of a radial wave (A). Excitation spread was computed on quadratical planar meshes composed of right-angled triangles. The mean error $\|e\|_1$ and the maximum error $\|e\|_\infty$ was evaluated for different numbers of nodes. The dependence of the computation time for one complete activation cycle on the number of nodes (B) was dominated by the linear part of $\mathcal{O}(N \log N)$.

The restitution curves of the different substrates (Figure 8.6B+D) in general and under the influence of drugs are discussed in detail in Section 6.1.2. Regarding the AFlut vulnerability, the WL is the decisive factor. Both different regions and different substrates exhibited distinct behavior at different BCLs. At short BCLs, CT was the region with the shortest WL opposed to long BCLs where it was the region with the longest BCL, e.g. (Figure 8.6E).

8.2.1 Activation Times

The fast marching algorithm and its implementation were verified and benchmarked by comparison to the analytical solution of a radial wave, quantitative comparison to the monodomain model on planar meshes with the same nodes, and qualitative comparison of the excitation pattern on a biatrial geometry. For a radial wave originating from a single node and spreading in an isotropic substrate, an analytical solution of the activation time map can be obtained. These analytical values were compared to the results yielded by the fast marching implementation on planar meshes composed of ordered triangles. The test mesh was of size 1 m × 1 m and a CV of 750 mm/s was assumed. The deviation was dependent on the number of nodes used to discretize the domain (Figure 8.7A). For node counts above 2000, both the maximum error and the

mean error remained stable indicating a converged solution. The implementation scaled as expected considering the algorithm complexity $\mathcal{O}(N \log N)$ with the linear part prevailing over the logarithmic part for relevant numbers of nodes (Figure 8.7B). The benchmark was performed on a single core of an *Intel Core i5* machine at a clock rate of 2.9 GHz. On this system, regular excitation patterns could be computed in real-time for models comprising up to 50,000 nodes.
Besides comparison to analytical solutions, monodomain simulations on planar patches served as a benchmark (Figure 8.8A+B). The time at which V_m exceeded –40 mV was used as the activation time. Each voxel of the structured grid used in the finite difference monodomain simulation was split into two triangles to obtain a triangular surface mesh for fast marching simulations. As the nodes of both meshes coincided, quantitative comparison was possible without the need for interpolation. The maximum deviation of activation times was 1.88% for ordered triangles (each voxel split by a diagonal from the bottom left to the top right, Figure 8.8C) and 1.78% for random split orientation (Figure 8.8E). The fast marching activation times were slightly later than the monodomain activation times on average. For moderately anisotropic substrates, the deviation depended on the assumed myocyte orientation. While the deviation was low for myocyte orientation coinciding with edges of all triangles (1.58%, Figure 8.8F), it was significantly higher for myocytes oriented 45° to the right-angled triangle edges (up to 23.3%, Figure 8.8D). The deviation was small in the direction of fast propagation and highest in the direction of slowest propagation, in which the fast marching activation times were later. The faster propagation in the monodomain simulation can be explained by the higher amount of activated tissue perpendicular to the myocyte orientation causing a higher source-to-sink ratio. This effect was not considered in the fast marching simulation as no anisotropic correction was implemented.

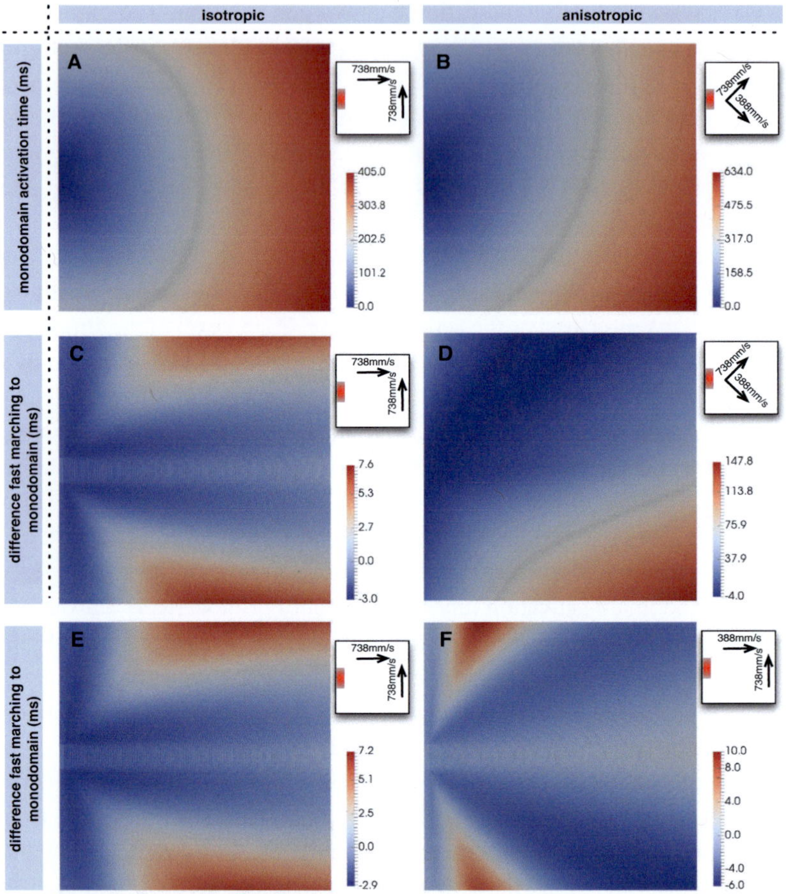

Figure 8.8: Monodomain activation times of almost radial waves in the isotropic (A) and an anisotropic case (B) on quadratic tissue patches with 30 cm side length. Fast marching activation was later for nodes along the diagonal in both ordered (C) and randomly oriented right-angled triangles (E). The deviation was larger for anisotropy 45° to the main triangle orientation axes (D) compared to myocyte orientation aligned with the right angled edges of the triangles (F). Excitation was triggered from the red area in the schematic representation in the top right corner of each panel. Note the different scales of the color bars.

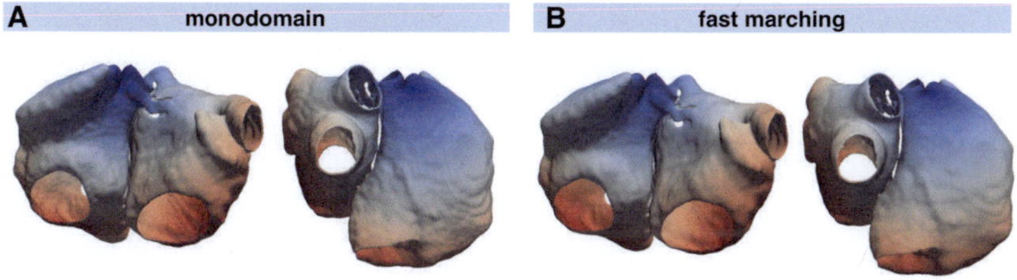

Figure 8.9: Comparison of monodomain activation times in a volumetric biatrial model (A) with fast marching activation times on a triangular surface mesh of the same subject embedded in three-dimensional space (B). Earliest activation (blue) was triggered from the junction of the SVC with the RAA.

A segmented magnetic resonance imaging (MRI) dataset was used to generate a volumetric structured grid for the monodomain simulation as well as a triangular mesh of the smoothed epicardial surface suitable for fast marching simulations. The activation patterns matched qualitatively as can be seen in Figure 8.9. Nearest neighbor comparison yielded an average activation time deviation of 4% and a maximum deviation of 8% between the fast marching and the monodomain simulations.

8.2.2 Flutter Loops and Geometric Snakes

Excitation propagation was calculated from several stimulus sites and sites of collision were detected using the activation vectors as shown in Figure 8.10A+B. From the sites of wavefront collision, the activation front was traced back to the stimulus site along the gradient of the activation time field. Combining the traces obtained by following the activation waves of both colliding waves yielded a set of initial loops for each stimulus node (Figure 8.10C). The WL condition Equation (8.3) was not fulfilled by several loops that could thus be neglected during the following steps (lighter colored loops in Figure 8.10C).

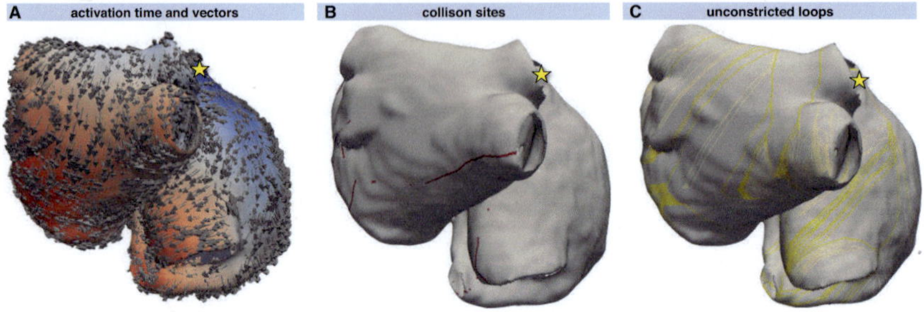

Figure 8.10: Activation time resulting from a stimulus at the junction of the SVC with the RAA (yellow star) ranging from early (blue) to late (red). The direction of the activation is indicated by arrows (A). Points of wavefront collisions were detected and are indicated by red dots in (B). (C) shows the loops composed of the two traces leading from the site collision to the stimulus site (yellow star). The yellow loops fulfill the WL condition Equation (8.3) whereas the light gray loops do not and were thus not considered for further steps.

A geometrical snake was initialized for each valid loop candidate as illustrated in Figure 8.11. Each node along the loop was surrounded by a micro-snake with segments covering all adjacent triangles (Figure 8.11A). By enforcing the constraints introduced in Section 8.1.2, the initial micro-snakes were merged into two distinct snakes: one snake on the outside of the loop nodes with consistently outwards-oriented snaxels and one inside-oriented snake on the inside of the loop nodes. The outwards-oriented snake could be identified as the longer one and disregarded. In this way, a consistently oriented snake adjacent to the loop nodes was constructed.

Figure 8.12 shows a geometrical snake initialized along a flutter loop candidate in the LA. The stimulus leading to that loop was applied between the two left PVs (yellow star in Figure 8.12A). The segment connecting the loop candidate with the stimulus location was shared by both half loops and disregarded before the snake was initialized. The initial RTT of 390 ms was reduced to 304 ms by iterating the snake according to Equation (8.7). The converged snake reflects myocyte orientation and CV heterogeneity (Figure 8.12F).

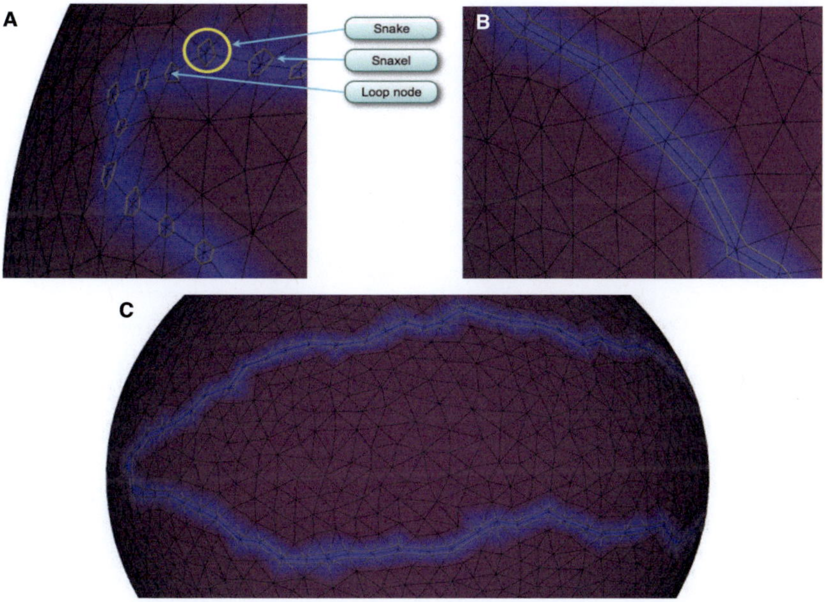

Figure 8.11: Initialization of a geometric snake along a loop (blue band). Initially, a micro-snake is established around each loop node (A). Snake segments are represented by thin grey tubes. Enforcing the constraints regarding the maximum number of snaxels per edge lead to two consistently oriented snakes (B), (C). Only the shorter snake was considered for constriction while the longer one was disregarded.

8.2.3 Vulnerability Maps

By triggering stimulation from different points, identifying loop candidates, and constricting them using geometrical snakes, AFlut vulnerability maps were generated as outlined in Figure 8.5. The vulnerability maps were sensitive to tissue anisotropy as indicated by the lower number of flutter paths in the isotropic model (Figure 8.13A) compared to the anisotropic case (Figure 8.13B). While the heterogeneous A and B values defining the CV according to Equation (8.1) were scaled in the isotropic case to match the activation time of the last element in the anisotropic case (158 ms), only 28.7% of all elements were covered by vulnerable paths in the isotropic case compared to 50.9% in the anisotropic case.

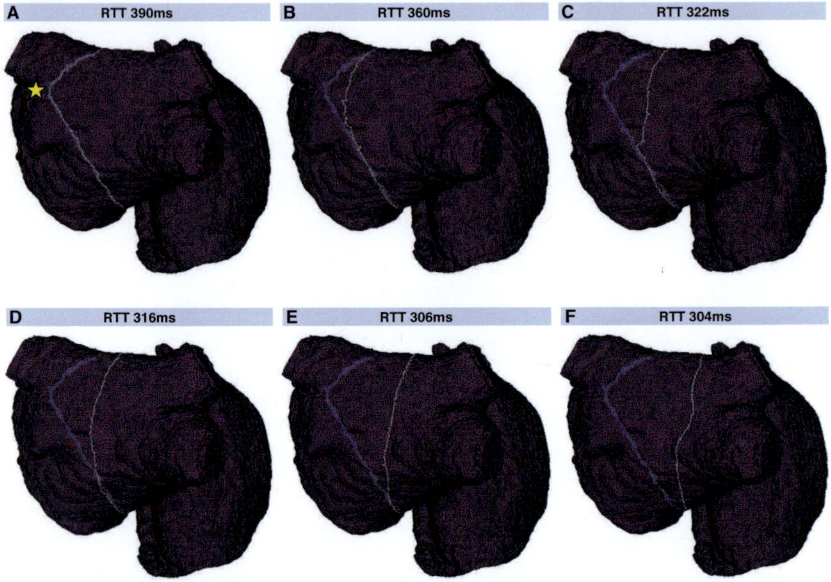

Figure 8.12: Evolution of a geometric snake covering the LA. Initially, the snake covered the loop found by the collision tracing algorithm (blue band) corresponding to a RTT of 390 ms (A). By iteratively constricting the snake (B-F), the shortest RTT of 304 ms considering heterogeneous CV and anisotropy was found. In this way, the influence of the particular choice of the stimulus site (yellow star in (A)) could be reduced.

In heterogeneous models regarding both CV and ERP, no vulnerable paths could be found in both isotropic and anisotropic setups with the CV scaled to obtain the same total activation time as in the anisotropic, heterogenous case.

The number of vulnerable paths and the share of RA myocardium covered by them was highly dependent on the CV. In the homogeneous anisotropic setup, the coverage increased from 0% at a CV of 475 mm/s to over 90% for CVs of 360 mm/s and more (Figure 8.14A). The degree of coverage did also depend on the number of different stimulus locations evaluated (Figure 8.14B). Considering all 19,296 RA nodes (minimum distance: 0 mm) yielded a coverage of 54.5% for a fixed CV of 425 mm/s. Requiring a minimum distance of 1 mm between stimulus points reduced their number to 8,254 without affecting the result significantly (50.9%). Considering less points yielded lower coverage rates (39.4% for 2 mm $\widehat{=}$ 2,136 nodes, 3.8% for 20 mm $\widehat{=}$ 19 nodes).

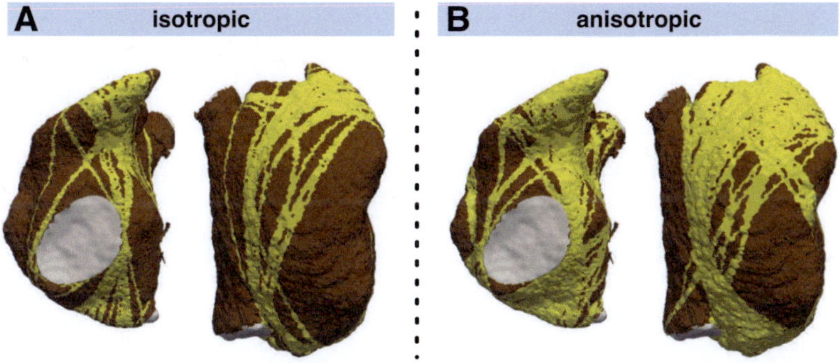

Figure 8.13: Influence of anisotropic conduction on a vulnerability map in the RA. Vulnerable paths are marked in yellow on the brown RA myocardium; the blood pool is indicated in gray. While the latest activation coincided in the isotropic (A) and anisotropic model (B), anisotropy lead to a higher number of vulnerable paths. The heterogeneous CV definitions are detailed in the text.

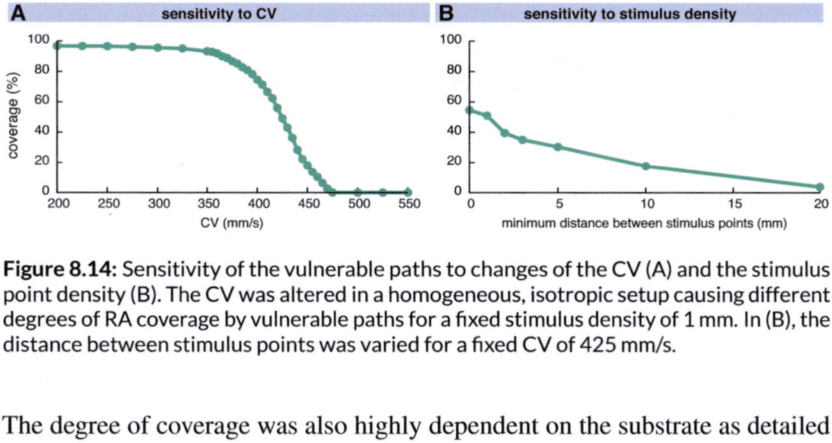

Figure 8.14: Sensitivity of the vulnerable paths to changes of the CV (A) and the stimulus point density (B). The CV was altered in a homogeneous, isotropic setup causing different degrees of RA coverage by vulnerable paths for a fixed stimulus density of 1 mm. In (B), the distance between stimulus points was varied for a fixed CV of 425 mm/s.

The degree of coverage was also highly dependent on the substrate as detailed in Table 8.2. 8,254 stimulus points with a minimum distance of 1 mm were considered using the CV and ERP values fitted from the monodomain model output using the biophysically detailed Courtemanche et al. cell model [47] given in Table 8.1. While the fitted exponential restitution of the ERP and the CV was modeled homogeneously across the RA, its heterogeneous anisotropy (k in Table 8.1) was kept.

Table 8.2: Degree of coverage of RA elements with paths vulnerable to AFlut for different substrates and antiarrhythmic drugs amiodarone (*amio*) and dronedarone (*drone*). In the right three columns, the A and B values determining the CV according to Equation (8.1) were scaled to match the activation time of the last element in the control substrate with no drug applied.

	Degree of coverage					
	Original CV			**Total activation time matched**		
	no drug	amio	drone	no drug	amio	drone
Control	18.1%	70.5%	0.0%	18.1%	0.0%	0.0%
cAF	96.0%	96.3%	95.6%	96.2%	96.1%	94.9%
N588K	93.2%	94.1%	0.0%	93.0%	77.8%	0.0%
L532P	96.2%	96.5%	34.5%	96.3%	96.0%	11.1%

Both the cAF substrate and the two human ether-à-go-go-related gene (hERG) mutations were more vulnerable to AFlut than the control model representing healthy myocytes. The higher degree of coverage under the influence of amiodarone observed for all substrates can be explained by the WL restitution (Figure 8.6F). The WL was shortened by the administration of amiodarone due to conduction slowing caused by the sodium channel inhibition. This effect was most pronounced in the control substrate and was reflected in the vulnerability maps as well (Figure 8.15).

In order to separate the effects of the different substrates and compounds on CV and ERP, the total activation time of the RA was matched with the activation of the last element in the control model and no drug (191 ms) in a second set of simulations (Figure 8.16), i.e. the A and B parameters determining the CV according to Equation (8.1) were scaled while keeping the anisotropy ratio k constant. In this way, only the effect on the repolarization (ERP) was considered leading to a reduction of vulnerable paths under the influence of amiodarone in all substrates and a more pronounced reduction under the influence of dronedarone compared to Figure 8.15.

Besides evaluating different substrates, distinct spatial heterogeneities were introduced in the RA model. The normal RA myocardium was parametrized with an isotropic CV of 700 mm/s and an ERP of 250 ms for all BCLs. A circular zone of slow conduction on the posterior wall was modeled (Figure 8.17A).

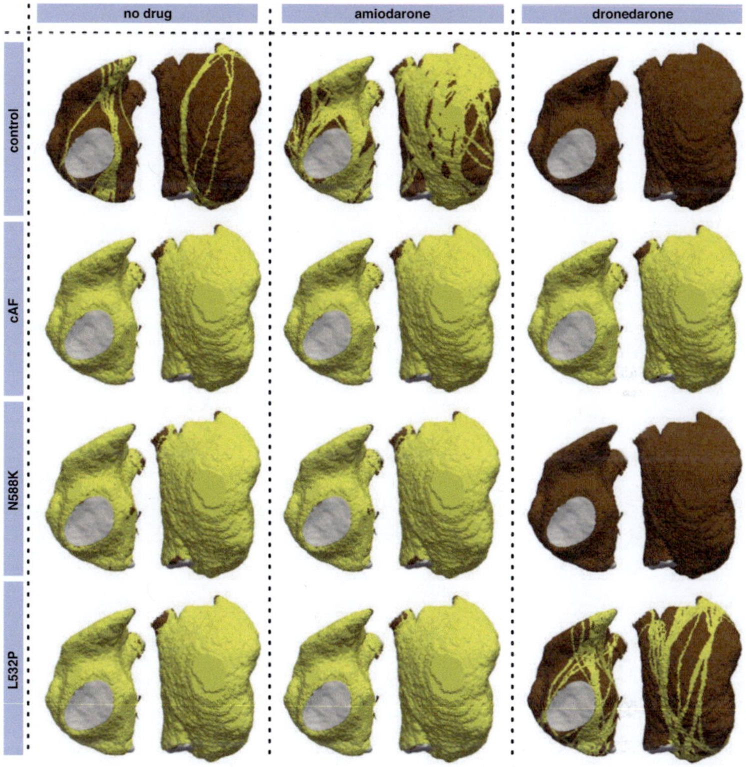

Figure 8.15: Vulnerability maps of the RA for combinations of different substrates and pharmacological agents. Besides a control substrate representing healthy myocytes, a cAF remodeled substrate (neglecting changes of cell-to-cell coupling), and two hERG mutations were evaluated. Standard concentrations of the antiarrhythmic agents amiodarone (2.3 μM) and dronedarone (0.21 μM) were administered in the center and right columns. Vulnerable paths are marked in yellow on the brown RA myocardium; the blood pool is indicated in gray.

Depending on the CVs inside and outside a circular zone of slow conduction, the wave might be faster bypassing the zone than propagating through it. Comparing the time the wave takes to bypass the circle with the time it takes to propagate through the zone of slow conduction yields a critical CV_{slow}/CV_{normal} ratio of $2/\pi \approx 0.63$. If the ratio is higher, the dominant path is through the zone of slow conduction. If it is lower, the bypassing wave is faster.

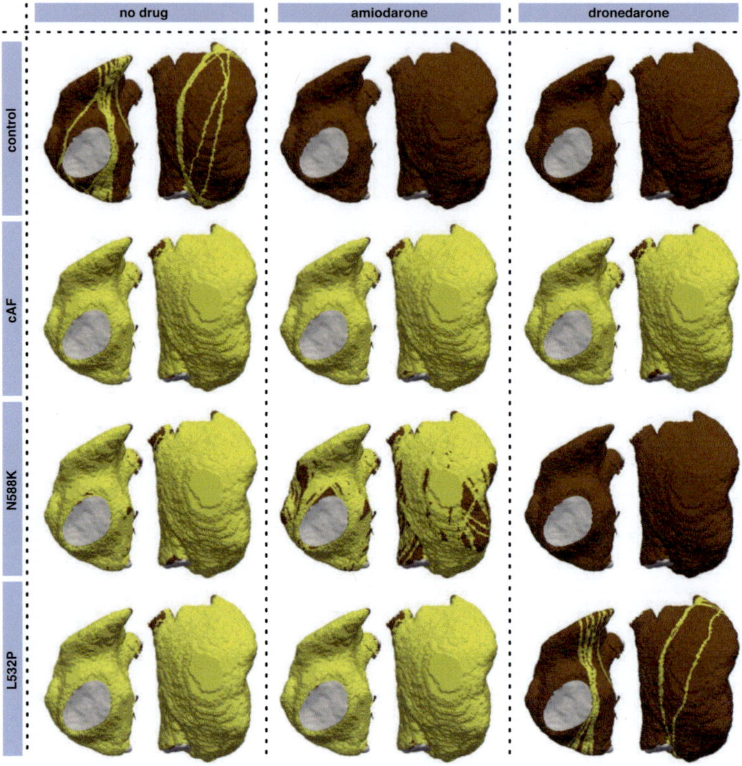

Figure 8.16: Vulnerability maps of the RA for combinations of different substrates and pharmacological agents. In contrast to Figure 8.15, only the ERP was modeled substrate-specific, thus only considering differences in repolarization.

Therefore, the zone of slow conduction within the surrounding tissue conducting at 704 mm/s was parametrized with a CV of 500 mm/s resulting in a ratio of 0.71 (Figure 8.18B), and 250 mm/s ($\widehat{=}$ 0.36, Figure 8.18C). In contrast to the control model (Figure 8.18A), the zones of slow conduction yielded additional flutter paths. For the CV of 500 mm/s in the zone of slow conduction, 24.1% of the RA were covered by vulnerable paths (Figure 8.18B) in contrast to 14.1% in the control case (Figure 8.18A). Additional flutter paths crossed the periphery of the zone of slow conduction and thereby prolonged the RTT.

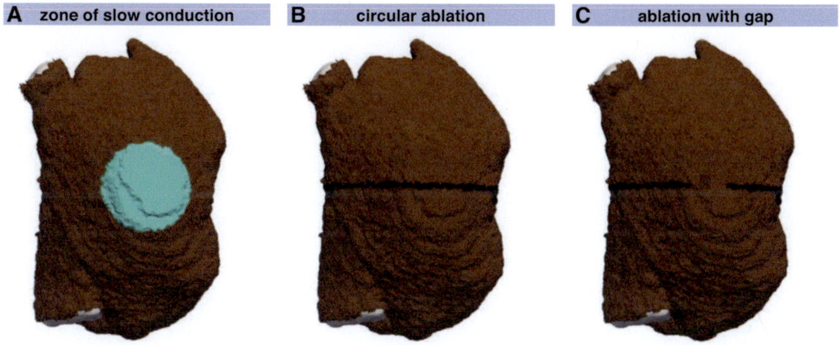

Figure 8.17: Substrate modifications introduced in the RA model: a zone of slow conduction (cyan in (A)), a circular ablation lesion (black in (B)+(C)), as well as a gap in the ablation lesion (C).

For the slower CV of 250 mm/s, the entire zone of slow conduction was covered by vulnerable paths yielding a total RA coverage of 47.8% (Figure 8.18C). The paths were not constricted to the faster route outside the zone as the route through the zone of slow conduction was optimal considering the field of view of the geometrical snake. When computing an inducability map (see Figure 8.5 and Discussion), the driving path would be running around the zone of slow conduction, though.

The second spatial substrate modification was an ablation lesion which encircled the RA completely from both sides of the TV (Figure 8.17B). Rather than being a clinically used ablation pattern, this scenario serves as an example separating the RA into two electrically isolated regions. The lesion was modeled as non-conductive, thus no flutter paths could cross it. In an additional scenario, a gap in the ablation lesion was assumed at the central posterior wall (Figure 8.17C and Figure 8.18E). In case of the complete lesion, no flutter paths were identified (Figure 8.18D) as the WL condition could not be fulfilled on any of the two separated, smaller substrates. The gap in the ablation lesion yielded numerous vulnerable paths running through the gap at various angles (Figure 8.18E). The flutter paths covered 42.9% of the RA in contrast to 14.1% in the control case.

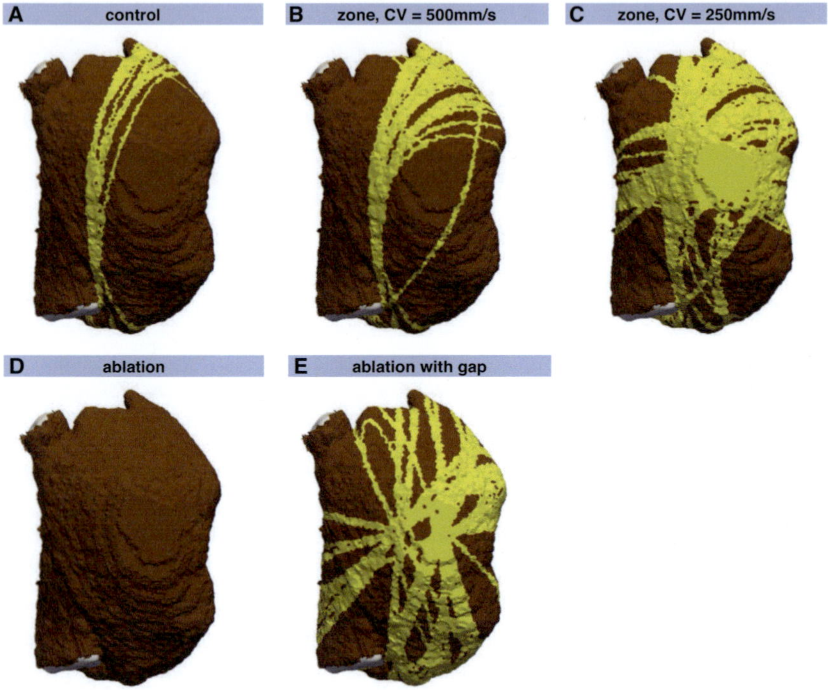

Figure 8.18: Vulnerability maps of the RA for different substrate modifications. Compared, to (A), a zone of slow conduction was assumed (cf. Figure 8.17A) in (B)+(C). A circular ablation lesion was introduced in (D) (cf. Figure 8.17B). In (E), a gap in the ablation lesion was modeled on the central posterior wall (cf. Figure 8.17C).

The time to compute a complete vulnerability map depends on the number of stimulus points considered and the number of loops candidates fulfilling the WL condition over time. The computation is faster, the fewer loop candidates there are and the earlier the constricted loops are disregarded because they no longer fulfill the WL condition. For the RA mesh consisting of 38,033 triangles, computation was timed on an *Intel Xeon E5-2697V2* machine with twelve cores at a base clock rate of 2.7 GHz. The control vulnerability map in Figure 8.18A with a coverage of 14.1% was computed within 4.0 min whereas it took 5.5 min to compute the vulnerability map for the RA including the zone of slow conduction causing a coverage of 47.8% (Figure 8.18C).

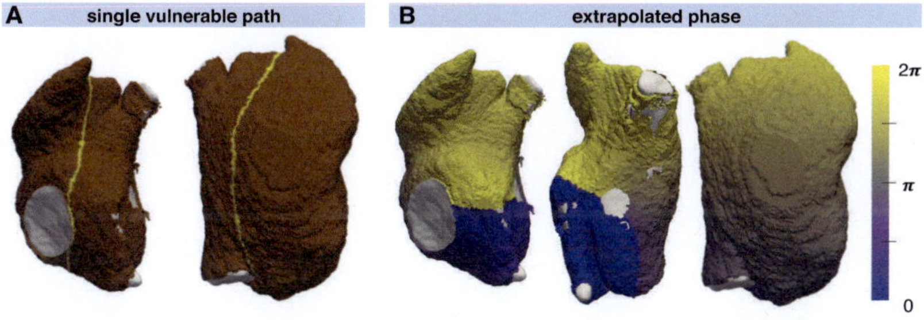

Figure 8.19: Individual vulnerable paths in the RA (A) were extrapolated to the whole RA in phase domain (B) by applying the eikonal-diffusion approach with the path from (A) as a Dirichlet boundary condition.

8.2.4 Phase Extrapolation

The vulnerable paths represented in the vulnerability maps and identified using the methods described above were extrapolated on the whole RA in terms of phase using the methods described in Section 8.1.3. Towards this end, the eikonal-diffusion based approach was employed. Each vulnerable path (Figure 8.19A) was extrapolated in phase space individually (Figure 8.19B). The eikonal-diffusion approach converged within 16 to 18 iterations for assumed CVs between $0.1\times$ and $2\times$ the ground truth value and assumed RTTs between $0.3\times$ and $3\times$ the ground truth value.

The phase map was then used to determine the initial state of a dynamic fast marching simulation. Figure 8.20 gives an example of how the dominant path determines the reentry driving AFlut. The reentry was initiated with the wavefront starting from the septal side of the TV running towards the CS region (Figure 8.19B). However, reentry around the TV could be sustained (Figure 8.20). Thus, the wavefront passing over to the posterior wall at the junction with the inferior vena cava (IVC) (cf. Figure 8.19B) and running upwards collided with the downwards wave passing over at the junction of the SVC with the RAA and ceased. As the ERP of the tricuspid valve ring (TVR) was shorter than that of the surrounding RA myocardium (cf. Figure 8.6A), the driving reentry circle around the TVR excited the remaining RA every other cycle (Figure 8.20A vs. Figure 8.20D).

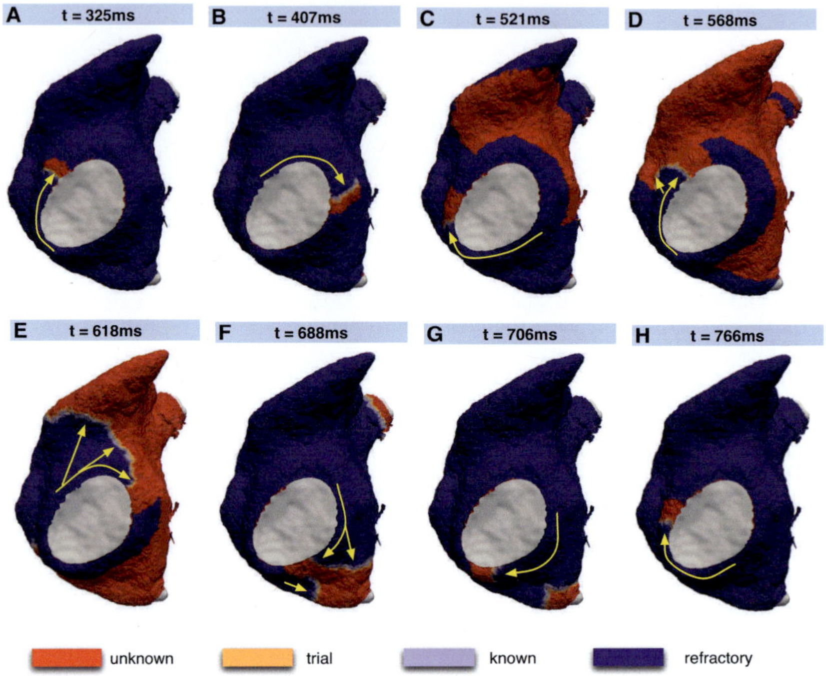

Figure 8.20: Dynamic fast marching simulation with AFlut around the TV. Every second cycle, tissue towards the RAA was non-refractory (D) and excited by the dominant flutter path (E). Wavefronts collided in the CS region (F) such that only the dominant flutter path around the TV was still active and driving reentry (H). The blood pool is indicated in gray.

8.3 Discussion

In this chapter, a workflow to identify vulnerable paths potentially sustaining AFlut was presented. The approach builds on fast marching simulations of excitation propagation and geometric snakes to constrict paths identified on the basis of wavefront collision sites. Throughout the whole pipeline, heterogeneous, anisotropic, and frequency-dependent tissue properties are considered in terms of CV and ERP.

The fast marching simulation was verified against analytical solutions for simple excitation patterns and against activation times determined in mon-

odomain simulations for more complex excitation patterns and computational domains. The maximum error was below 5% with respect to the analytical solution for node distances below 2.8 mm considering physiologic CVs. The implementation allows real-time simulations of activation times for models up to 50,000 nodes on a standard desktop machine. Regarding the monodomain simulation, the deviation was higher for high anisotropy ratios resulting in wavefronts with differing curvature. This issue is discussed further in the Limitations section below (8.3.1).
The geometrical snake approach presented by Bischoff and Kobbelt [444, 445] was implemented and adapted to the excitation propagation application scenario considering heterogeneous, anisotropic, and frequency-dependent tissue properties. Applying the geometric snake approach to loop candidates identified as circular paths from an initial stimulus point via a site of wavefront collision back to the initial stimulus yielded AFlut vulnerability maps. The number and the location of the identified vulnerable flutter paths was sensitive to anisotropy (Figure 8.13), the substrate properties regarding CV and repolarization, as well as modification of these parameters due to pharmacological compounds (Figure 8.15 and Figure 8.16), zones of slow conduction or ablation lesions (Figure 8.18), and most importantly the assumed CV (Figure 8.14). Anisotropic substrates were more vulnerable than isotropic tissue when matching the total activation time of the RA due to the concentration of flutter paths along the fast-conducting bundles. The WL is a crucial parameter as can be seen by the higher number of vulnerable paths identified for the cAF and hERG mutated substrates compared to control. While dronedarone reduced the AFlut vulnerability, amiodarone rendered the substrate more vulnerable due to the reduced WL caused by the slowed CV (cf. Figure 8.6). When only considering the effect on repolarization, thus altering ERP to represent the influence of the drug, amiodarone exhibited antiarrhythmic properties as well. The effect was less pronounced than for dronedarone, though. Zones of slow conduction increased the number and the density of vulnerable paths as the cycle length increases both by conducting through the slow zone and by bypassing it. While ablation lesions isolating different regions completely rendered the RA invulnerable to AF, a small gap in the lesion increased the number of vulnerable paths threefold compared to control. This effect can be explained by the narrow isthmus formed by the gap in the lesion. Moreover, shortcuts leading to wavefront collision and ceasing the reentrant activation

are cut off by the lesion, thus stabilizing the reentry. The assumed CV had the biggest effect on the number of vulnerable paths and the degree of RA coverage by them. A CV slowing by 25% rendered an invulnerable RA model highly vulnerable with a flutter path coverage of over 90%. This finding highlights the importance of a reliable CV estimation to draw relevant conclusions from personalized models using the method presented here. The CV of the individual patient has to be measured in a spatially resolved, and preferably frequency-dependent, manner. Weber et al. proposed a method to estimate local CV and its restitution based on a cosine fit method [455, 456]. The advent of new electro-anatomical mapping systems and catheters with improved signal quality, in particular the *Rhythmia*^{TM} mapping system and the *Orion*^{TM} catheter from *Boston Scientific, Natick, MA, USA*, as well as sophisticated signal processing approaches gives rise to hope for such CV mapping in the near future [457, 458].
The computation of a single activation sequence was faster than real-time, a complete vulnerability map took several minutes, however. Most of the computational cost was due to the constriction of the loop candidates using the geometrical snake approach. While the time spent to calculate excitation propagation accounted for only a minor share, less complex alternatives to the fast marching algorithm exist. Graph-based approaches, such as the A* algorithm [161, 173, 459] or the fastest route algorithm [460] are however only faster if the activation time at only a subset of nodes is needed. Cellular automata (e.g. [461]) on the other hand do not consider quadratic approximation of activation times. The computational complexity of the geometrical snake implementation could be reduced by optimizing the number of neighbors considered for the calculation of the snaxel velocity (Equation (8.7)) and the convergence criteria. Indeed, the approach considering $N = 30$ neighbors with decreasing weight could be approximated by a spatial multi-grid approach starting with distant neighbors in early iterations and focussing on closer nodes at later iterations. When aiming at an interactive modification of the substrate, e.g. by introducing virtual ablation lesions, results from previous evaluation can be reused for regions not affected by the last modification. Moreover, intermediate results could be precomputed, thus trading memory footprint in for reduced computation time. This potential for optimizations makes interactive assessment of ablation therapy in almost real-time seem achievable.

While several other studies mentioned in the introduction of this chapter assessed ablation patterns regarding the prevention or termination of AF, this is the first work to assess the vulnerability to AFlut based on an individualized anatomical model besides a very recent work by Zahid et al. with substantially increased computational effort [440] to the best of my knowledge (see also review in [11]). Child et al. introduced the reentry vulnerability index (RVI) as a quantitative metric based on the difference between activation and repolarization intervals at pairs of spatial locations [462]. The RVI correlates with exit sites of scar-related reentrant arrhythmia as commonly observed in the ventricles [463]. However, it aims at predicting functional lines of block rather than providing a comprehensive map of vulnerable paths based on the individual geometrical properties. The same holds for a study by Wallman et al. quantifying the arrhythmogeneity of scar and left-to-right heterogeneity in the ventricles [464].

Lines et al. proposed a method to replicate clinically mapped atrial tachycardias *in silico* [442]. Trächtler et al. used the fast marching implementation presented here for a similar *in silico* reproduction of clinical cases [465, 466]. While both methods allow to test ablation strategies regarding the termination of the specific reentry, they do not allow to draw conclusions regarding the vulnerability to AFlut along other paths. Thus, these approaches do not provide the means to optimize AF ablation aiming at the prevention of post-ablational AFlut.

The method presented here could be further developed regarding two aspects. First, the extrapolated phase map obtained by the eikonal-diffusion approach could not only be used to initialize a fast marching simulation but also to replicate the flutter path in a monodomain simulation. Matene et al. proposed a suitable approach [290], which they used to initiate AF by extrapolating phase singularities [467, 468]. By initiating the same flutter loop in both the fast marching and the monodomain environment, the fast marching approach could be validated with respect to macro-reentry. Second, the dominant flutter paths sustaining reentry in the dynamic simulations could be tracked and compared to the paths used to extrapolate the initial state. In this way, not only a map of vulnerable flutter paths but also a map of inducible flutter paths could be computed.

The complete pipeline could be validated using clinical cases once tools for a spatially resolved CV estimation become available. The anatomical model of the individual patient built from MRI data would be augmented with a priori knowledge and LA breakthrough measurements using the methods presented in Chapter 7. CV and ERP would be parametrized using intracardiac measurements complemented with model-based assumptions. Preferably, the subjects should be recruited from patients undergoing ablation of AFlut that developed after AF ablation. If a gap in the ablation lesion is identified during the second procedure, the lesions placed during the AF ablation procedure as well as the gap in it would be included as further a priori knowledge. The clinically observed flutter path should then be found in the vulnerability (and potentially inducability) map. Moreover, the ablation terminating the flutter in the clinical setting should also remove the specific vulnerable path from the map.

8.3.1 Limitations

The implementation of the fast marching algorithm used in this work does consider anisotropic CV but does not consider recursive anisotropic correction as proposed by Sermesant et al. [176]. In [162], the authors of [176] showed that the computation time is higher by a factor of $\approx$1.6 when considering anisoptropic correction. While the influence of the anisotropic correction has never been evaluated systematically, it should not be too relevant for moderate anisotropy values. For the application presented in this chapter, subtle differences of the activation sequence do not play a role for the final result as fast marching activation times serve only as the input for subsequent processing. Another limitation of the presented method is that it is restricted to monoatrial flutter paths. The reason for this can be seen in Figure 8.21 in which a biatrial loop candidate was constricted using the geometrical snakes approach. While a shortcut within the LA exists, it cannot be considered by the snake as it is constrained by the IACs and can thus not cross the septum. However, the method could be extended to identify shortcuts within the two atria by also considering monoatrial loops in addition.

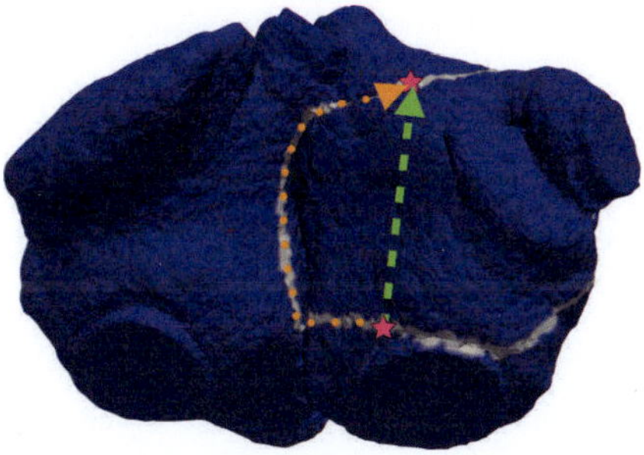

Figure 8.21: Limitation of geometrical snakes concerning biatrial loops. While a shortcut between the two purple stars exists (dashed green line), the snake cannot constrict further and remains on the dotted orange line due to the discrete IACs.

The final constricted biatrial loop could be used to initialize additional monoatrial loops comprising the segment of the biatrial loop and shortest connection between the two open ends at the IACs. When computing inducability maps instead of vulnerability maps, this limitations is not relevant since reentry along a loop as in Figure 8.21 could not be induced if it could not be induced as a monoatrial loop as well.

Regarding the dynamic simulation of AFlut, the missing representation of electrotonic coupling is a limitation. A situation as depicted in Figure 8.20 with a consistent 2:1 conduction pattern would hardly be possible in a monodomain simulation. The longer action potentials (APs) of the RA tissue surrounding the TVR would delay repolarization and recovery from refractoriness of the TVR myocytes. The driving flutter path around the TV would thus be slowed resulting in a 1:1 conduction pattern, eventually.

The biggest hurdle is the sparsity of the available clinical data to characterize an individual's substrate and the associated uncertainty. The importance of a reliable CV estimation is highlighted by the fact that a CV uncertainty of Δc corresponds to scaling of the atrium by a factor of $\sqrt{\Delta c}$. Considering that the minimal WL needed to sustain reentry is defined by the product of CV and ERP, uncertainty of ERP plays an important role as well [469, 470]. Improved electro-anatomic mapping systems providing better signal quality and simultaneous mapping using a multitude of electrodes, as well as advanced signal processing methods make it seem probable to have suitable data available in the near future. Moreover, the uncertainty in the data can be taken into account by probabilistic modeling using Bayesian inference and compressed sensing methods [471].

8.3.2 Conclusion

In this chapter, a comprehensive method to analyze the vulnerability to AFlut was presented. The individual anatomy as well as electrophysiology in terms of CV, ERP, and their frequency-dependence was taken into account. This tool provides the means to evaluate potential ablation strategies *in silico* regarding their arrhythmic potential for AFlut before actually applying them in the electrophysiology lab. In this way, this work can be one piece in the puzzle to overcome the *learning by burning* paradigm [472, 473] and eventually reduce the number of patients suffering from post-ablational AFlut.

PART IV

UNDERSTANDING THE BODY SURFACE P-WAVE

CHAPTER 9

Contribution of the Left and the Right Atrium to the P-Wave

As outlined in Chapter 2, atrial rhythm disorders are progressive diseases. Thus, they are more likely to be treated effectively, the earlier they are detected. In the best case, patients at risk to develop atrial rhythm disorders can be identified before the onset of the arrhythmia. Adequate preventive measures can then prevent or at least postpone the outbreak in a large share of patients. The P-wave in the body surface electrocardiogram (ECG) has long been used to gain insight into anatomy, function and dysfunction of the atria [474, 475]. As a 12-lead ECG is routinely acquired non-invasively as part of a large number of examinations, ECG-derived measures represent ideal risk markers due to their availability and low associated costs [476]. These properties render ECG-based markers more attractive than alternatives like ultrasound, magnetic resonance imaging (MRI), electroanatomical mapping, or ECG imaging. Therefore, clinicians aim to stratify arrhythmia risk based on P-wave markers [477, 478]. The assessment of morphological features of the P-wave is recommended in current guidelines for ECG interpretation [479] regarding the diagnosis of atrial abnormalities such as left or right atrial enlargement. The anatomy and physiology of the left atrium (LA) are of particular interest regarding the risk to develop atrial fibrillation (AF).

Nevertheless, we are lacking mechanistic understanding of left and right atrial contribution to the P-wave to date despite a multitude of empirical studies correlating P-wave features with properties of the LA and right atrium (RA) [480–482].

Some literature sources state that the P-waves originating from left and right atrial sources are almost simultaneous, thus fused into a single peak [479]. Others argue that the left and right atrial P-wave can be almost perfectly separated in the time domain due to the delayed activation of the LA [483]. The question which parts of the atria contribute to the P-wave during different temporal phases and the projection onto different leads is of great importance to evaluate the theoretical limits regarding the diagnostic potential of specific P-wave markers. Even though many aspects of AF induced remodeling affect atrial repolarization, which is reflected in the atrial T-wave not normally visible in the ECG, anatomical alterations, fibrosis and gap junction remodeling can potentially be reflected in the P-wave. Thus, the answer to the aforementioned question will foster our understanding and eventually help to identify patients at risk early before severe remodeling sets in. Optimized preventive and therapeutic measured can then relieve part of the burden related to atrial arrhythmias from both patients and healthcare system.

The study presented in this chapter uses an *in silico* approach to separate the contributions of the LA and the RA to the P-wave in a perfectly controlled environment. The analysis is conducted on a population of eight individualized anatomical models.

The P-wave was investigated *in silico* in several aspects before. A double layer can serve as a source model for the P-wave as shown in [484], however anisotropic conductivity tensors are required [485]. While Lu et al. presented a reasonable P-wave obtained using a generic, homogeneous thorax model [486], other studies showed that at least the blood and the lungs with their respective properties need to be considered [177, 487]. Colman et al. analyzed the effect of acetylcholine on the P-wave using a detailed cellular model and a simplified torso [488] and assessed the accuracy of a clinically used algorithm to locate atrial focal points [489]. In contrast to all aforementioned studies, Krueger et al. conducted finite element computations instead of using the boundary element method to investigate P-wave genesis and alterations related to hemodialysis [23, 490]. Several computational studies assessed P-waves during AF [491–494], however I am not aware of any work distinguishing between RA and LA contribution besides two very recent studies [495, 496] published after this study was submitted as a conference paper [497].

Parts of this work have been published as a conference contribution [497] and are currently under review [498] as a journal paper and a conference contribution [499].

9.1 Methods

9.1.1 Cohort of Anatomical Models

In earlier work [23, 183], anatomical models of eight individuals were constructed at IBT based on magnetic resonance images. The MRI studies were approved by the institutional review boards of the centers where the data were acquired and participating patients and volunteers gave informed consent. The study population characteristics are summarized in Table 9.1. The imaging data were segmented using a combination of automatic and manual approaches [183]. For the atrial wall, a homogeneous thickness of 2.5–3 mm had to be assumed due to the poor MRI contrast. The segmented atria were then converted to a structured grid with an isotropic voxel resolution of 0.33 mm resulting in between 5.4×10^5 and 2.6×10^6 elements for excitation propagation simulations. The segmented torsos were converted to a tetrahedral mesh using the CGAL library [500] resulting in between 1.1×10^6 and 2.9×10^6 elements. These existing volumetric bi-atrial models were augmented with tissue labels as a basis for a heterogeneous electrophysiological model and myocyte orientation allowing for anisotropic conduction using the approach described in Chapter 7. In order to control right-to-left atrial conduction, the initially isolated atria were connected via four discrete interatrial connections (IACs): Bachmann's bundle (BB), middle posterior connection (MPC), lower posterior connection (LPC), and at the coronary sinus (CS) [32, 33].

Table 9.1: Characteristics of the eight patients and volunteers (*subjects*) used to build the *in silico* models. Abbreviations: Heart rate (HR), control (Ctl), long-QT syndrome (LQT).

Subject	#1	#2	#3	#4	#5	#6	#7	#8
Age (years)	47	19	26	50	27	25	38	66
Weight (kg)	52	66	79	79	100	70	90	100
Diagnosis	Ctl	LQT2	Ctl	LQT1	Ctl	Ctl	Ctl	AF
HR (1/min)	81	76	69	62	70	53	86	62
PWD (ms)	95	95	107	91	103	97	99	176
RA blod volume (ml)	98	52	117	88	132	99	72	155
LA blod volume (ml)	55	27	63	79	81	87	53	136
RA myocardium (1×10^3 mm^3)	26	12	27	38	52	21	36	38
LA myocardium (1×10^3 mm^3)	19	10	25	32	26	19	29	34

Table 9.2: Relative values $\hat{g}_x$ of ion channel conductivities representing regional heterogeneities [158] with respect to the original Courtemanche et al. model of human atrial myocytes [47]. Monodomain conductivity perpendicular to myocyte orientation $\sigma_\perp$ with relation to the working myocardium (87 mS/m) and anisotropy factor. Italic values differ from normal myocardium.

Anatomical structure	$\hat{g}_{Kr}$	$\hat{g}_{to}$	$\hat{g}_{Ca,L}$	$\sigma_\perp/\sigma_{\perp,RA/LA}$ (%)	anisotropy
RA / LA	1.0	1.0	1.0	100	3.75
Crista Terminalis	1.0	1.0	*1.67*	100	*6.56*
Atrial appendages	1.0	*0.68*	*1.06*	100	3.75
Atrio-ventricular rings	1.0	*1.53*	*0.67*	100	3.75
Pectinate muscles	1.0	1.0	1.0	*66*	*10.52*
Bachmann's Bundle	1.0	1.0	1.0	*116*	*9.0*
Inferior isthmus	1.0	1.0	1.0	*86*	*1.0*

9.1.2 Electrophysiological Modeling

Ionic currents in the voxels representing atrial myocytes were computed using a heterogeneous version of the Courtemanche et al. membrane model [47, 158]. As introduced in Section 3.1, the ion currents are calculated according to Ohm's law by multiplying the difference between the transmembrane voltage V_m and the respective Nernst potential E_X with the maximum conductivity g_X and the open probability of the channel. Based on prior work [158], the maximum conductivities g_X of several channels were altered by multiplication with a factor $\hat{g}_X$ as given in Table 9.2 to account for regional heterogeneity.

Besides maximum ion channel conductivities, also monodomain tissue conductivity and its anisotropy regarding myocyte orientation was modeled heterogeneously according to Table 9.2. After initialization of the cell models in a single cell environment to establish steady-state, stimulation was triggered from the junction of the superior vena cava (SVC) and the right atrial appendage (RAA) (cf. EAS3 in Section 10.1). Excitation propagation was calculated by the monodomain reaction-diffusion solver *acCELLerate* [169, 170] using a finite element method on regular hexahedral grids and explicit Euler integration with constant time stepping of 20 μs.
The sources of the extracellular potential within the torso and on the body surface that are measured during ECG acquisition are the impressed currents stemming from the gradient of V_m as introduced in Section 3.4. These currents were masked in order to separate the LA from the RA P-wave.
In order to obtain the parts of the P-wave stemming from the RA, the sources in the LA were muted by setting $\sigma_i \nabla V_m$ to 0 in all LA elements and vice versa. The conductivity tensors σ were set according to the data by Gabriel & Gabriel [501] and the reduced bidomain formulation (Section 3.4, [177]) was solved with a temporal resolution of 1 ms once for the LA sources and once for the RA sources. Thanks to the linearity of the problem, the regular P-wave could be obtained by the superposition of the LA and the RA P-waves. The vectorcardiogram (VCG) was derived from the 12-lead ECG using the inverse Dower matrix [61]. The electrical axis of the atria α was calculated using the P-wave amplitudes in leads aVF and I:

$$\alpha = \arctan\left(\frac{2}{\sqrt{3}}\frac{aVF}{I}\right) \tag{9.1}$$

9.2 Results

Figure 9.1 shows the activation time maps yielded by the monodomain simulations. After the stimulus at the junction between the SVC and the RAA, the excitation spread predominantly along the fast conducting bundles, such as the crista terminalis (CT). The last elements were activated 76–112 ms after the stimulus. The characteristics of the resulting P-waves are given in Table 9.3.

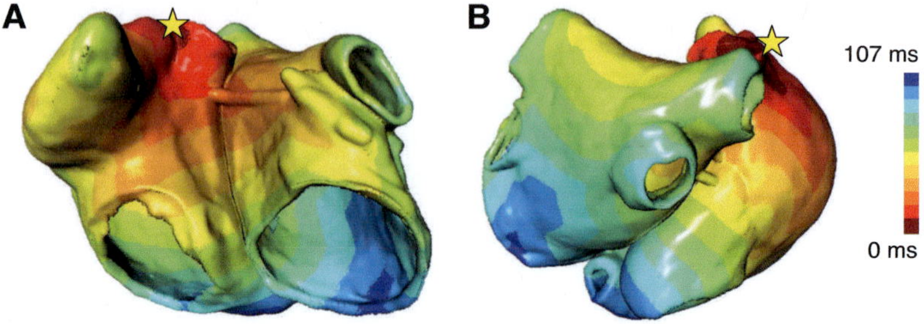

Figure 9.1: Local activation times resulting from the excitation propagation simulation using model #5. Excitation originated from the junction of the SVC and the RAA indicated by the yellow star. Anterior view in (A), posterior view in (B).

Table 9.3: Characteristics of the simulated P-waves using the eight *in silico* models and excitation origin at the junction between the superior vena cava and the right atrial appendage (cf. EAS3 in Section 10.1).

Model	#1	#2	#3	#4	#5	#6	#7	#8
PWD (ms)	91	76	83	87	100	105	78	112
Max. amplitude lead	II	III	II	II	V_1	II	II	II
Amplitude II (mV)	0.26	0.14	0.18	0.22	0.35	0.22	0.27	0.18
Axis α (°)	73.1	65.0	66.9	65.2	60.3	77.7	64.5	71.0
Positive I	√	√	√	√	√	√	√	√
Positive II	√	√	√	√	√	√	√	√
Negative aVR	√	√	√	√	√	√	√	√
Monophasic I	√	√	√	√	√	x	√	√
Biphasic V_1	√	√	√	x	√	x	√	x

The P-wave duration (PWD) differed by between ± 25 ms between the measured and the simulated P-waves for subjects #1 to #7 with a mean PWD of 91.5 ms in the simulations. The fact that no patient-specific substrate model was employed in this study explains the shorter simulated P-wave for the AF subject #8 (–64 ms). Potential AF-induced conduction slowing was not included in the model because the focus of this study was on inter-individual anatomical rather than electrophysiological differences. The P-waves in Einthoven leads I, II were upright in all models and negative in Goldberger lead aVR. In Wilson lead V_1, the P-wave was biphasic for all models except #4, #6, and #8 for which no significant initial positive phase was present.

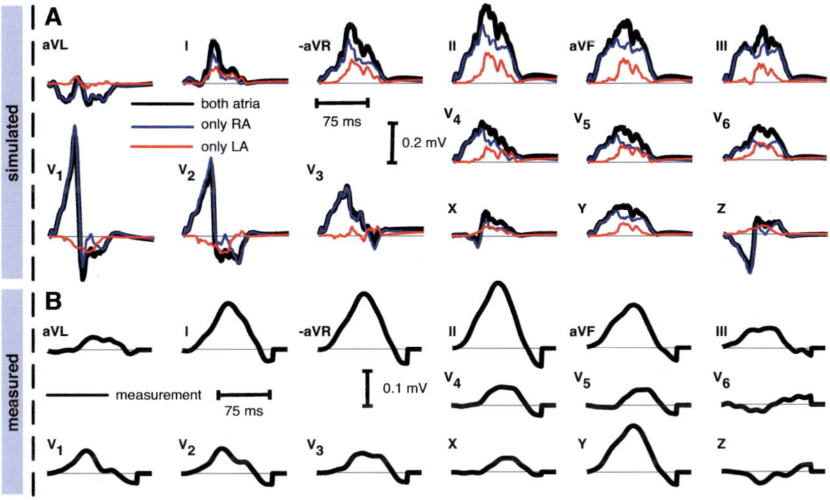

Figure 9.2: ECGs obtained through simulation using model #5 (A) and measurement in subject #5 (B). The iso-potential line is indicated by a thin grey line. In (A), the blue traces correspond to the right atrial P-wave whereas the the red ones stem from sources in the LA. LA and RA P-waves add up to the regular P-wave represented by the black traces.

As an example, the simulated 12-lead ECG and VCG signals are shown for model #5 in Figure 9.2A. No filters were applied to the simulated signals. Common filters used in clinical ECG systems did not affect the simulated P-wave morphology significantly, though (data not shown). Comparing the simulated with the measured signal (see Figure 9.2B) shows fair correspondence. It has to be kept in mind that the computational model was only personalized in terms of anatomy and not in terms of electrophysiological properties. Despite gross correspondence, the polarity in lead aVL is different as well as the morphology in VCG lead X, which was biphasic in the simulation but not in the measurement. The high amplitude of the positive phase in lead V_1 is caused by the depolarization of the RAA, which is oriented almost perpendicular to the sternum, thus in line with V_1, and close to the chest (Figure 9.3). Hence, the activation of the RAA caused a high positive signal amplitude in V_1 with a sharp drop once the RAA was fully activated.

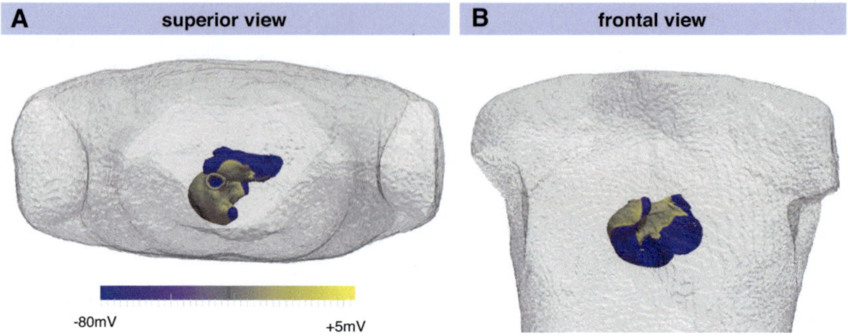

Figure 9.3: Superior (A) and frontal (B) view of the V_m distribution of the atria embedded in the semi-transparent torso of model #5 at 43 ms after the initial stimulus corresponding to the time of the maximum signal downslope at the transition from the positive to the negative phase in lead V_1 in Figure 9.2A. The RAA is aligned with the axis from V_1 to Wilson's central terminal and close to the chest as can be seen in the superior view (A). Thus, the activation of the RAA causes the high positive signal amplitude in V_1 with a sharp drop once the RAA is fully activated.

The separate contributions of the LA and the RA can be seen in Figure 9.2A, e.g., and are summarized for the whole cohort of models using the P-wave area in lead II in Figure 9.4. The median contribution of the RA to the P-wave integral was 79% and thus much larger than that of the LA (24%). The RA and LA values do not add up to 100% due to the non-linearity of the median operator. Looking at the different temporal phases of the P-wave separately reveals that the first third was dominated by RA sources in all models. The LA contributed with only 6% to the P-wave integral of that phase. For the second and last temporal third, the LA share was 30% and 34%, respectively. Considering the different ECG and VCG leads separately (Figure 9.5) reveals that the RA P-wave was strongest projected onto Einthoven lead II, while the LA P-wave was most pronounced in Wilson lead V_2. The RA P-wave dominated strongest in lead III with the median RA/LA P-wave area ratio being 3.3. The relative share of the LA was biggest in lead I in which the signal was however still dominated by the RA with a median factor of 1.1.

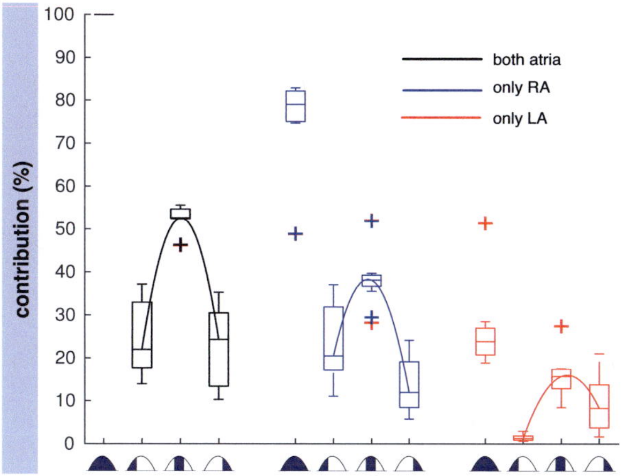

Figure 9.4: Contribution to the entire P-wave area in lead II separated by the two atria and three temporal phases. The regular P-wave (black) is composed of sources in the RA (blue) and LA (red). The entire P-wave duration (left column in each group) is composed of three temporal thirds (columns 2, 3, 4 in each group). Cubic splines were used to interpolate the time course of the median values during the three temporal thirds. Box plots represent n=8 models; values were normalized for each model.

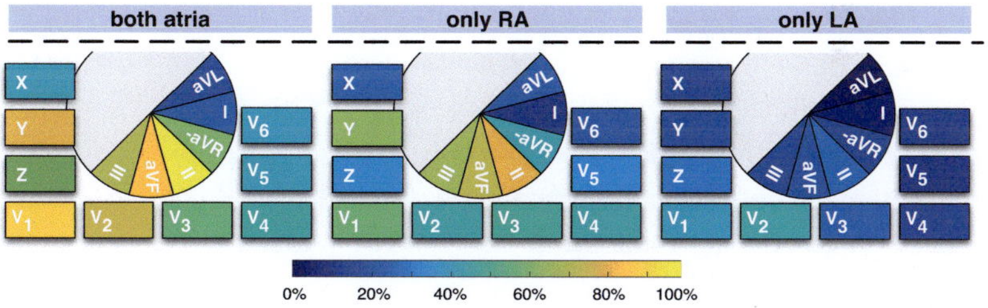

Figure 9.5: Projection intensity of the combined and separated simulated P-waves onto the different ECG and VCG leads. The color encodes the median (n=8) integral of absolute values (P-wave area), which were normalized to the maximum lead in the regular P-wave for each model (V_1 for #5, II for all other models). Values for the LA and the RA add up to the value for both atria.

9.3 Discussion

In this study, a cohort of eight anatomically personalized models comprising both atria and the subject's torsos was used to gain insight into the genesis of the P-wave with a particular focus on the distinct contributions of the two atria. The *in silico* approach employed gave the unique opportunity to separate the P-waves stemming from the RA and the LA, which is not possible *in vivo*.
The LA share of the P-wave integral of absolute values (P-wave area) was between 19% and 51% with a median value of 24% in this study. These results are in line with a recent study using a dipole-current source approach [495] published after the results of the study presented here were submitted as a conference contribution [497]. The signal originating from the LA was small and the P-wave was mostly dominated by the RA even during late phases of the P-wave (cf. Figure 9.4), which is in line with the very sparse experimental data [502]. The fact that LA sources do interfere with RA sources during the whole P-wave and that the P-wave is mostly dominated by RA sources explains some of the difficulties experienced in P-wave-based LA assessment [479, 503–508]. This is reflected in current guidelines [479] by the recommendation to only diagnose a left atrial abnormality (LAAb) and restrain from diagnosing a specific abnormality.
The P-waves obtained using the computational models and their derived indices were within the clinically observed ranges [509, 510]. Comparison of the simulated with the measured P-waves showed gross correspondence, particularly when considering that the impact of differences beyond anatomical variability of the atria and the torso variability was not included in the models. In particular, electrophysiological variability in terms of intrinsic inter-individual variability, disease related remodeling, as well as variability of conduction velocity and its anisotropy were not accounted for. The modeling approach focussing on the influence of gross anatomical variability did not reproduce the considerably longer measured PWD for the AF subject #8 because the potentially AF-remodeled substrate was not considered in the simulation. On the other hand, the chosen approach allowed to focus on the variability in the P-wave and related markers solely induced by anatomical differences in a controlled environment without additional influencing factor. Therefore, the fact that subject #8 had the largest LA did translate to the longest simulated

PWD in the model cohort. The remaining seven subjects had structurally healthy atria.
Lemery et al. performed a simultaneous mapping and ECG study in 35 patients with a history of symptomatic AF [502]. Earliest LA activation was conducted via BB at 31 ± 13 ms after earliest activation of the RA in 31 of the 35 patients and via non-specified IACs in the four remaining patients. These results are in line with the simulation results for common sites of earliest activation (cf. EAS3 to EAS5 in Section 10.1). The tendency towards later activation in the measurement can be explained by potential AF-induced conduction slowing in the study population. While Lemery et al. did annotate a standard P-wave with activation times of anatomical structures in the RA and the LA, they could not distinguish the contributions of simultaneously activated regions and thus not establish a clear separation of RA and LA sources.
After the results of this study were published in a conference paper, Ferrer et al. conducted a finite element modeling study using a detailed atrial and thorax model [496]. Their results show gross correspondence to the results presented here, particularly regarding lead V_1, which plays an important role in the next chapter. In Einthoven lead II, their left and right atrial P-waves are somewhat more distinct in the time domain, which might be explained by their choice of IACs. Only the CS connection and BB were included and BB touched on the LA more distant to the septum than in our model. The contribution to the P-wave was further differentiated by separating 21 distinct regions. The main contributors in the RA were the RAA, the lateral wall and the right atrial septum. In the LA, the LAA and the posterior wall contributed to the largest extent.
In the study presented in this Chapter, the Courtemanche et al. cell model [47] was chosen for the computation of ion kinetics because of its suitability proven in a benchmark [156]. The heterogeneous variants of the Courtemanche et al. model caused regional differences (heterogeneity) in the action potential (AP) plateau and early repolarization. These were reflected in ECG signals deviations from zero after the end of the P-wave in the PQ-segment particularly in the precordial leads. This phenomenon was described before both for clinical measurements [511] and in computer simulations [512, 513].

9.3.1 Limitations

The size of the virtual cohort of n=8 models is small compared to most *in vivo* studies. However, a model population carries a significant advantage over using a single model result: the effect of characteristics specific to a single subject can be minimized by assessing a distribution of results. The results for models #2 and #8 that deviate from the other six models highlight that the evaluation of a single model may be misleading. As a lot of modeling studies base their conclusions on a single anatomical model [484, 486–488, 490–494, 514] or two models [515], the virtual cohort of eight models is an important step forward and larger than most *in silico* cohort with only few exceptions for ventricular studies (e.g. [516, 517]) and even fewer for applications in the atria [23, 438, 440, 518]. Considering that only anatomical variability of the subjects used to build the models was considered in this study gives confidence that the study cohort covers a good share of the general population's variability. The P-wave amplitude in the simulations was larger than in the measured signals, particularly in leads V_1 and V_2 in model #5. This effect might be due to an overestimation of the extent of fast-conducting bundles in the RA, which were introduced by the rule-based algorithm outlined in Chapter 7. Another possible source of error is the assumed homogeneous wall thickness that might lead to an over- or underestimation of RA myocardial mass, particularly in the RAA causing the high positive amplitude in leads V_1 and V_2. In addition, the intracellular and extracellular conductivities carry uncertainty [177, 519]. Moreover, subject #5 had the largest RA in the cohort in terms of myocardial wall volume. Thus, the results regarding the relative contribution of the LA and the RA should not be compromised by the variability in P-wave amplitude that can be attributed to variability in myocardial volume and the proximity of the atria to the precordial wall.

9.3.2 Conclusion

While markers based on the P-wave in the ECG carry the great advantage of being routinely acquired due to the non-invasiveness and the low associated costs, the findings of this study highlight important limitations. The results obtained in the cohort of eight *in silico* models suggest that the contribution of the LA to the P-wave is less than one third. Also a temporal discrimination was not possible to the extent described in some textbooks which attribute the last temporal third of the P-wave almost exclusively to the LA [510]. LA activation was reflected in the middle third of the P-wave to the greatest extent rather than the terminal third. The domination of the P-wave by sources from the RA helps to understand the difficulties experienced in P-wave-based assessment of the LA [479, 520]. In conclusion, this study fosters our understanding of P-wave genesis and the spatio-temporal projection of atrial activation on the body surface potentials.

CHAPTER 10

Effect of Earliest Activated Site and Interatrial Connections

P-wave morphology in the body surface electrocardiogram (ECG) has been shown to correlate with the risk to develop atrial fibrillation (AF) empirically [39, 72, 521]. In particular, P-wave terminal force in lead V_1 (PTF-V_1) has been suggested as a surrogate marker [475, 522]. A possible mechanism linking elevated PTF-V_1 and the higher AF risk is left atrial enlargement (LAE). However, this link could not be established mechanistically and, most importantly, the sensitivity and specificity of the marker is unsatisfying [505]. Therefore, an additional contributor is analyzed in this study by testing the hypothesis that the location of the excitation origin (the earliest activated site (EAS) in the right atrium (RA)) and its relative proximity to conducting interatrial connections (IACs) influences PTF-V_1 to a significant extent.

The EAS corresponds to the location where the atrial myocardium captures the stimulus generated by the sinus node (SN). The EAS is known to express significant variability both between individuals and over time within an individual [39] influenced by e.g. the degree of vagal stimulation. The IACs vary as well tremendously in terms of their presence, location, and conductive properties [32].

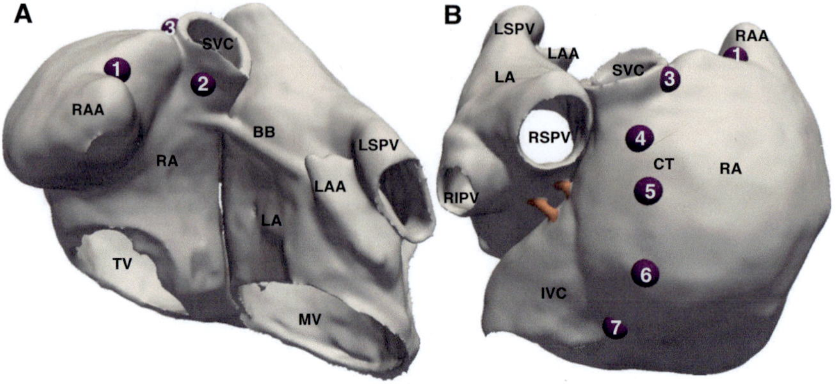

Figure 10.1: Position of the earliest activated sites EAS1 to EAS7 in the RA exemplary visualized on bi-atrial model #5. Anterior view in (A), posterior view in (B). Besides the EAS, RAA, LAA, TV, MV, SVC, IVC, left (L) and right (R), superior (S) and inferior (I) pulmonary veins (PV), CT and BB are indicated for orientation.

In this study, the influence of the EAS and the presence / intactness of the posterior IACs on PTF-V_1 is analyzed using the virtual cohort of anatomically individualized computational models introduced in the previous chapter. Nguyên et al. recently investigated the effect of the position and orientation of the ventricles on ECG morphology using computational models of two subjects [515]. While the genesis of the P-wave and the effect of different influencing factors have been studied *in silico* before as described in Chapter 9, the effect of a shift of the EAS and its relation to the conductive properties of the IACs has not been studied before.
Parts of this work are currently under review as a journal paper [498] and a conference contribution [499].

10.1 Methods

This study was conducted using the set of eight anatomical models introduced in Chapter 9. Excitation propagation was triggered from different positions on the epicardial surface around the SN region along the CT to study the effect of a shift of the EAS caused by e.g. effects mediated by the autonomic nervous system [39]. EASs ordered from anterior/superior positions to more

posterior/inferior positions were defined as follows (see Figure 10.1): EAS1 was located midway between the tip of the RAA and its junction with the SVC, EAS2 at the superior part of the anterior wall, and EAS3 at the junction of the RAA and the SVC. EAS4 to EAS7 were uniformly distributed along the CT between EAS3 and the junction of the IVC and the RA (EAS7).
The standard setup comprised four IACs (BB, coronary sinus (CS), middle posterior connection (MPC), and lower posterior connection (LPC)). Because the two posterior connections (MPC and LPC) are known to be fragile [32], they were modeled non-conductive in a second set of simulations (see Figure 10.1B).
The P-waves obtained through monodomain simulations and subsequent forward calculation of the ECG as described in Chapter 9 were analyzed on the body surface potential map (BSPM) and the ECG level. Two variants of P-wave terminal force in lead V_1 were employed: the classical definition by the product of the duration and the amplitude of the negative P-wave as proposed by Morris et al. [475] (referred to as PTF) and the integral of the negative P-wave (referred to as $PTF_{integral}$). $PTF_{integral}$ was calculated as the sum of signed values of the respective part of the P-wave multiplied with the time between samples. Beginning and end of the P-wave as well as its negative part were annotated manually.

10.2 Results

10.2.1 ECG Morphology Analysis

The general properties of the simulated P-waves considering all four IACs and EAS3 corresponding to the site where the SN is modeled most often were already presented and discussed in Chapter 9 (see particularly Table 9.3 and Figure 9.2).

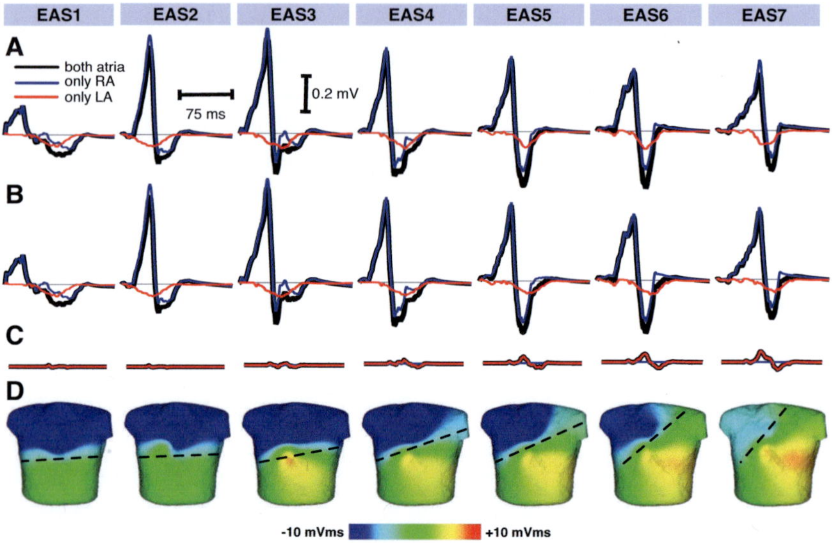

Figure 10.2: P-waves in ECG lead V_1 (A-B) and body surface potential integral maps (D) in model #5 for varying earliest activates sites EAS1 to EAS7 in the RA. The left (red) and blue (right) atrial P-waves add up to the regular P-wave represented by the black traces. The iso-potential line is indicated by a thin grey line. Four IACs were present in (A), whereas the two posterior connections (MPC and LPC) were non-conductive in (B). The difference of ECGs caused by the non-conductive posterior IACs shown in (C) reveals that only the LA P-wave is affected and a more pronounced effect for more inferior EASs. The dashed line in (D) indicates the perceived iso-potential line, which rotates counter-clockwise from EAS1 to EAS7.

The influence of a shift of the EAS on the ECG signal in Wilson lead V_1 is shown in Figure 10.2A for model #5. Looking at the regular P-wave stemming from both atria, the amplitude of the first (positive) phase increased monotonically from EAS1 to EAS3 and declined monotonically from EAS3 to EAS7. The driver of this effect was the RA which contributed almost exclusively to that phase. The P-wave integral BSPM (see Figure 10.2D for model #5) revealed a counter-clockwise rotation of the iso-potential line for EAS2 to EAS7.

Table 10.1: Interatrial connections conducting LA breakthrough for simulations with varying earliest activated sites EAS1 to EAS7 in the RA. For the IACs via which breakthrough occurred, the time is given.

Model	#1 (ms)	#2 (ms)	#3 (ms)	#4 (ms)	#5 (ms)	#6 (ms)	#7 (ms)	#8 (ms)
EAS1	BB: 29 MPC: 46	BB: 31 MPC: 42	BB: 34 MPC: 46	BB: 31 MPC: 43	BB: 33 MPC: 56	BB: 28 MPC: 46	BB: 27 MPC: 62	BB: 25
EAS2	BB: 9 MPC: 25	BB: 11 MPC: 23	BB: 13 MPC: 26	BB: 8 MPC: 22	BB: 7 MPC: 31	BB: 8	BB: 13 MPC: 48	BB: 8 MPC: 30
EAS3	BB: 18 MPC: 32	BB: 19 MPC: 31	BB: 20 MPC: 32	BB: 22 MPC: 28	BB: 19 MPC: 35	BB: 18 MPC: 26	BB: 26 MPC: 42	BB: 16
EAS4	BB: 26 MPC: 35	BB: 25 MPC: 33	MPC: 28 BB: 29	MPC: 27 BB: 30 CS: 65	BB: 27 MPC: 35	MPC: 28 BB: 29	BB: 31 MPC: 44	BB: 21 MPC: 42
EAS5	BB: 35 MPC: 40	BB: 31 MPC: 33	MPC: 28 BB: 36 CS: 75	MPC: 30 BB: 36 CS: 63	BB: 34 MPC: 36 CS: 69	MPC: 32 BB: 38 CS: 81	BB: 39 MPC: 44	BB: 27 MPC: 41 CS: 56
EAS6	MPC: 41 BB: 45 CS: 71	MPC: 35 BB: 37	MPC: 30 BB: 43 CS: 71	MPC: 33 BB: 44 CS: 55	MPC: 36 BB: 41 CS: 62	MPC: 35 BB: 45 CS: 74	MPC: 40 BB: 48 CS: 96	BB: 34 MPC: 39 CS: 50
EAS7	LPC: 45 BB: 57 CS: 59	MPC: 38 BB: 42	MPC: 35 BB: 53 CS: 60	LPC: 37 BB: 52 CS: 47	MPC: 33 BB: 48 CS: 55	LPC: 36 BB: 57 CS: 61	MPC: 37 BB: 60 CS: 84	MPC: 33 BB: 39 CS: 45

10.2.2 Left Atrial Breakthrough

Earliest LA breakthrough was conducted via BB in most cases as can be seen in Figure 10.3A and detailed in Table 10.1. Later, secondary breakthrough via posterior IACs or the CS occurred in most cases. The more the stimulus site was shifted from EAS3 towards EAS7 (inferior), the more often the posterior IACs were the path via which earliest LA breakthrough was conducted. Breakthrough via the CS was also observed more frequent and more early for more inferior EASs: no CS breakthrough for EAS1 to EAS3 vs. CS breakthrough in seven out of eight models for EAS7. Regarding EAS more inferior than EAS3 (EAS4 to EAS7), earliest breakthrough was conducted via a posterior IAC in three to seven out of eight models. For EAS7, earliest breakthrough occurred via the LPC in three models and the MPC in the remaining five models. In model #8 with the largest atrial volume, earliest breakthrough occurred via a connection other than BB only for EAS7. The anatomical properties of model #2 impeded CS breakthrough for all EASs.

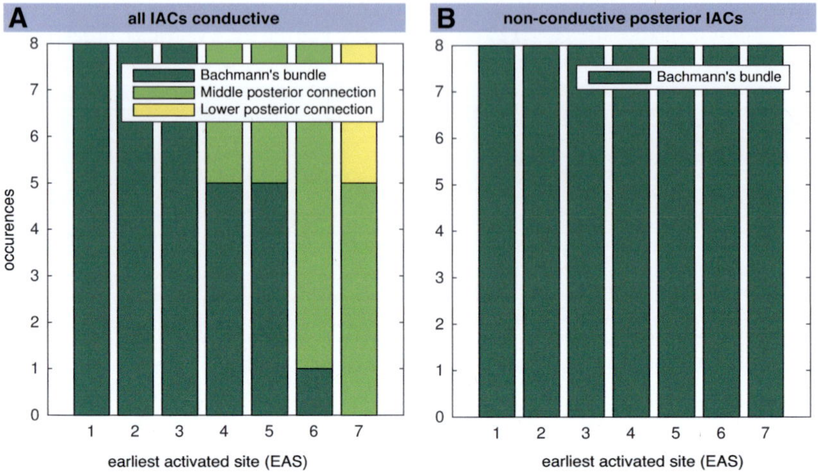

Figure 10.3: Distribution of the IAC conducting the earliest LA breakthrough for varying earliest activated sites EAS1 to EAS7 in the RA in the model population (n=8). In (A), four IACs were present, whereas the two posterior IACs (MPC and LPC) were non-conductive in (B).

10.2.3 P-Terminal Force in Lead V_1

Two variants of P-wave terminal force in lead V_1 were evaluated: the classical definition using the product of the duration and the amplitude of the negative P-wave phase (PTF-V_1, Figure 10.4A) and the integral of that phase ($PTF_{integral}$-V_1, Figure 10.4B). The highest absolute values for both measures were observed for EAS1 on the superior part of the anterior RA caused by a short initial positive P-wave deflection followed by a longer negative phase (see e.g. Figure 10.2A). Median PTF-V_1 was –20.0 mVms for EAS1; median $PTF_{integral}$-V_1 was –9.4 mVms. The EASs on the posterior wall of the RA (EAS2 to EAS7) yielded a U-shaped PTF-V_1 curve with median absolute values increasing from the center of the RAA (EAS2: –8.3 mVms) via the junction of the SVC and the RAA (EAS3: –14.0 mVms) down the CT (EAS4: –15.6 mVms, EAS5: –16.1 mVms). For more inferior EAS, PTF decreased again in terms of absolute values (EAS6: –13.0 mVms) up to –8.7 mVms for EAS7 located at the junction between the IVC and the RA.

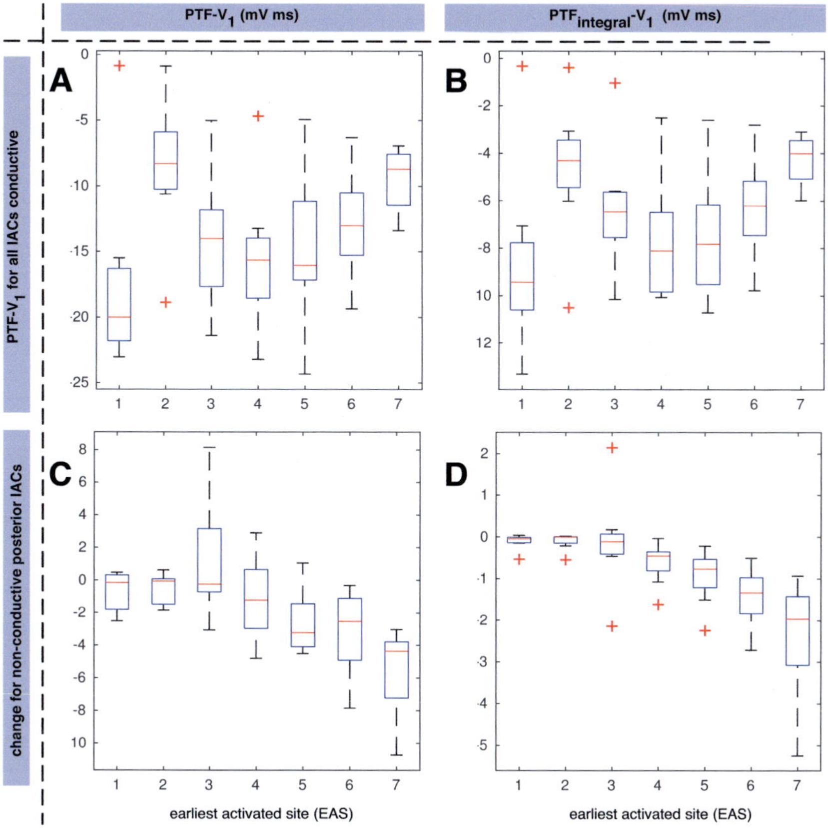

Figure 10.4: P-wave terminal force (PTF-V_1, (A+C)) and P-wave integral terminal force (PTF$_{integral}$-V_1, (B+D)) for varying earliest activated sites EAS1 to EAS7 in the RA. In (A+B), four IACs were present, (C+D) show the difference when the two posterior connections were non-conductive. Note the different scales of the panels.

Looking at the integral instead of the product of the duration and the maximum amplitude yielded a qualitatively similar curve. The absolute values were smaller by an average factor of 2.1 as expected for approximately sinusoidal negative P-wave terminals. However, the intermodel variability was significantly smaller for PTF$_{integral}$ than for PTF. All outliers and most of the whiskers in the box plots in Figure 10.4A+B were caused by models #2 and

#8. Model #2 was the smallest in terms of RA and LA blood volume and showed an almost linear decrease of PTF-V_1 from –0.9 mVms for EAS1 to –7.4 mVms for EAS7. Model #8 (being the largest model in the cohort) on the other hand showed the reverse behavior with a decrease in terms of absolute values from –22.0 mVms for EAS1 to –8.5 mVms for EAS7.

10.2.4 Influence of Posterior Interatrial Connections

The posterior IACs were modeled as non-conductive in a second set of simulations. This was reflected in the fact that earliest LA breakthrough was always conducted via BB (see Figure 10.3B). BB and CS breakthrough times given in Table 10.1 were unaffected by non-conductive posterior IACs, breakthrough via the posterior IACs did not occur as a matter of course.
The part of the P-wave originating from sources in the LA was affected by the absence of the posterior IACs for EAS3 to EAS7 (see Figure 10.2B+C). While the morphology regarding the polarity and the number of phases was not affected, the amplitude was altered. Taking into consideration the comparatively small contribution of the LA to the overall P-wave shown in Chapter 9, the effect on PTF-V_1 (Figure 10.4C) and $PTF_{integral}$-V_1 (Figure 10.4D) is remarkable. Non-conductive posterior IACs caused higher absolute PTF-V_1 on average with an increasing effect amplitude from EAS1 to EAS7. When evaluating $PTF_{integral}$-V_1, the interindividual spread was significantly lower yielding a very consistent relation (Figure 10.4D).

10.3 Discussion

The study presented in this chapter investigates the effect of a variation of the EAS in the RA on body surface potentials, particularly on the ECG-derived marker PTF in Wilson lead V_1. While this marker is commonly used to quantify left atrial abnormalities (LAAbs) [521], the present study tested the hypothesis that the marker is also affected by contributors in the RA. In particular, significant variability in the origin of sinus excitation exists both on the interindividual and the intraindividual level.

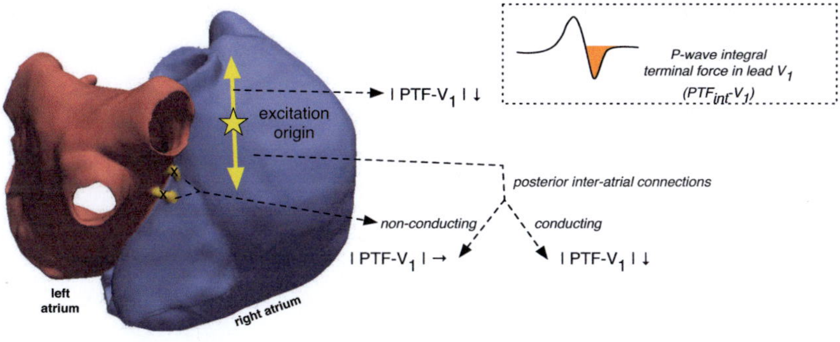

Figure 10.5: In conclusion, the results presented in this chapter show that a shift of the EAS towards both more superior/anterior and more inferior locations causes lower absolute values of PTF-V_1. If the posterior IACs are non-conductive, a shift towards more inferior locations does not affect PTF-V_1 significantly.

In dogs, it has been shown that the EAS is shifted towards inferior regions of the SN complex under vagal stimulation. On the other hand, an acceleration of the heart rate causes a shift towards more superior/anterior regions [39, 523, 524]. In humans, common EAS are found between the mid-septal region and the junction of the SVC with the RAA [42]. The set of EAS in this study was extended to also cover a more inferior position (EAS7) which may correspond to EAS under pronounced vagal stimulation (very low heart rates), an anterior position (EAS2), and a position in the center of the RAA roof (EAS1) corresponding to the common electrode location used for permanent atrial pacing.

The presented results show that the precise location of the EAS in the RA affects PTF-V_1 significantly. This P-wave marker exhibited a U-shaped course for EASs from anterior/superior positions to posterior/inferior positions (EAS2 to EAS7). This progression indicates a reduced leftwards-pointing component (opposite to the vector pointing from Wilson's central terminal to V_1) for both very anterior/superior and posterior/inferior excitation origins and the strongest leftwards-oriented component for intermediate positions (EAS4 to EAS5). EAS1 in the center of the RAA roof did not fit in this scheme. EAS1 yielded the highest PTF-V_1 values, which can be explained by the preferred excitation direction pointing towards the LA, thus away from V_1 with respect to Wilson's central terminal, evolving after the short time when the RAA tip is excited. Less RAA tissue behind the EAS towards the RAA tip could contribute to a rightwards-oriented vector for EAS1 compared to the other EAS. PTF-V_1 turned out to be very sensitive to rather small changes in the location of excitation origin (or rather excitation capture) reflected by the fact that EASs in close vicinity to each other yielded markedly different PTF-V_1 (e.g. an average factor of 2.0 between EAS2 and EAS4).

The mostly negative P-waves in leads V_1 and V_2 observed for EAS1 are in line with the clinically observed P-waves in patients with atrial pacing electrodes in this region. The finding that shifting the excitation origin from EAS4/EAS5 towards more anterior/superior positions decreases absolute PTF-V_1 values is in line with the findings by Yokota et al.: PTF-V_1 (referred to as the maximal LA component in their work) decreased during exercise in healthy subjects [525]. However, an earlier study in men with seemingly healthy hearts found that the probability of abnormally high PTF-V_1 values increases after exercise [507]. These equivocal findings can possibly be explained by the experimental protocol. In [507], the ECGs were acquired 5 min after rather than during exercise, which may have caused an overcompensation resulting in vagal stimulation. Vagal stimulation in turn corresponds to higher absolute PTF values in [525] and the study presented here. The results on the BSPM level are in fair agreement with an *in vivo* study [185]. For pacing in positions close to EAS2 to EAS6, they also report a counter-clockwise rotation of the iso-potential line as shown in Figure 10.2D.

The *in silico* approach employed in this study allowed to asses how the intactness of the posterior IACs influence the ECG, which is not feasible *in vivo*. While gross ECG morphology was unaltered by rendering the posterior IACs non-conductive, PTF-V_1 absolute values were increased. Non-conductive posterior IACs translated to a very consistent effect when evaluating the integral of the negative phase in lead V_1 (Figure 10.4D) instead of the product of amplitude and duration (Figure 10.4C). The effect was most pronounced for posterior/inferior EASs, which can be explained by the LA breakthrough sites. A larger share of earliest LA breakthrough conducted via one of the posterior IACs in the model cohort (Figure 10.3A) correlated with a higher difference in PTF between simulations with conductive and non-conductive IACs (Figure 10.4C+D). When the LA could not be activated via the posterior IACs due to their non-conductance, PTF remained stable for EAS4 to EAS7.

Thus, the recruitment of the posterior IACs explains the decrease in absolute PTF-V_1 values for the most inferior excitation origins (EAS6 and EAS7). The significant interindividual variability in both PTF markers for EAS4 and EAS5 can be explained by the variability in the crucial IAC conducting earliest LA breakthrough (BB vs. posterior IACs), which was also largest for these EAS. Earliest LA breakthrough was never conducted via the CS connections. Indeed, no LA breakthrough was conducted via this IAC for EAS more superior than EAS5. While this indicates a subordinate role of the CS IAC during sinus rhythm, it may play a more important role during less organized excitation patterns characterizing atrial arrhythmias and maintain biatrial reentry.
Regarding the two variants of PTF, $\text{PTF}_{integral}$-V_1 was the more conclusive marker showing more consistent trends (Figure 10.5). The reason for this can be found in the fact that PTF-V_1 on the other hand is only determined by the maximum value in terms of amplitude. This maximum value can be determined by the activation of only a small share of the atrial myocardium neglecting all the rest. The integral value contrariwise covers the activation of all tissue during the negative phase of the P-wave instead of being based on the amplitude of just one time instant. This makes the integral marker also less prone to noise artifacts for normally distributed noise. Therefore, it is less prone to artifacts and future studies should consider to evaluate this more robust and conclusive integral marker.
In Chapter 9, it was shown that the P-wave is mostly dominated by sources originating in the RA and the LA contributes to the integral with a median value of only 24%. Also during late phases of the P-wave, the LA signals interfere with those stemming from the RA and do not dominate the P-wave signal. These findings explain the limited, however consistent, effects of conduction failure of the posterior IACs on the ECG.

10.3.1 Limitations

The limitations discussed in the previous chapter (Section 9.3.1) regarding the size of the model cohort and P-wave amplitudes also apply to the study presented in the current chapter. Moreover, we modeled four IACs and focussed on the effect of the intactness of the posterior IACs. While additional IACs might be present (particularly on the anterior side) their vicinity to BB makes

it unlikely to alter the activation pattern dramatically [33]. IACs other than the MPC and LPC might become dysfunctional as well, e.g. BB [35, 526, 527]. However, the posterior IACs are most vulnerable to conduction block due to their thin and fragile nature [35]. Thus, the focus was on these IACs in this study leaving the influence of the others for future work.
Futhermore, the rule-based annotation of myocyte orientation may introduce a bias.

10.3.2 Conclusion

The advantage of the P-wave as a tool to assess electrical function is the ease of acquisition. Recently, it re-raised excitement as an accessible surrogate of atrial activation [476] and proved to be valuable for AF prediction [478, 528–530]. Regarding the LA, the P-wave is most commonly used to assess LAAb (particularly LAE) based on PTF. While some studies showed good correlation between P-wave markers and LA size [480, 482], others showed poor correlation [504, 506, 508].
The study presented in this chapter confirms the hypothesis that P-wave morphology, and in particular PTF, is affected by a shift of the EAS and its relative proximity to intact IACs. As both the excitation origin and the IACs express significant intraindividual and interindividual variability in terms of presence, location and conductive properties, their effect can explain the limits of PTF-based assessment of LA anatomy: differences in PTF-V_1 are not of purely anatomical origin but also an electrical phenomenon.
The presented results highlight the need to be aware of the limits regarding our current understanding of further factors influencing the P-wave, its morphology, and related markers. Only by pushing and overcoming these limits by integrating the P-wave into extended research aiming at a mechanistic understanding of arrhythmogenesis, healthcare practitioners will eventually be put in a position to fully leverage the potential of the P-wave in terms of AF prevention.

CHAPTER 11

Influence of Left Atrial Anatomical Properties

The previous chapter introduced the general idea of ECG-based assessment of left atrial anatomy. Biomarkers based on the P-wave carry the advantage of being easy to acquire. This fact and the empirical observation that e.g. abnormal P-wave terminal force (PTF) in Wilson lead V_1 is associated with a higher risk to develop atrial fibrillation (AF) renders the P-wave particularly interesting. A common explanation for both the higher AF risk and increased PTF-V_1 is left atrial enlargement (LAE). On the one hand, a larger atrium provides a larger substrate that can sustain and accommodate reentry with longer wavelengths, thus rendering it more vulnerable to AF. On the other hand, the increase in left-myocardial volume causes a more pronounced leftwards-pointing excitation vector once left atrium (LA) breakthrough occurred. However, when actually comparing PTF-V_1 with LA size, the correlation is rather poor with one possible explanation being the influence of the earliest activated site (EAS) in the right atrium (RA) and conductive properties of the posterior interatrial connections (IACs) as presented in Chapter 10. Besides, P-wave abnormalities can be caused by e.g. atrial hypertension, atrial hypertrophy, atrial overload, atrial strain, partial or complete interatrial conduction block, intraatrial conduction slowing, as well as impaired ventricular distensibility [479]. Therefore, current guidelines advise to use the term left atrial abnormality (LAAb) rather than committing to a specific cause when basing the diagnosis solely on the

P-wave [479, 531]. In earlier times, also the terms *P-mitrale*, *P-congenitale*, and *P-pulmonale* were used to refer to abnormal P-waves [479].
Several empirical studies investigated correlates of LAE and P-wave abnormalities. Besides being a predictor for AF [532–535] and consequently stroke [536], LAE indicates left ventricular dysfunction in general [537] and is a predictor for congestive heart failure [532], cardiac mortality [536, 538], and combined cardiovascular events [539–541]. Therefore, it is desirable to assess LA size non-invasively based on P-wave markers as part of routine examinations.
Historically, the ratio of the P-wave duration (PWD) and the length of the P-R-segment was the first ECG marker to estimate LA size [542]. However, it showed to correlate poorly with LA size in more recent studies for common threshold values of 1.6 [481, 543, 544]. PTF-V_1 was soon used more frequently after it was defined as the product of the amplitude and the duration of the negative phase of the P-wave in Wilson lead V_1 in 1964 by Morris et al. [475]. They established an association between abnormal PTF-V_1 and (mitral or aortic) valve disease, which in turn is associated with LAE. PTF-V_1 absolute values of 4 mVms or more are considered abnormal [481, 482, 506, 543–546]. Other markers are the P-wave area in lead II approximated as the product of the duration and the amplitude multiplied by 0.5 [505, 543, 547], P-wave axis $<30°$, or the positive PTF in lead aVL [531]. Another common marker is the PWD [546], usually measured in Einthoven lead II, which is considered prolonged for values >105 ms [481], >110 ms [506, 531, 543–545], or (more recently) >120 ms [479, 528]. PWD, however, is also used to quantify conduction delay [480, 548]. While a notched P-wave is intuitively caused by interatrial conduction delay [479], it has also been suggested and used as a marker for LAE quantification with a threshold of 40 ms for the duration of the notch in lead II [479, 506, 544, 545].
This multitude of ECG markers used to assess LA size has proven to be suboptimal in a number of studies prohibiting their use to diagnose LAE as a specific LAAb [479, 508, 531]. Truong et al. evaluated the correlation of P-wave markers with LA volume determined through cardiac computed tomography [505]. Sensitivity, specificity, positive and negative predictive values, and accuracy are given in Table 11.1.

Table 11.1: Statistic evaluation of P-wave markers for LAE with respect to LA size determined by computed tomography. Abbreviations: positive predictive value (PPV), negative predictive value (NPV), P-wave duration (PWD), P-R-segment duration (PRd), P-wave area (PWA). Data from [505].

	sensitivity	specificity	PPV	NPV	accuracy
PWD > 110 ms	71%	55%	61%	66%	63%
PWD/PRd > 1.6	81%	27%	53%	59%	54%
PWA in II > 4 mVms	73%	19%	47%	41%	46%
PTF-V_1 > 4 mVms	49%	54%	51%	51%	51%
notched P-wave in II	19%	85%	57%	51%	53%
biphasic P-wave in V_1	26%	76%	52%	51%	51%

The best overall accuracy of 63% was obtained by PWD > 110 ms. Other studies, partly based on echocardiography as a reference measure, reported equivocal results regarding sensitivity and specificity [506, 543].

The reasons for the rather poor performance of the presented ensemble of P-wave markers and a mechanistic link between anatomical properties and features of the P-wave are not understood, to date. A controlled *in vivo* study is hard to design because LA size cannot be adjusted in a single patient. Therefore, this study investigates the effect of LA hypertrophy on the P-wave in the body surface ECG *in silico*. The computational approach being applied allows to dissect the effect of LA wall thickening in a controlled environment: different degrees of hypertrophy can be simulated in the same subject's model. Moreover, a method to analyze the effect of LA dilation *in silico* is presented as a tool to analyze a second potential anatomical cause for LAAb.

Parts of this work are based on a supervised student's project [549] and is currently under review for conference publication [550, 551].

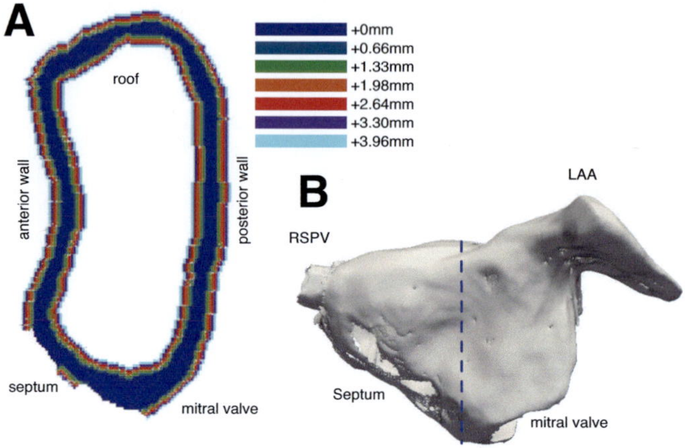

Figure 11.1: Cross section through the LA wall of model #3 with different levels of wall thickening coded by the color (A). The cross section is aligned along the dashed blue line in (B).

11.1 Methods

11.1.1 Left Atrial Hypertrophy

The LA wall was thickened in four anatomical models to investigate the effect of LA hypertrophy. The models #2 to #5 introduced in Section 9.1.1 were used for this purpose. The voxel-based bi-atrial models covering the two atria, the trunks of the great vessels, and the blood within the atria had an isotropic resolution of 0.33 mm. The additional wall thickness due to hypertrophy was modeled equally and homogeneously on the endocardial and the epicardial side in steps of one voxel. Therefore, wall thickness was increased up to the initial value plus 3.96 mm in steps of 0.66 mm yielding seven different models variants (Figure 11.1). The dilation of one voxel layer was implemented such that voxels adjacent to LA voxels that were not RA voxels were marked as LA voxels. Reapplying this operation added one more voxel layer and so forth. By posing an additional adjacency constraint that requires or prohibits neighborhood to LA blood, the method can also be used to model purely endocardial or purely epicardial hypertrophy, respectively.

Myocyte orientation in the atria and distinct tissue classes were annotated in the dilated models using the approach presented in Chapter 7.
Numerical field calculation in the torso was conducted on tetrahedral meshes as introduced in Section 3.4. These meshes were built from the segmented imaging data that were provided in a voxel-based format. As the torso model was of lower resolution than the 0.33 mm-resolved atria, the bi-atrial models including the hypertrophic LA wall and augmented inter-atrial connections were transferred to the torso model by nearest neighbor interpolation. During this mapping step, it was ensured that the two atria are separated and share no nodes except from the IACs. Then, a tetrahedral torso mesh was generated for each model and each degree of hypertrophy using the *CGAL* library [500]. The myocyte orientation was included in the torso mesh, as well. Excitation propagation was simulated using *acCELLerate* as described in Section 9.1.2 followed by a forward calculation of the body surface potentials.

11.1.2 Left Atrial Dilation

LA dilation was induced by LA pressure overload in the anatomical model #3 using the cardiac continuum mechanics simulation environment *CardioMechanics* [15, 552]. *CardioMechanics* requires a tetrahedral atrial mesh with a significantly lower resolution than used for the electrophysiology simulations. Therefore, the atrial surfaces were extracted from the voxel model and smoothed using the *VTK* library [409]. After the resolution of the surface meshes was adjusted using *Blender* [553], they were filled with tetrahedra using the *Gmsh* meshing software [554].
For the dilation of the atria, pressure was applied on the closed surface formed by the conjunction of the LA endocardium and the vessel and valve orifices. As boundary conditions, the septal region and the valve plane were fixated in order to prevent dilation into the RA and the ventricles. The pressure on the endocardial surface was then gradually increased causing the enclosed volume to balloon from an initial value of 54 ml to 154 ml while keeping the volume of the myocardial wall constant. The mechanics simulation was not performed on the whole torso model but only on the atrial model due to the number of computational elements.

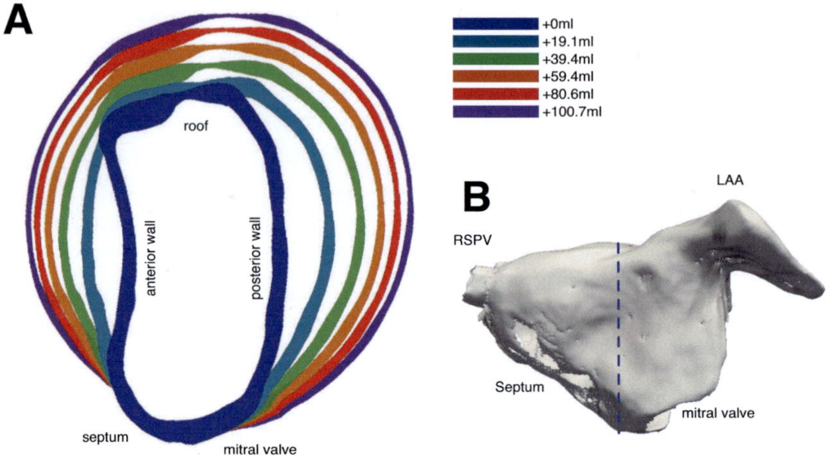

Figure 11.2: Cross section through the LA wall of model #3 with different levels of dilation coded by the color and induced by pressure overload (A). The cross section is aligned along the dashed blue line in (B).

The triangular surface mesh of the dilated, low resolution atrial model were subsequently up-sampled using a subdivision filter and filled with tetrahedra of smaller size for the simulation of electrophysiological excitation propagation. For the calculation of electrical fields within the torso, the dilated LA has to be integrated into the torso. Therefore, the surfaces of the lung had to be deformed to make room for the dilated LA as can be seen in Figure 11.3. A reduction of the lung volume due to increased LA size appeared reasonable due to the high compliance of the lung tissue.

The models of dilated left atria within a subject-specific torso can be used to simulate excitation propagation, as well as the electrical fields stemming from the currents impressed by the gradient of the transmembrane voltages using a finite element approach. A suitable approach was recently implemented [168] at IBT providing the means for a combined active/passive tissue bidomain simulation. While the extracellular domain is defined within the whole torso, the intracellular domain can be restricted to the active tissue within the atria, thus reducing computational cost.

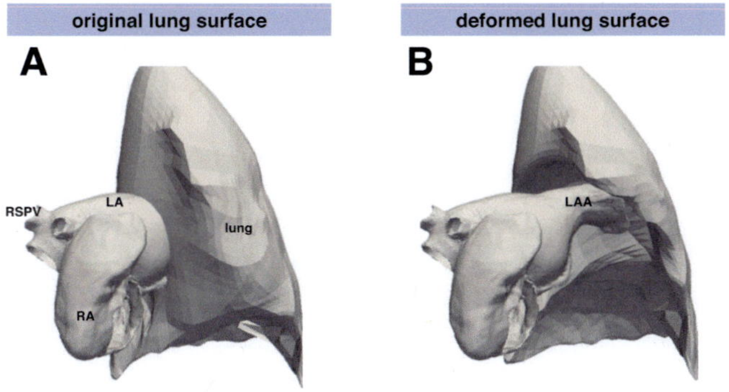

Figure 11.3: The dilated LA intersects with the lobes of the left lung as segmented using the imaging data (A). Therefore, the volume of the left lung was manually reduced to make room for the dilated LA (B). Figure modified from [549].

However, the implementation has not been fully validated regarding the simulation of atrial body surface potentials, i.e. P-waves, prohibiting to draw clinically relevant conclusions based on the simulation output. For this reason, only the effect of LA hypertrophy on the ECG but not the effect of LA dilation is assessed in the remainder of this chapter.

11.2 Results

The LA wall was thickened to seven different degrees in four anatomically personalized models. The generation of tetrahedral torso meshes using *CGAL* however failed in eight of the 28 cases. Therefore, some values are missing in Figure 11.4, which shows the effect of LA hypertrophy on different P-wave markers.

PWD (Figure 11.4A) was almost unaffected by LA wall thickening even though the latest activated regions were located in the LA for all non-hypertrophic models. For models #2, #3, and #5, the maximum difference in PWD for different wall thicknesses was 2 ms; for model #4, it was 9 ms. The P-wave area under the curve in lead II (Figure 11.4B) correlated with increased wall thickness due to an increase in amplitude.

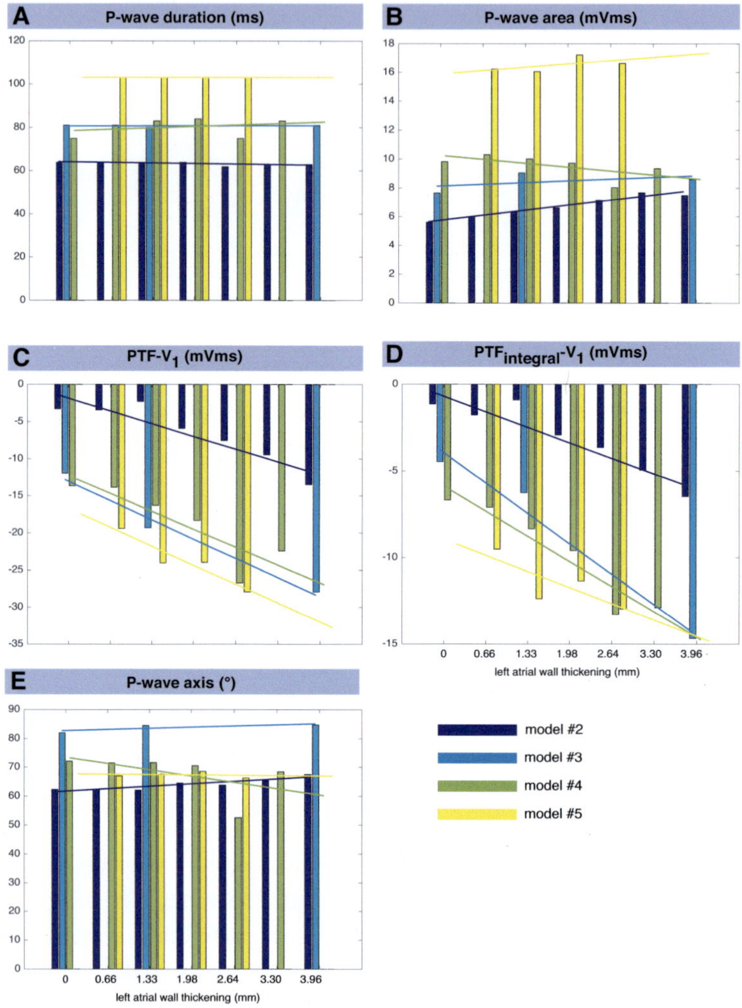

Figure 11.4: Effect of LA hypertrophy (wall thickening) on different P-wave markers. P-wave duration (A) and P-wave area (integral) (B) were measured in Einthoven lead II. P-wave terminal force in lead V_1 measured by the product of amplitude and duration (C) as well as the integral (D) of the negative phase of the P-wave. P-wave axis (E) was determined based on leads aVF and I. Missing values were due to failure of torso mesh generation. Lines indicate a linear regression of the marker values for each model.

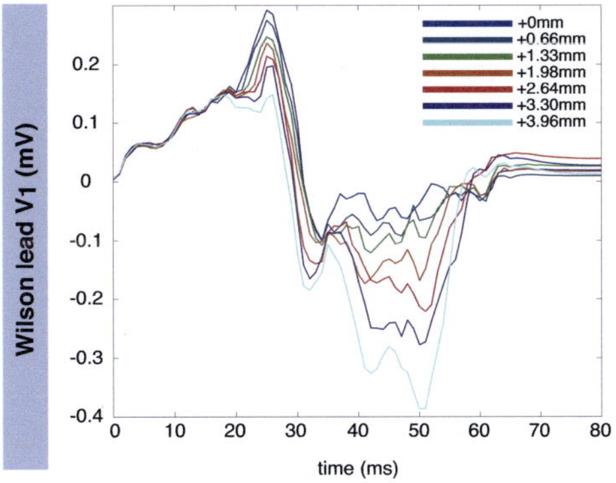

Figure 11.5: P-waves in Wilson lead V_1 for different degrees of LA wall thickening in model #2.

This relation was not consistent across models, however, with Pearson correlation coefficients ranging from 0.63 for model #4 to 0.98 for model #2. P-wave axis α was determined based on the amplitudes in leads aVF and I:

$$\alpha = \arctan\left(\frac{2}{\sqrt{3}}\frac{aVF}{I}\right). \tag{11.1}$$

The axis did not show a consistent dependency on the degree of wall thickening with a positive correlation for models #2 and #3 and a negative correlation for models #4 and #5 (Figure 11.4E). The ECG in lead V_1 (Figure 11.5) reveals that during the early P-wave, no change was present because the LA was not yet activated. Once the LA got activated, the voltage in V_1 tended to lower values for higher degrees of hypertrophy. Thus, the amplitude of the (late) positive phase decreased while the amplitude of the subsequent negative phase increased. This translates to a strong and consistent correlation between LA wall thickness and PTF-V_1 with a mean correlation coefficient of –0.93 and a mean slope of –3.49 mVms/mm wall thickening (Figure 11.4C). Evaluating the integral of the negative phase of the P-wave in lead V_1 (PTF$_{integral}$-V_1) instead of the product of the duration and the amplitude (PTF-V_1) yielded comparable results with mean values of –0.95 for the correlation coefficient and a slope of –1.26 mVms/mm wall thickening (Figure 11.4D).

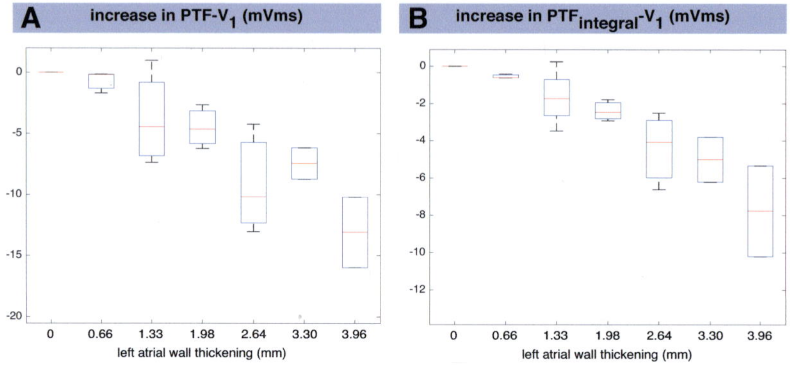

Figure 11.6: Difference in PTF in Wilson lead V_1 with respect to the non-hypertrophic baseline model (A). In (B), the integral of the negative phase of the P-wave was considered instead of the product of the amplitude and the duration. Box plots represent up to four anatomical models (cf. Figure 11.4). The missing baseline value for model #5 was linearly extrapolated.

The distribution of the increase in PTF-V_1 (Figure 11.6A) and $PTF_{integral}$-V_1 (Figure 11.6B) with respect to the value obtained using the non-hypertrophic baseline models yielded a monotonic, rather robust relation, as well.

11.3 Discussion

The results obtained through computational modeling using a cohort of 4 anatomical models suggest that PWD is unaffected by LA hypertrophy and the effect on P-wave axis is highly dependent on the individual anatomy of the patient. PTF-V_1 seems to be a sensitive marker for LA wall thickening and was superior to evaluating the integral of the whole P-wave as only the amplitude of the negative P-wave was increased by a thickened LA wall whereas the amplitude of the positive phase was decreased towards its end. The evaluation of the integral of the negative phase of the P-wave in lead V_1 ($PTF_{integral}$-V_1) was more conclusive than considering the product of amplitude and duration (classical definition of PTF-V_1). This observation is in line with the results regarding the effect of the earliest activated site in the RA and the posterior IACs presented in Chapter 10. The LA wall thickness has not been correlated with measured P-wave indices in clinical studies, so far. Thus, the findings of this study cannot be compared to sensitivity values observed in the general population *in vivo*. In patients with a history of AF, the posterior LA wall was slightly thinner than in patients in sinus rhythm [24]. However, this observation does not allow to draw conclusions regarding the risk to develop AF. The difference might as well develop under AF conditions rather than being decisive for AF initation.

A limitation of the presented study is the assumption of homogeneous hypertrophy across the LA which might not be the case *in vivo* as well as the assumption that the RA is not affected at all. Besides, the lowest degree of hypertrophy considered in this study was 0.66 mm, thus already more than 20% of the initial thickness of the LA myocardial wall. More subtle changes could be investigated using this methodology, in general. However, only a restriction to endocardial or epicardial hypertrophy could achieve an increase of 10% wall thickness without the need to resample the voxel dataset. This resampling process would potentially introduce interpolation artifacts requiring additional validation. An additional limitation regarding the P-wave amplitude is the fact that hypertrophy might be accompanied by fibrosis leading to a reduction of the source currents per volume. The limitations mentioned and discussed in Chapter 9 and Chapter 10 apply to the study presented in this chapter as well.

LAE is commonly defined as an increased total volume of the LA rather than an increased myocardial volume. The method presented in Section 11.1.2 will allow to investigate the effect of dilation in the near future. Intuitively, one would assume that the P-wave is prolonged by LA dilation while the signal amplitude (positive as well as negative) rather decreases. How pronounced these effects actually are remains to be seen. Particularly regarding PTF-V_1, the question is if the two counteracting effects balance each other or if e.g. the prolongation outweighs the decrease in amplitude leading to increased absolute PTF-V_1 values. Conceptually, LAE could also be a combination of dilation and hypertrophy. For the ventricles, it is known that they respond to pressure overload in two phases. First, the increased pressure is compensated by hypertrophic remodeling. If the condition persists or worsens, the system decompensates and the ventricles dilate [48]. The same might be true for atrial pressure overload underpinned by the observation that the atrial wall is thinner in AF patients compared to the healthy population (2.1-2.5 mm vs. 2.3-2.9 mm) [24]. The two-stage mechanism could explain the contradicting findings regarding the sensitivity and specificity of PTF-V_1 with respect to the diagnosis of LAE [481, 482, 506, 543–546]. In that case, PTF-V_1 would be increased during the hypertrophic phase and potentially abate towards more moderate values once decompensation, and thus dilation, sets in. In conclusion, it was shown that the P-wave markers PTF-V_1, and even more so $PTF_{integral}$-V_1, are sensitive to changes in LA wall thickness. The observations that the P-wave is drawn towards negative voltages in lead V_1 and that the PWD is unaffected provide mechanistic explanations why the aforementioned markers are superior to others. The interplay of LA hypertrophy and dilation might cause the poor empirical correlation of LA size and PTF-V_1.

CHAPTER 12

Conclusion

In this thesis, important aspects of human atrial patho-electrophysiology have been investigated using computational models. The studies span from the level of single ion channels up to investigations of the P-wave on the body surface ECG level. The presented results pave the way for tailoring therapies in different ways. Once basic patho-mechanisms are elucidated and understood, physicians can apply mechanism-specific therapy. Moreover, computational models representing subpopulations of patients provide the means to tailor and optimize therapies in a group-specific way. Last but not least, models of the individual patient can be used to evaluate therapeutic options in a patient-specific way if all the essential data needed to parametrize the model to the individual patient for the specific question at hand are available. Figure 12.1 gives an overview of the studies presented in this thesis, the corresponding modeling scales, the kinds of tailored therapies improved by the developed methods and derived insights, as well as the way via which they can be translated into benefits for the patient in clinical practice (comprehension of mechanisms, improved diagnosis, and improved therapy).

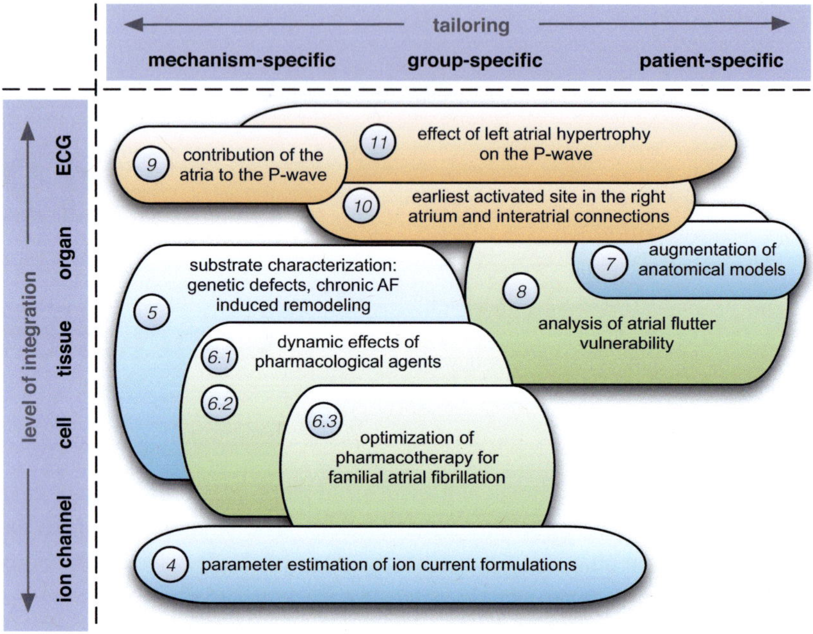

Figure 12.1: Classification of the projects presented in this thesis regarding the level of integration and regarding the type of tailored therapy benefiting from the results. Colors indicate the area of improvement: diagnosis (orange), model development and comprehension of patho-mechanisms (blue), and atrial fibrillation therapy (green). Numbers refer to the corresponding chapters of this thesis.

First, a method to incorporate altered ion channel behavior caused by genetic mutations or the influence of pharmacological agents into mathematical models in an accurate, robust, and reliable way was presented. The newly proposed hybrid scheme comprising both gradient-based and derivative-free, population-based algorithms proved to yield optimal results within a wide range of ion current formulations and noise conditions. Using the proposed hybrid optimization method, experimental data can be routinely transferred into computational models, thus it is an important tool to exploit and leverage today's and tomorrow's high-throughput patch clamp methods. A comprehensive multi-scale assessment of the effect of changes on the ion channel is imperative as the biophysical systems of interest are mostly complex and non-linear. Besides establishing a method of high practical relevance, the study serves as an example how synthetic data derived from models provide the means to evaluate novel methods under controlled conditions.

Next, the parameter estimation approaches were utilized to include the effects of two mutations of the human ether-à-go-go-related gene (hERG) into computational models. These substrates of familial atrial fibrillation (AF) were assessed on multiple levels of integration regarding their arrhythmic potential. While both mutations affect the same gene, they cause qualitatively different effects suggesting more offensive approaches for subjects carrying the L532P mutation compared to N588K. The consequences of the mutations on higher levels of integration in terms of AP morphology changes, refractory behavior, as well as rotor initiation and sustainment capacity allow to identify individuals harboring a genetic substrate predisposing to AF. By aiding risk stratification and paving the way for genotype-guided therapeutic strategies, the findings presented here help to bridge the gap from bench to bedside.

Moreover, the Courtemanche et al. model was adapted to reflect remodeling induced by chronic atrial fibrillation (cAF). The adapted model reproduces experimentally observed findings and provides mechanistic descriptions how remodeling increases susceptibility to reentry through shortened wavelength facilitating the initiation and maintenance of atrial arrhythmias according to the *AF begets AF* paradigm. The adapted model provides the means to evaluate tailored therapeutic strategies for cAF patients *in silico*.

Thirdly, the substrate models of cAF remodeling and the two hERG mutations were used to characterize the specific effects of amiodarone and dronedarone under consideration of circadian changes of the heart rate and the drug concentration. The study shows how atrial electrophysiology is differentially affected by the two compounds in a concentration-dependent and heart rate-dependent manner. A newly proposed arrhythmia score aggregating several biomarkers from the cellular and tissue level peaks to critical values for dronedarone but not for amiodarone. The insights gained from in silico modeling regarding AP alternans as a proarrhythmic mechanism provide possible explanations for the superior efficacy of amiodarone over dronedarone in the treatment of AF. As the drug effects differ significantly in a cAF remodeled substrate, the responder rate could be improved by considering the atrial substrate in tailored therapies.

By integrating experimental data regarding the effects of vernakalant from different scales into a computational model, the understanding of the cellular mode of action of vernakalant was advanced. Furthermore, relevant gaps in the current knowledge and experimental data were identified. By highlighting them, this study has the potential to fuel and direct future wet-lab and computational research on this aspiring antiarrhythmic agent. As such, it serves as an example how the interplay between experimentalists and modelers can lead to mutual benefit and cross-fertilize and speed up research.

The last study regarding pharmacotherapy aimed at the restoration of the wild-type action potential (AP) in mutant myocytes by designing hypothetical multi-channel blockers, as well as by optimizing the concentration of existing compounds. The results serve as a proof of concept and provide insight into the pharmacodynamic response of hERG mutant myocytes rendering patients vulnerable to AF. As such, they may aid in the design and advancement of tailored therapeutic and preventive approaches considering the atrial substrate. Future work could extend the presented approaches to account for variance and uncertainty using probabilistic modeling as recently proposed [555].

Furthermore, a mesh-type agnostic method to augment anatomical models with a priori knowledge regarding myocyte orientation, anatomical structures, interatrial connections (IACs), and standard ablation patterns was presented based on a coherent and consistent set of rules. The algorithm can be applied to all common data structures used in computational modeling of cardiac electrophysiology and biomechanics. Furthermore, the implementation is flexible regarding the resolution of the underlying mesh. The object-oriented design of the software using modern software engineering methods yields an extendable piece of software with maintainable code.

Building on the augmented anatomical models, a pipeline to assess the vulnerability of atrial flutter was established. The individual anatomy as well as electrophysiology in terms of CV, ERP, and their frequency-dependence is taken into account. This tool provides the means to evaluate potential ablation strategies *in silico* regarding their arrhythmic potential for AFlut before actually applying them in the electrophysiology lab. In this way, this work can be one piece in the puzzle to overcome the *learning by burning* paradigm and eventually reduce the number of patients suffering from post-ablational AFlut. The advent of electro-anatomical mapping systems providing high signal quality gives rise to the hope that the method can be validated and applied to clinical cases in the near future.

Finally, the genesis of P-wave in the body surface electrocardiogram (ECG) was studied regarding the influence of several contributors. First, the distinct contributions of the left atrium (LA) and the right atrium (RA) to the P-wave in the different ECG leads were separated in a time-resolved manner. While biomarkers based on the P-wave in the ECG carry the great advantage of being routinely acquired due to the non-invasiveness and the low associated costs, the findings of this study highlight important limitations. The results obtained in the cohort of eight *in silico* models suggest that the contribution of the LA to the P-wave is less than one third. The domination of the P-wave by sources from the RA helps to understand the difficulties experienced in P-wave-based assessment of the LA.

Moreover, the hypothesis that P-wave morphology, and in particular P-wave terminal force (PTF) in lead V_1, is affected by a shift of the earliest activated site (EAS) and its relative proximity to intact IACs was confirmed. As both the excitation origin and the IACs express significant intraindividual and interindividual variability in terms of presence, location and conductive properties, their effect can explain the limits of PTF-based assessment of LA anatomy: differences in PTF-V_1 are not of purely anatomical origin but also an electrical phenomenon.

Besides the factors mentioned above, the anatomical properties of the LA contribute to PTF-V_1. It was shown that LA hypertrophy increases PTF through higher ECG amplitudes but does not change P-wave duration. The presented findings show that PTF-V_1 is a sensitive marker for LA wall thickening and elucidate why it is superior to P-wave area. The interplay of LA hypertrophy and dilation might be the reason for the poor empirical correlation of LA size and PTF-V_1. Therefore, the presented method to investigate LA dilation leveraging computational models carries great potential. The presented results highlight the need to be aware of the limits regarding our current understanding of further factors influencing the P-wave, its morphology, and related markers. Only by pushing and overcoming these limits by integrating the P-wave into extended research aiming at a mechanistic understanding of arrhythmogenesis, healthcare practitioners will eventually be put in a position to fully leverage the potential of the P-wave in terms of AF prevention.

In conclusion, the studies presented in this thesis advanced the state of the art in computational modeling of atrial patho-electrophysiology in several aspects. Novel methods to transfer experimental data into models, to quantify the effects of pharmacological agents and optimize them, to augment anatomical models with a priori knowledge, and to assess vulnerability to atrial flutter were presented. Moreover, the boundary regarding our understanding of basic mechanisms was pushed. This includes the differential mode of action of amiodarone and dronedarone regarding the atrial substrate and circadian changes of heart rate and drug concentration, as well as the contributors to P-wave morphology and terminal force. Summing up, this thesis presents methods paving the way to tailor AF therapy under consideration of the specific pathomechanisms, the distinct properties of subpopulations, and patient-individual characteristics. By translating the methods and insights into clinical practice, appropriate and more efficient therapy can be delivered in shorter time. In this way, not only the socio-economical costs of AF but foremost the individual patient's burden can be reduced eventually.

APPENDIX **A**

Parameter Estimation

A.1 Ion Current Formulations

Here, the I_{Kr}, I_{Kur}, and I_{Ks} ion current formulations from Courtemanche et al. [47] used in this study are given. The estimated parameters are highlighted in red in the equations. Their classification as additive or multiplicative together with their values in the original formulation and the corresponding wide and narrow range are given in Table A.1–Table A.3.
The intracellular potassium concentration $[K]_i$ was estimated for all currents:

$$E_K = \frac{R \cdot T}{F \cdot z_K} \ln \frac{[K]_o}{[K]_i} \; . \tag{A.1}$$

A.1.1 I_{Kr}

$$I_{Kr} = g_{Kr} x_r \frac{1}{1 + \exp\left(\frac{V_m + x_{r,m3}}{x_{r,m4}}\right)} (V_m - E_K) \; , \tag{A.2}$$

with x_r being the gating variable. Its steady state value $x_{r\infty}$, the two rate constants α_{x_r} and β_{x_r} and the time constant τ_{x_r} are defined as follows:

$$x_{r\infty} = \frac{1}{1+\exp\left(\frac{V_m + x_{r,m1}}{x_{r,m2}}\right)} , \tag{A.3}$$

$$\tau_{x_r} = \frac{1}{(\alpha_{x_r} + \beta_{x_r}) \cdot x_{r,KQ10}} , \tag{A.4}$$

$$\alpha_{x_r} = \frac{x_{r,a1}\,(V_m + x_{r,a2})}{1-\exp\left(\frac{V_m + x_{r,a2}}{x_{r,a3}}\right)} , \tag{A.5}$$

$$\beta_{x_r} = 7.3898 \times 10^{-5} \frac{V_m + x_{r,b1}}{\exp\left(\frac{V_m + x_{r,b1}}{x_{r,b2}}\right) - 1} . \tag{A.6}$$

A.1.2 I_{Kur}

$$I_{Kur} = g_{Kur} u_a^3 u_i \left(V_m - E_K\right) , \tag{A.7}$$

$$g_{Kur} = g_{Kur1} + \frac{g_{Kur2}}{1+\exp\left(\frac{V_m + g_{Kur3}}{g_{Kur4}}\right)} , \tag{A.8}$$

$$\alpha_{u_a} = u_{a,a1} \left[\exp\left(\frac{V_m + u_{a,a2}}{u_{a,a3}}\right) + \exp\left(\frac{V_m + u_{a,a4}}{u_{a,a5}}\right)\right]^{-1} , \tag{A.9}$$

$$\beta_{u_a} = 0.65 \left[u_{a,b1} + \exp\left(\frac{V_m + u_{a,b2}}{u_{a,b3}}\right)\right]^{-1} , \tag{A.10}$$

$$\tau_{u_a} = \frac{1}{(\alpha_{u_a} + \beta_{u_a}) \cdot \mathrm{u}_{a,KQ10}} , \tag{A.11}$$

$$u_{a,\infty} = \left[1 + \exp\left(\frac{V_m + u_{a,m1}}{u_{a,m2}}\right)\right]^{-1} , \tag{A.12}$$

$$\alpha_{u_i} = u_{i,a1}\left[u_{i,a2} + \exp\left(\frac{V_m + u_{i,a3}}{u_{a,a4}}\right)\right]^{-1}, \tag{A.13}$$

$$\beta_{u_i} = \exp\left(\frac{V_m + u_{i,b1}}{u_{i,b2}}\right), \tag{A.14}$$

$$\tau_{u_i} = \frac{1}{(\alpha_{u_i} + \beta_{u_i}) \cdot \mathrm{u}_{i,KQ10}}, \tag{A.15}$$

$$u_{i,\infty} = \left[1 + \exp\left(\frac{V_m + u_{i,m1}}{u_{i,m2}}\right)\right]^{-1}. \tag{A.16}$$

A.1.3 I_{Ks}

$$I_{Ks} = g_{Ks} x_s^2 (V_m - E_K), \tag{A.17}$$

$$x_{s\infty} = \frac{1}{\sqrt{1 + \exp\left(\frac{V_m + x_{s,m1}}{x_{s,m2}}\right)}}, \tag{A.18}$$

$$\tau_{x_s} = \frac{0.5}{(\alpha_{x_r} + \beta_{x_r}) \cdot \mathrm{x}_{s,KQ10}}, \tag{A.19}$$

$$\alpha_{x_s} = \frac{x_{s,a1}(V_m + x_{s,a2})}{1 - \exp\left(\frac{V_m + x_{s,a2}}{x_{s,a3}}\right)}, \tag{A.20}$$

$$\beta_{x_s} = 3.5 \times 10^{-5} \frac{(V_m + x_{s,b1})}{\exp\left(\frac{V_m + x_{s,b1}}{x_{s,b2}}\right) - 1}. \tag{A.21}$$

Table A.1: I_{Kr} parameters: besides the parameter names and units, their classification as additive (±) or multiplicative (*), the standard Courtemanche et al. value [47] and the parameter ranges for the parameter estimation are given.

Parameter	Unit	Type	Standard value	Narrow range	Wide range
$x_{r,a1}$	1	*	3×10^{-4}	3×10^{-5}..3×10^{-3}	3×10^{-6}..3×10^{-2}
$x_{r,a2}$	mV	±	14.1	-45.9..74.1	-105.9..134.1
$x_{r,a3}$	mV	*	-5	-50..-0.5	-500..-0.05
$x_{r,b1}$	mV	±	3.3328	-63.33..56.67	-123.33..116.67
$x_{r,b2}$	mV	*	5.1237	0.51237..51.237	0.05123..512.37
$x_{r,KQ10}$	1	*	1.0	0.1..10.0	0.01..100.0
$x_{r,m1}$	mV	±	14.1	-45.9..74.1	-105.9..134.1
$x_{r,m2}$	mV	*	-6.5	-65.0..-0.65	-650.0..-0.065
$x_{r,m3}$	mV	±	15.0	-45.0..75.0	-105.0..135.0
$x_{r,m4}$	mV	*	22.4	2.24..224.0	0.224..2240.0
g_{Kr}	nS/pF	*	0.0294118	0.0029..0.2942	0.0003..2.94
$[K]_i$	mM	*	138.99	13.899..1389.94	1.38994..13899.4

A.2 Experimental Protocols

In this section, the details of the experimental protocols used to acquire wet-lab I_{Kr}, I_{Kur}, and I_{Ks} current traces in the group of Eberhard Scholz at University Hospital Heidelberg are given.

All currents were recorded using a *Warner OC-725A* (*Warner Instruments, Hamden, CT, USA*) amplifier, low-pass filtered at 1 to 2 kHz (-3dB, four-pole Bessel filter) and digitized at 5 to 10 kHz (*Digidata 1322A, Axon Instruments, Union City, CA, USA*). The currents recorded in different cells were normalized to their maximum value, averaged, and scaled to the average maximum value.

A.2.1 hERG measurements

Human ether-à-go-go-related gene (hERG; alternative nomenclature KCNH2) encodes the α-subunit of the Kv11.1 protein carrying the rapid delayed rectifier potassium current (I_{Kr}).

Table A.2: I_{Kur} parameters: besides the parameter names and units, their classification as additive (±) or multiplicative (*), the standard Courtemanche et al. value [47] and the parameter ranges for the parameter estimation are given.

Parameter	Unit	Type	Standard value	Narrow range	Wide range
$u_{a,a1}$	1	*	0.65	0.065..6.5	0.0065..65.0
$u_{a,a2}$	mV	±	10.0	-50..70	-110..130
$u_{a,a3}$	mV	*	-8.5	-85..-0.85	-850.0..-0.085
$u_{a,a4}$	mV	±	-30.0	-90.0..30.0	-150.0..90.0
$u_{a,a5}$	mV	*	-59.0	-590..-5.9	-5900.0..-0.59
$u_{a,b1}$	1	±	2.5	-57.5..62.5	-117.5..122.5
$u_{a,b2}$	mV	±	82.0	22.0..142.0	-38.0..202.0
$u_{a,b3}$	mV	*	17.0	1.7..170.0	0.17..1700.0
$u_{a,m1}$	mV	±	30.3	-29.7..90.3	-89.7..150.3
$u_{a,m2}$	mV	*	-9.6	-96.0..-0.96	-960.0..-0.096
$u_{a,KQ10}$	1	*	3.0	0.3..30.0	0.03..300.0
$u_{i,a1}$	1	*	1.0	0.1..10.0	0.01..100.0
$u_{i,a2}$	1	±	21.0	-39.0..81.0	-99.0..141.0
$u_{i,a3}$	mV	±	-185.0	-245.0..-125.0	-305.0..-65.0
$u_{i,a4}$	mV	*	-28.0	-280.0..-2.8	-2800.0..-0.28
$u_{i,b1}$	mV	±	-158.0	-218.0..-98.0	-278.0..-38.0
$u_{i,b2}$	mV	±	-16.0	-160.0..-1.6	-1600.0..-0.16
$u_{i,m1}$	mV	±	-99.45	-159.45..-39.45	-219.45..20.55
$u_{i,m2}$	mV	*	27.48	2.748..274.8	0.2748..2748.0
$u_{i,KQ10}$	1	*	3.0	0.3..30.0	0.03..300.0
g_{Kur1}	nS/pF	±	0.005	-59.95..60.0	-119.9..120.0
g_{Kur2}	nS/pF	*	0.05	0.005..0.5	0.0005..5.0
g_{Kur3}	mV	±	-15.0	-75.0..45.0	-135.0..105.0
g_{Kur4}	mV	*	-13.0	-130.0..-1.3	-1300.0..-0.13
$[K]_i$	mM	*	138.9	13.89..1389.9	1.389..13899

Wildtype hERG channels were expressed in Xenopus oocytes after injection of 46 nl cRNA solution per oocyte. After 3 to 4 days incubated at a temperature of 16° C, double micro-electrode voltage clamp experiments were performed in $n = 8$ cells. The tip resistances of the micro-electrodes were in the range of 1 to 5 MΩ. The voltage clamp recordings were performed at room temperature (23 to 25° C). The bathing solution consisted of 5 mM KCl, 100 mM NaCl, 1.5 mM $CaCl_2$, 2 mM $MgCl_2$, and 10 mM HEPES (pH adjusted to 7.4 with NaOH) and the pipette solution contained 3 M KCl. The applied voltage clamp protocol and the corresponding current traces are depicted in Figure 4.1C.

Table A.3: I_{Ks} parameters: besides the parameter names and units, their classification as additive (±) or multiplicative (*), the standard Courtemanche et al. value [47] and the parameter ranges for the parameter estimation are given.

Parameter	Unit	Type	Standard value	Narrow range	Wide range
$x_{s,a1}$	1	*	4×10^{-5}	$4\times10^{-6}..4\times10^{-4}$	$4\times10^{-7}..4\times10^{-3}$
$x_{s,a2}$	mV	±	-19.9	-79.9..40.1	-139.9..100.1
$x_{s,a3}$	mV	*	-17.0	-170.0..-1.7	-1700.0..-0.17
$x_{s,b1}$	mV	±	-19.9	-79.9..40.1	-139.9..100.1
$x_{s,b2}$	mV	*	9.0	0.9..90.0	0.09..900.0
$x_{s,KQ10}$	1	*	2.0	0.2..20.0	0.02..200.0
$x_{s,m1}$	mV	±	-19.9	-79.9..40.1	-139.9..100.1
$x_{s,m2}$	mV	*	-12.7	-127.0..-1.27	-1270.0..-0.127
g_{Ks}	nS/pF	*	0.12941176	0.0129..1.294	0.00129 12.94
$[K]_i$	mM	*	138.994	13.899..1389.94	1.3899..13899.4

A.2.2 KCNA5 measurements

KCNA5 encodes the Kv1.5 protein carrying the ultra-rapid delayed rectifier potassium current (I_{Kur}). Wildtype KCNA5 was transfected into chinese hamster ovary (CHO) cell using *Fugene* reagent (*Promega, Madison, WI, USA*) (3 μg DNA per bowl). The CHO cells were incubated at 37° C in minimum essential medium α and an atmosphere of 95% humidified air and 5% CO_2. The medium was supplemented with 100 μg/ml streptomycin sulphate, 10% fetal bovine serum, and 100 U/ml penicillin G sodium. Resistances ranged between 38 and 98 MΩ. The bathing solution consisted of 140 mM NaCl, 5 mM KCl, 1 mM $MgCl_2*6H_2O$, 10 mM HEPES, 1.8 mM $CaCl_2*2H_2O$, and 10 mM glucose monohydrate. pH was adjusted to 7.4 using NaOH. The pipette solution contained 100 mM K aspartate, 20 mM KCl, 2 mM $MgCl_2*6H_2O$, 1 mM $CaCl_2*2H_2O$, 10 mM HEPES, 10 mM EGTA, and 2 mM Na_2ATP. pH was adjusted to 7.2 using KOH; patch clamp recordings were performed at a temperature of 37° C in $n = 3$ cells. The applied voltage protocol and the corresponding current traces are depicted in Figure 4.1D.

A.2.3 KCNQ1+KCNE1 measurements

KCNQ1 encodes the α-subunit of the Kv7.1 protein carrying the slow delayed rectifier potassium channel (I_{Ks}), KCNE1 encodes the β-subunit of Kv7.1. KCNQ1 was co-expressed with KCNE1 in Xenopus oocytes after injection of 46 nl cRNA solution per oocyte. Double micro-electrode voltage clamp experiments were performed at room temperature (20 to 25° C) 2 days after injection in $n = 5$ cells. The tip resistances of the micro-electrodes were in the range of 1 to 5 MΩ. The bathing solution consisted of 5 mM KCl, 100 mM NaCl, 1.5 mM $CaCl_2$, 2 mM $MgCl_2$, and 10 mM HEPES (pH adjusted to 7.4 with NaOH). The current and voltage electrodes were filled with 3 M KCl solution. The applied voltage protocol and the corresponding current traces are depicted in Figure 4.1E.

References

[1] A. J. Camm, P. Kirchhof, G. Y. H. Lip, et al., "Guidelines for the management of atrial fibrillation: The task force for the management of atrial fibrillation of the european society of cardiology (ESC)," *Europace*, vol. 12, no. 10, pp. 1360–1420, 2010.

[2] Y. Miyasaka, M. E. Barnes, B. J. Gersh, et al., "Time trends of ischemic stroke incidence and mortality in patients diagnosed with first atrial fibrillation in 1980 to 2000: Report of a community-based study," *Stroke*, vol. 36, no. 11, pp. 2362–2366, 2005.

[3] S. E. Wolowacz, M. Samuel, V. K. Brennan, et al., "The cost of illness of atrial fibrillation: a systematic review of the recent literature," *Europace*, vol. 13, no. 10, pp. 1375–1385, 2011.

[4] B. P. Krijthe, A. Kunst, E. J. Benjamin, et al., "Projections on the number of individuals with atrial fibrillation in the European Union, from 2000 to 2060," *Eur Heart J*, vol. 34, no. 35, pp. 2746–2751, 2013.

[5] D. Swancutt, R. Hobbs, D. Fitzmaurice, et al., "A randomised controlled trial and cost effectiveness study of systematic screening (targeted and total population screening) versus routine practice for the detection of atrial fibrillation in the over 65s: (SAFE)," *BMC Cardiovasc Disord*, vol. 4, p. 12, 2004.

[6] G. Lin, H. H. Lu, Y. Shen, et al., "Meta-analysis of the therapeutic effects of various methods for the treatment of chronic atrial fibrillation," *Exp Ther Med*, vol. 6, no. 2, pp. 489–496, 2013.

[7] M. Schmidt, U. Dorwarth, D. Andresen, et al., "German ablation registry: Cryoballoon vs radiofrequency ablation in paroxysmal atrial fibrillation - one-year outcome data," *Heart Rhythm*, vol. 13, no. 4, pp. 836–844, 2016.

[8] A. Chugh, H. Oral, K. Lemola, et al., "Prevalence, mechanisms, and clinical significance of macroreentrant atrial tachycardia during and following left atrial ablation for atrial fibrillation," *Heart Rhythm*, vol. 2, no. 5, pp. 464–471, 2005.

[9] O. Dössel, M. W. Krueger, F. M. Weber, et al., "Computational modeling of the human atrial anatomy and electrophysiology," *Med Biol Eng Comput*, vol. 50, no. 8, pp. 773–799, 2012.

[10] N. A. Trayanova, "Mathematical approaches to understanding and imaging atrial fibrillation: Significance for mechanisms and management," *Circ Res*, vol. 114, no. 9, pp. 1516–1531, 2014.

[11] V. Jacquemet, "Lessons from computer simulations of ablation of atrial fibrillation," *J Physiol*, 2016, epub ahead of print.

[12] N. A. Trayanova and K. C. Chang, "How computer simulations of the human heart can improve anti-arrhythmia therapy," *J Physiol*, 2015, epub ahead of print.

[13] R. L. Winslow, N. Trayanova, D. Geman, et al., "Computational medicine: Translating models to clinical care," *Sci Transl Med*, vol. 4, no. 158, p. 158rv11, 2012.

[14] A. McCulloch, "Systems biophysics: Multiscale biophysical modeling of organ systems," *Biophys J*, vol. 110, no. 5, pp. 1023–1027, 2016.

[15] T. Fritz, "Biomechanical modeling of the human heart - modeling of the ventricles, the atria and the pericardium and the inverse problem of cardiac mechanics," PhD thesis, Institute of Biomedical Engineering, Karlsruhe Institute of Technology (KIT), Karlsruhe, 2015.

[16] R. M. Anderson, *The gross physiology of the cardiovascular system*. Tucson: Racquet Press, 1993.

[17] D. Sánchez-Quintana, J. A. Cabrera, V. Climent, et al., "Anatomic relations between the esophagus and left atrium and relevance for ablation of atrial fibrillation," *Circulation*, vol. 112, no. 10, pp. 1400–1405, 2005.

[18] C. Stöllberger, G. Ernst, E. Bonner, et al., "Left atrial appendage morphology: Comparison of transesophageal images and postmortem casts," *Z Kardiol*, vol. 92, no. 4, pp. 303–308, 2003.

[19] S. Y. Ho and D. Sánchez-Quintana, "The importance of atrial structure and fibers," *Clin Anat*, vol. 22, no. 1, pp. 52–63, 2009.

[20] D. Sánchez-Quintana, R. H. Anderson, J. A. Cabrera, et al., "The terminal crest: Morphological features relevant to electrophysiology," *Heart*, vol. 88, no. 4, pp. 406–411, 2002.

[21] K. Wang, S. Y. Ho, D. G. Gibson, et al., "Architecture of atrial musculature in humans," *Br Heart J*, vol. 73, no. 6, pp. 559–565, 1995.

[22] J. Papez, "Heart muculature of the atria," *Am J Anat*, vol. 27, no. 3, pp. 255–285, 1920.

[23] M. W. Krüger, *Personalized multi-scale modeling of the atria: Heterogeneities, fiber architecture, hemodialysis and ablation therapy*, Karlsruhe Transactions on Biomedical Engineering, vol. 19. Karlsruhe: KIT Scientific Publishing, 2012.

[24] P. G. Platonov, V. Ivanov, S. Y. Ho, et al., "Left atrial posterior wall thickness in patients with and without atrial fibrillation: Data from 298 consecutive autopsies," *J Cardiovasc Electrophysiol*, vol. 19, no. 7, pp. 689–692, 2008.

[25] B. Hall, V. Jeevanantham, R. Simon, et al., "Variation in left atrial transmural wall thickness at sites commonly targeted for ablation of atrial fibrillation," *J Interv Card Electrophysiol*, vol. 17, no. 2, pp. 127–132, 2006.

[26] R. H. Anderson and A. C. Cook, "The structure and components of the atrial chambers," *Europace*, vol. 9 S6, pp. vi3–vi9, 2007.

[27] R. Lemery, L. Soucie, B. Martin, et al., "Human study of biatrial electrical coupling: Determinants of endocardial septal activation and conduction over interatrial connections," *Circulation*, vol. 110, no. 15, pp. 2083–2089, 2004.

[28] F. Saremi, S. Channual, S. Krishnan, et al., "Bachmann bundle and its arterial supply: Imaging with multidetector CT - implications for interatrial conduction abnormalities and arrhythmias," *Radiology*, vol. 248, no. 2, pp. 447–457, 2008.

[29] R. Lemery, G. Guiraudon, and J. P. Veinot, "Anatomic description of Bachmann's bundle and its relation to the atrial septum," *Am J Cardiol*, vol. 91, no. 12, pp. 1482–1485, 2003.

[30] J. P. Veinot and R. Lemery, "Innovations in cardiovascular pathology anatomic and electrophysiologic determinants associated with ablation of atrial arrhythmias," *Cardiovasc Pathol*, vol. 14, no. 4, pp. 204–213, 2005.

[31] M. Chauvin, D. C. Shah, M. Haïssaguerre, et al., "The anatomic basis of connections between the coronary sinus musculature and the left atrium in humans," *Circulation*, vol. 101, no. 6, pp. 647–652, 2000.

[32] P. G. Platonov, L. Mitrofanova, V. Ivanov, et al., "Substrates for intra-atrial and interatrial conduction in the atrial septum: Anatomical study on 84 human hearts," *Heart Rhythm*, vol. 5, no. 8, pp. 1189–1195, 2008.

[33] S. Y. Ho, D. Sanchez-Quintana, J. A. Cabrera, et al., "Anatomy of the left atrium: Implications for radiofrequency ablation of atrial fibrillation," *J Cardiovasc Electrophysiol*, vol. 10, no. 11, pp. 1525–1533, 1999.

[34] S. I. Sakamoto, T. Nitta, Y. Ishii, et al., "Interatrial electrical connections: The precise location and preferential conduction," *J Cardiovasc Electrophysiol*, vol. 16, no. 10, pp. 1077–1086, 2005.

[35] P. G. Platonov, "Interatrial conduction in the mechanisms of atrial fibrillation: from anatomy to cardiac signals and new treatment modalities," *Europace*, vol. 9 S6, pp. vi10–vi16, 2007.

[36] F. F. Bukauskas, "Molecular organization, gating, and function of gap junction channels," in *Cardiac Electrophysiology: From Cell to Bedside*, D. P. Zipes and J. Jalife, Eds. Philadelphia: Elsevier Saunders, 2014, ch. 8, pp. 85–94.

[37] C. V. Desimone, A. Noheria, N. Lachman, et al., "Myocardium of the superior vena cava, coronary sinus, vein of marshall, and the pulmonary vein ostia: Gross anatomic studies in 620 hearts," *J Cardiovasc Electrophysiol*, vol. 23, no. 12, pp. 1304–1309, 2012.

[38] H. Nathan and M. Eliakim, "The junction between the left atrium and the pulmonary veins: An anatomic study of human hearts," *Circulation*, vol. 34, no. 3, pp. 412–422, 1966.

[39] P. G. Platonov, "P-wave morphology: Underlying mechanisms and clinical implications," *Ann Noninvasive Electrocardiol*, vol. 17, no. 3, pp. 161–169, 2012.

[40] N. Chandler, O. Aslanidi, D. Buckley, et al., "Computer three-dimensional anatomical reconstruction of the human sinus node and a novel paranodal area," *Anat Rec*, vol. 294, no. 6, pp. 970–979, 2011.

[41] D. Sánchez-Quintana, J. A. Cabrera, J. Farré, et al., "Sinus node revisited in the era of electroanatomical mapping and catheter ablation," *Heart*, vol. 91, no. 2, pp. 189–94, 2005.

[42] J. P. Boineau, T. E. Canavan, R. B. Schuessler, et al., "Demonstration of a widely distributed atrial pacemaker complex in the human heart," *Circulation*, vol. 77, no. 6, pp. 1221–1237, 1988.

[43] R. B. Schuessler, J. P. Boineau, and B. I. Bromberg, "Origin of the sinus impulse," *J Cardiovasc Electrophysiol*, vol. 7, no. 3, pp. 263–274, 1996.

[44] W. J. Meek and J. A. E. Eyster, "Experiments on the origin and propagagation of the impulse in the heart: Iv. the effect of vagal stimulation and of cooling on the location of the pacemaker within the sino-auricular node," *Am J Physiol*, vol. 34, pp. 368–383, 1914.

[45] O. Monfredi, H. Dobrzynski, T. Mondal, et al., "The anatomy and physiology of the sinoatrial node - a contemporary review," *PACE - Pacing Clin Electrophysiol*, vol. 33, no. 11, pp. 1392–1406, 2010.

[46] B. Hille, *Ionic channels of excitable membranes*. Sunderland: Sinauer Associates, 2001.

[47] M. Courtemanche, R. J. Ramirez, and S. Nattel, "Ionic mechanisms underlying human atrial action potential properties: insights from a mathematical model," *Am J Physiol*, vol. 275, no. 1 Pt 2, pp. 1522–1539, 1998.

[48] R. F. Schmidt and F. Lang, *Physiologie des Menschen - mit Pathophysiologie*, R. F. Schmidt, F. Lang, and M. Heckmann, Eds. Heidelberg: Springer, 2007.

[49] S. Brady, G. Siegel, R. W. Albers, et al., *Basic neurochemistry: molecular, cellular and medical aspects*. Philadelphia: Lippincott-Raven, 2005.

[50] D. C. Bartos, E. Grandi, and C. M. Ripplinger, "Ion channels in the heart," *Compr Physiol*, vol. 5, no. July, pp. 1423–1464, 2015.

[51] L. Sherwood, *Human physiology: From cells to systems*. Belmont: Brooks/Cole, 2007.

[52] D. Durrer, R. T. van Dam, G. E. Freud, et al., "Total excitation of the isolated human heart," *Circulation*, vol. 41, no. 6, pp. 899–912, 1970.

[53] Y. Wang and Y. Rudy, "Electrocardiographic imaging of normal human atrial repolarization," *Heart Rhythm*, vol. 6, no. 4, pp. 582–583, 2009.

[54] J. E. Saffitz, H. L. Kanter, K. G. Green, et al., "Tissue-specific determinants of anisotropic conduction velocity in canine atrial and ventricular myocardium," *Circ Res*, vol. 74, no. 6, pp. 1065–1070, 1994.

[55] R. De Ponti, S. Y. Ho, J. A. Salerno-Uriarte, et al., "Electroanatomic analysis of sinus impulse propagation in normal human atria," *J Cardiovasc Electrophysiol*, vol. 13, no. 1, pp. 1–10, 2002.

[56] D. Harrild and C. Henriquez, "A computer model of normal conduction in the human atria," *Circ Res*, vol. 87, no. 7, pp. E25–E36, 2000.

[57] G. Seemann, C. Höper, F. B. Sachse, et al., "Heterogeneous three-dimensional anatomical and electrophysiological model of human atria," *Philos Trans A Math Phys Eng Sci*, vol. 364, no. 1843, pp. 1465–1481, 2006.

[58] C. Tobón, C. Ruíz, J. F. Rodríguez, et al., "Vulnerability for reentry in a three dimensional model of human atria: A simulation study," *IEEE Eng Med Biol Soc EMBC*, pp. 224–227, 2010.

[59] M. S. Spach, P. C. Dolber, and J. F. Heidlage, "Influence of the passive anisotropic properties on directional differences in propagation following modification of the sodium conductance in human atrial muscle. a model of reentry based on anisotropic discontinuous propagation," *Circ Res*, vol. 62, no. 4, pp. 811–832, 1988.

[60] J. Malmivuo and R. Plonsey, *Bioelectromagnetism: Principles and applications of bioletric and biomagnetic fields*. New York/Oxford: Oxford University Press, 1995.

[61] J. Carlson, R. Havmöller, A. Herreros, et al., "Can orthogonal lead indicators of propensity to atrial fibrillation be accurately assessed from the 12-lead ECG?" *Europace*, vol. 7, no. S2, pp. 39–48, 2005.

[62] G. Lee, P. Sanders, and J. Kalman, "Catheter ablation of atrial arrhythmias: State of the art," *Lancet*, vol. 380, no. 9852, pp. 1509–1519, 2012.

[63] B. Surawicz and T. Knilans, *Chou's electrocardiography in clinical practice: Adult and pediatric*, 6th ed. Philadelphia: Elsevier Health Sciences, 2008.

[64] B. Olshansky, K. Okumura, P. G. Hess, et al., "Demonstration of an area of slow conduction in atrial flutter," *J Am Coll Cardiol*, vol. 16, no. 7, pp. 1639–1648, 1990.

[65] G. R. Villacastín J, Pérez-Castellano N, Moreno J, "Left atrial flutter after radiofrequency catheter ablation of focal atrial fibrillation," *J Cardiovasc Electrophysiol*, vol. 14, no. 4, pp. 417–421, 2003.

[66] A. B. Biviano, E. J. Ciaccio, J. Fleitman, et al., "Atrial tachycardias after atrial fibrillation ablation manifest different waveform characteristics: Implications for characterizing tachycardias," *J Cardiovasc Electrophysiol*, vol. 26, no. 11, pp. 1187–1195, 2015.

[67] T. Yamada and G. N. Kay, "Atrial flutter following pulmonary vein isolation: What is the mechanism?" *J Cardiovasc Electrophysiol*, vol. 24, no. 10, pp. 1186–1188, 2013.

[68] R. Kobza, G. Hindricks, H. Tanner, et al., "Late recurrent arrhythmias after ablation of atrial fibrillation: Incidence, mechanisms, and treatment," *Heart Rhythm*, vol. 1, no. 6, pp. 676–683, 2004.

[69] P. Jaïs, D. C. Shah, M. Haïssaguerre, et al., "Mapping and ablation of left atrial flutters," *Circulation*, vol. 101, no. 25, pp. 2928–2934, 2000.

[70] J. Granada, W. Uribe, P.-H. Chyou, et al., "Incidence and predictors of atrial flutter in the general population," *J Am Coll Cardiol*, vol. 36, no. 7, pp. 2242–2246, 2000.

[71] A. Natale, K. H. Newby, E. Pisano, et al., "Prospective randomized comparison of antiarrhythmic therapy versus first-line radiofrequency ablation in patients with atrial flutter," *J Am Coll Cardiol*, vol. 35, no. 7, pp. 1898–1904, 2000.

[72] A. J. Camm, G. Y. H. Lip, R. De Caterina, et al., "2012 focused update of the ESC guidelines for the management of atrial fibrillation," *Eur Heart J*, vol. 33, no. 21, pp. 2719–2747, 2012.

[73] M. Zoni-Berisso, F. Lercari, T. Carazza, et al., "Epidemiology of atrial fibrillation: European perspective," *Clin Epidemiol*, vol. 6, pp. 213–220, 2014.

[74] E. J. Benjamin, P. a. Wolf, R. B. D'Agostino, et al., "Impact of atrial fibrillation on the risk of death the Framingham heart study," *Circulation*, vol. 98, no. 10, pp. 946–952, 1998.

[75] R. Nieuwlaat, A. Capucci, A. J. Camm, et al., "Atrial fibrillation management: A prospective survey in ESC member countries - the euro heart survey on atrial fibrillation," *Eur Heart J*, vol. 26, no. 22, pp. 2422–2434, 2005.

[76] J. Andrade, P. Khairy, D. Dobrev, et al., "The clinical profile and pathophysiology of atrial fibrillation: Relationships among clinical features, epidemiology, and mechanisms," *Circ Res*, vol. 114, no. 9, pp. 1453–1468, 2014.

[77] U. Schotten, S. Verheule, P. Kirchhof, et al., "Pathophysiological mechanisms of atrial fibrillation: A translational appraisal," *Physiol Rev*, vol. 91, no. 1, pp. 265–325, 2011.

[78] U. Schotten, D. Dobrev, P. G. Platonov, et al., "Current controversies in determining the main mechanisms of atrial fibrillation," *J Intern Med*, 2016, epub ahead of print.

[79] M. Haïssaguerre, P. Jais, and D. C. Shah, "Spontaneous initiation of atrial fibrillation by ectopic beats originating in the pulmonary veins," *N Engl J Med*, vol. 339, no. 10, pp. 659–666, 1998.

[80] A. Burashnikov and C. Antzelevitch, "Late-phase 3 EAD: A unique mechanism contributing to initiation of atrial fibrillation," *PACE - Pacing Clin Electrophysiol*, vol. 29, no. 3, pp. 290–295, 2006.

[81] R. P. Katra and K. R. Laurita, "Cellular mechanism of calcium-mediated triggered activity in the heart," *Circ Res*, vol. 96, no. 5, pp. 535–542, 2005.

[82] P. G. A. Volders, A. Kulcsar, M. A. Vos, et al., "Similarities between early and delayed afterdepolarizations induced by isoproterenol in canine ventricular myocytes," *Cardiovasc Res*, vol. 34, no. 2, pp. 348–359, 1997.

[83] O. Berenfeld and J. Jalife, "Mechanisms of atrial fibrillation rotors, ionic determinants, and excitation frequency," *Cardiol Clin*, vol. 32, no. 4, pp. 495–506, 2014.

[84] A. T. Winfree, "Spiral waves of chemical activity," *Science*, vol. 175, no. 4022, pp. 634–636, 1972.

[85] S. M. Narayan, D. E. Krummen, K. Shivkumar, et al., "Treatment of atrial fibrillation by the ablation of localized sources: CONFIRM (conventional ablation for atrial fibrillation with or without focal impulse and rotor modulation) trial," *J Am Coll Cardiol*, vol. 60, no. 7, pp. 628–636, 2012.

[86] K. Tanaka, S. Zlochiver, K. L. Vikstrom, et al., "Spatial distribution of fibrosis governs fibrillation wave dynamics in the posterior left atrium during heart failure," *Circ Res*, vol. 101, no. 8, pp. 839–847, 2007.

[87] G. Moe and J. Abildskov, "Atrial fibrillation as a self-sustaining arrhythmia independent of focal discharge," *Am Heart J*, vol. 58, no. 1, pp. 59–70, 1959.

[88] G. Moe, "A conceptual model of atrial fibrillation," *J Electrocardiol*, vol. 1, no. 2, pp. 145–146, 1960.

[89] J. N. Weiss, A. Garfinkel, H. S. Karagueuzian, et al., "Chaos and the transition to ventricular fibrillation: A new approach to antiarrhythmic drug evaluation," *Circulation*, vol. 99, no. 21, pp. 2819–2826, 1999.

[90] G. Lee, S. Kumar, A. Teh, et al., "Epicardial wave mapping in human long-lasting persistent atrial fibrillation: transient rotational circuits, complex wavefronts, and disorganized activity," *Eur Heart J*, vol. 35, no. 2, pp. 86–97, 2014.

[91] M. A. Allessie, N. M. S. de Groot, R. P. M. Houben, et al., "Electropathological substrate of long-standing persistent atrial fibrillation in patients with structural heart disease: longitudinal dissociation," *Circ Arrhythm Electrophysiol*, vol. 3, no. 6, pp. 606–615, 2010.

[92] N. M. S. de Groot, R. P. M. Houben, J. L. Smeets, et al., "Electropathological substrate of longstanding persistent atrial fibrillation in patients with structural heart disease: epicardial breakthrough," *Circulation*, vol. 122, no. 17, pp. 1674–1682, 2010.

[93] H. Sun, R. Gaspo, N. Leblanc, et al., "Cellular mechanisms of atrial contractile dysfunction caused by sustained atrial tachycardia," *Circulation*, vol. 98, no. 7, pp. 719–727, 1998.

[94] M. C. E. F. Wijffels, C. J. H. J. Kirchhof, R. Dorland, et al., "Electrical remodeling due to atrial fibrillation in chronically instrumented conscious goats: Roles of neurohumoral changes, ischemia, atrial stretch, and high rate of electrical activation," *Circulation*, vol. 96, no. 10, pp. 3710–3720, 1997.

[95] V. Algalarrondo and S. Nattel, "Potassium channel remodeling in heart disease," *Card Electrophysiol Clin*, 2016, epub ahead of print.

[96] A. J. Workman, K. A. Kane, and A. C. Rankin, "Cellular bases for human atrial fibrillation," *Heart Rhythm*, vol. 5, no. 6-2, pp. S1–S6, 2008.

[97] H. Sun, D. Chartier, N. Leblanc, et al., "Intracellular calcium changes and tachycardia-induced contractile dysfunction in canine atrial myocytes," *Cardiovasc Res*, vol. 49, no. 4, pp. 751–761, 2001.

[98] S. Nattel, A. Maguy, S. Le Bouter, et al., "Arrhythmogenic ion-channel remodeling in the heart: Heart failure, myocardial infarction, and atrial fibrillation," *Physiol Rev*, vol. 87, no. 2, pp. 425–456, 2007.

[99] M. C. Wijffels, C. J. Kirchhof, R. Dorland, et al., "Atrial fibrillation begets atrial fibrillation: a study in awake chronically ins trumented goats," *Circulation*, vol. 92, no. 7, pp. 1954–1968, 1995.

[100] T. J. Cha, J. R. Ehrlich, L. Zhang, et al., "Atrial tachycardia remodeling of pulmonary vein cardiomyocytes: Comparison with left atrium and potential relation to arrhythmogenesis," *Circulation*, vol. 111, no. 6, pp. 728–735, 2005.

[101] L. Yue, J. Feng, R. Gaspo, et al., "Ionic remodeling underlying action potential changes in a canine model of atrial fibrillation," *Circ Res*, vol. 81, no. 4, pp. 512–525, 1997.

[102] D. R. V. Wagoner, A. L. Pond, P. M. Mccarthy, et al., "Outward K^+ current densities and Kv1.5 expression are reduced in chronic human atrial fibrillation," *Circ Res*, vol. 80, pp. 772–781, 2006.

[103] A. J. Workman, K. A. Kane, and A. C. Rankin, "The contribution of ionic currents to changes in refractoriness of human atrial myocytes associated with chronic atrial fibrillation," *Cardiovasc Res*, vol. 52, no. 2, pp. 226–235, 2001.

[104] N. Voigt, A. Friedrich, M. Bock, et al., "Differential phosphorylation-dependent regulation of constitutively active and muscarinic receptor-activated $I_{K,ACh}$ channels in patients with chronic atrial fibrillation," *Cardiovasc Res*, vol. 74, no. 3, pp. 426–437, 2007.

[105] D. Dobrev, E. Wettwer, A. Kortner, et al., "Human inward rectifier potassium channels in chronic and postoperative atrial fibrillation," *Cardiovasc Res*, vol. 54, no. 2, pp. 397–404, 2002.

[106] D. Dobrev, A. Friedrich, N. Voigt, et al., "The G protein-gated potassium current $I_{K,ACh}$ is constitutively active in patients with chronic atrial fibrillation," *Circulation*, vol. 112, no. 24, pp. 3697–3706, 2005.

[107] N. Gaborit, M. Steenman, G. Lamirault, et al., "Human atrial ion channel and transporter subunit gene-expression remodeling associated with valvular heart disease and atrial fibrillation," *Circulation*, vol. 112, no. 4, pp. 471–481, 2005.

[108] R. Bosch and X. Zeng, "Ionic mechanisms of electrical remodeling in human atrial fibrillation," *Cardiovasc Res*, vol. 44, pp. 121–131, 1999.

[109] D. Dobrev, E. Graf, E. Wettwer, et al., "Molecular basis of downregulation of G-protein-coupled inward rectifying K^+ current $I_{K,ACh}$ in chronic human atrial fibrillation: decrease in GIRK4 mRNA correlates with reduced $I_{K,ACh}$ and muscarinic receptor-mediated shorte," *Circulation*, vol. 104, no. 21, pp. 2551–2557, 2001.

[110] M. Skasa, E. Jungling, E. Picht, et al., "L-type calcium currents in atrial myocytes from patients with persistent and non-persistent atrial fibrillation," *Basic Res Cardiol*, vol. 96, no. 2, pp. 151–159, 2001.

[111] T. Christ, P. Boknik, S. Wöhrl, et al., "L-type Ca^{2+} current downregulation in chronic human atrial fibrillation is associated with increased activity of protein phosphatases," *Circulation*, vol. 110, no. 17, pp. 2651–2657, 2004.

[112] N. Voigt, A. W. Trafford, U. Ravens, et al., "Abstract 2630: Cellular and molecular determinants of altered atrial Ca^{2+} signaling in patients with chronic atrial fibrillation," *Circulation*, vol. 120, no. 18, pp. S667–S668, 2009.

[113] N. Voigt, N. Li, Q. Wang, et al., "Enhanced sarcoplasmic reticulum Ca^{2+} leak and increased Na^+-Ca^{2+} exchanger function underlie delayed afterdepolarizations in patients with chronic atrial fibrillation," *Circulation*, vol. 125, no. 17, pp. 2059–2070, 2012.

[114] J. B. Grammer, R. F. Bosch, V. Kühlkamp, et al., "Molecular remodeling of Kv4.3 potassium channels in human atrial fibrillation," *J Cardiovasc Electrophysiol*, vol. 11, no. 6, pp. 626–633, 2000.

[115] T. Christ, E. Wettwer, N. Voigt, et al., "Pathology-specific effects of the $I_{Kur}/I_{to}/I_{K,ACh}$ blocker AVE0118 on ion channels in human chronic atrial fibrillation," *Br J Pharmacol*, vol. 154, no. 8, pp. 1619–1630, 2008.

[116] R. Caballero, M. G. de la Fuente, R. Gomez, et al., "In humans, chronic atrial fibrillation decreases the transient outward current and ultrarapid component of the delayed rectifier current differentially on each atria and increases the slow component of the delayed rectifier current in both," *J Am Coll Cardiol*, vol. 55, no. 21, pp. 2346–2354, 2010.

[117] M. C. Brandt, L. Priebe, T. Böhle, et al., "The ultrarapid and the transient outward K^+ current in human atrial fibrillation. their possible role in postoperative atrial fibrillation," *J Mol Cell Cardiol*, vol. 32, no. 10, pp. 1885–1896, 2000.

[118] L.-P. Lai and S. K. S. Huang, "Changes in the mRNA levels of delayed rectifier potassium channels in human atrial fibrillation," *Cardiology*, vol. 92, no. 4, pp. 1–8, 2000.

[119] B. J. Brundel, I. C. Van Gelder, R. H. Henning, et al., "Ion channel remodeling is related to intraoperative atrial effective refractory periods in patients with paroxysmal and persistent atrial fibrillation," *Circulation*, vol. 103, no. 5, pp. 684–690, 2001.

[120] S. Oh, K.-B. Kim, H. Ahn, et al., "Remodeling of ion channel expression in patients with chronic atrial fibrillation and mitral valvular heart disease," *Korean J Intern Med*, vol. 25, no. 4, pp. 377–385, 2010.

[121] B. J. Brundel, I. C. Van Gelder, R. H. Henning, et al., "Alterations in potassium channel gene expression in atria of patients with persistent and paroxysmal atrial fibrillation: differential regulation of protein and mRNA levels for K^+ channels," *J Am Coll Cardiol*, vol. 37, no. 3, pp. 926–932, 2001.

[122] S. Neef, N. Dybkova, S. Sossalla, et al., "Camkii-dependent diastolic sr Ca^{2+} leak and elevated diastolic Ca^{2+} levels in right atrial myocardium of patients with atrial fibrillation," *Circ Res*, vol. 106, no. 6, pp. 1134–1144, 2010.

[123] U. Schotten, M. Greiser, D. Benke, et al., "Atrial fibrillation-induced atrial contractile dysfunction: A tachycardiomyopathy of a different sort," *Cardiovasc Res*, vol. 53, no. 1, pp. 192–201, 2002.

[124] A. J. Workman, K. A. Kane, and A. C. Rankin, "Characterisation of the Na,K pump current in atrial cells from patients with and without chronic atrial fibrillation," *Cardiovasc Res*, vol. 59, no. 3, pp. 593–602, 2003.

[125] S. Sossalla, B. Kallmeyer, S. Wagner, et al., "Altered Na^+ currents in atrial fibrillation. effects of ranolazine on arrhythmias and contractility in human atrial myocardium," *J Am Coll Cardiol*, vol. 55, no. 21, pp. 2330–2342, 2010.

[126] H. S. Duffy and A. L. Wit, "Is there a role for remodeled connexins in AF?No simple answers," *J Mol Cell Cardiol*, vol. 44, no. 1, pp. 4–13, 2008.

[127] A. Loewe, "Arrhythmic potency of human electrophysiological models adapted to chronic and familial atrial fibrillation," Master Thesis, Institute of Biomedical Engineering, Karlsruhe Institute of Technology (KIT), Karlsruhe, 2013.

[128] E. M. Vaughan Williams, "A classification of antiarrhythmic actions reassessed after a decade of new drugs," *J Clin Pharmacol*, vol. 24, no. 4, pp. 129–147, 1984.

[129] A. Loewe, Y. Lutz, M. Wilhelms, et al., "In-silico assessment of the dynamic effects of amiodarone and dronedarone on human atrial patho-electrophysiology," *Europace*, vol. 16, no. S4, pp. iv30–iv38, 2014.

[130] J. Y. Le Heuzey, G. M. De Ferrari, D. Radzik, et al., "A short-term, randomized, double-blind, parallel-group study to evaluate the efficacy and safety of dronedarone versus amiodarone in patients with persistent atrial fibrillation: The DIONYSOS study," *J Cardiovasc Electrophysiol*, vol. 21, no. 6, pp. 597–605, 2010.

[131] L. A. Siddoway, "Amiodarone: Guidelines for use and-monitoring," *Am Fam Physician*, vol. 68, no. 11, pp. 2189–2196, 2003.

[132] N. Gassanov, M. Dietlein, E. Caglayan, et al., "Amiodaron-induzierte Schilddrüsenfunktionsstörungen," *DMW - Dtsch Medizinische Wochenschrift*, vol. 135, no. 16, pp. 807–811, 2010.

[133] I. Kodama, "Amiodarone: Ionic and cellular mechanisms of action of the most promising class III agent," *Am J Cardiol*, vol. 9149, no. 99, pp. 20r–28r, 1999.

[134] N. Butte, B. W. Böttiger, and P. Teschendorf, "Amiodaron zur Therapie perioperativer kardialer Rhythmusstörungen: Ein Breitspektrumantiarrhythmikum?" *Anaesthesist*, vol. 57, no. 12, pp. 1183–1192, 2008.

[135] R. L. Page, B. Hamad, and P. Kirkpatrick, "Dronedarone," *Nat Rev Drug Discov*, vol. 8, pp. 769–770, 2009.

[136] S. Kathofer, D. Thomas, and C. A. Karle, "The novel antiarrhythmic drug dronedarone: Comparison with amiodarone," *Cardiovasc Drug Rev*, vol. 23, no. 3, pp. 217–230, 2005.

[137] R. Bogdan, H. Goegelein, and H. Ruetten, "Effect of dronedarone on Na^+, Ca^{2+} and HCN channels," *Naunyn-Schmied Arch Pharmacol*, vol. 383, no. 4, pp. 347–356, 2011.

[138] N. Penugonda, A. Mohmand-Borkowski, and J. F. Burke, "Dronedarone for atrial fibrillation: How does it compare with amiodarone?" *Cleve Clin J Med*, vol. 78, no. 3, pp. 179–185, 2011.

[139] R. Tadros, S. Nattel, and J. G. Andrade, "Dronedarone: Basic pharmacology and clinical use," *Card Electrophysiol Clin*, 2016, epub ahead of print.

[140] F. Buccelletti, P. Iacomini, G. Botta, et al., "Efficacy and safety of vernakalant in recent-onset atrial fibrillation after the european medicines agency approval: systematic review and meta-analysis," *J Clin Pharmacol*, vol. 52, no. 12, pp. 1872–1878, 2012.

[141] A. J. Camm, A. Capucci, S. H. Hohnloser, et al., "A randomized active-controlled study comparing the efficacy and safety of vernakalant to amiodarone in recent-onset atrial fibrillation," *J Am Coll Cardiol*, vol. 57, no. 3, pp. 313–321, 2011.

[142] P. R. Kowey, P. Dorian, L. B. Mitchell, et al., "Vernakalant hydrochloride for the rapid conversion of atrial fibrillation after cardiac surgery - a randomized, double-blind, placebo-controlled trial," *Circ Arrhythmia Electrophysiol*, vol. 2, no. 6, pp. 652–659, 2009.

[143] C. M. Pratt, D. Roy, C. Torp-Pedersen, et al., "Usefulness of vernakalant hydrochloride injection for rapid conversion of atrial fibrillation," *Am J Cardiol*, vol. 106, no. 9, pp. 1277–1283, 2010.

[144] I. G. Stiell, J. S. Roos, K. M. Kavanagh, et al., "A multicenter, open-label study of vernakalant for the conversion of atrial fibrillation to sinus rhythm," *Am Heart J*, vol. 159, no. 6, pp. 1095–1101, 2010.

[145] A. J. Camm, E. Toft, C. Torp-Pedersen, et al., "Efficacy and safety of vernakalant in patients with atrial flutter: A randomized, double-blind, placebo-controlled trial," *Europace*, vol. 14, no. 6, pp. 804–809, 2012.

[146] D. Fedida, "Vernakalant (RSD1235): a novel, atrial-selective antifibrillatory agent," *Expert Opin Investig Drugs*, vol. 16, no. 4, pp. 519–532, 2007.

[147] A. Luik, A. Radzewitz, M. Kieser, et al., "Cryoballoon versus open irrigated radiofrequency ablation in patients with paroxysmal atrial fibrillation: The prospective, randomized, controlled, noninferiority FreezeAF study," *Circulation*, vol. 132, no. 14, pp. 1311–1319, 2015.

[148] S. Magnani, D. Muser, W. Chik, et al., "Adjunct ablation strategies for persistent atrial fibrillation-beyond pulmonary vein isolation," *J Thorac Dis*, vol. 7, no. 2, pp. 178–184, 2015.

[149] A. Verma, C.-Y. Jiang, T. R. Betts, et al., "Approaches to catheter ablation for persistent atrial fibrillation," *N Engl J Med*, vol. 372, no. 19, pp. 1812–1822, 2015.

[150] S. M. Narayan, K. Shivkumar, D. E. Krummen, et al., "Panoramic electrophysiological mapping but not electrogram morphology identifies stable sources for human atrial fibrillation: Stable atrial fibrillation rotors and focal sources relate poorly to fractionated electrograms," *Circ Arrhythmia Electrophysiol*, vol. 6, no. 1, pp. 58–67, 2013.

[151] M. Haïssaguerre, M. Hocini, A. Denis, et al., "Driver domains in persistent atrial fibrillation," *Circulation*, vol. 130, no. 7, pp. 530–538, 2014.

[152] A. L. Hodgkin and A. F. Huxley, "A quantitative description of membrane current and its application to conduction and excitation in nerve," *Bull Math Biol*, vol. 52, no. 1-2, pp. 25–71, 1990.

[153] J.-M. Dubois, G. Ouanounou, and B. Rouzaire-Dubois, "The Boltzmann equation in molecular biology," *Prog Biophys Mol Biol*, vol. 99, no. 2-3, pp. 87–93, 2009.

[154] D. P. Zipes, *Cardiac electrophysiology: From cell to bedside*, 6th ed. Philadelphia: Elsevier Saunders, 2014.

[155] H. Hettmann, "Benchmarking electrophysiological models of human atrial myocytes," Bachelor Thesis, Institute of Biomedical Engineering, Karlsruhe Institute of Technology (KIT), Karlsruhe, 2012.

[156] M. Wilhelms, H. Hettmann, M. M. Maleckar, et al., "Benchmarking electrophysiological models of human atrial myocytes," *Front Physiol*, vol. 3, no. 487, 2013.

[157] C. H. Luo and Y. Rudy, "A dynamic model of the cardiac ventricular action potential. I. simulations of ionic currents and concentration changes," *Circ Res*, vol. 74, no. 6, pp. 1071–1096, 1994.

[158] M. W. Krueger, A. Dorn, D. U. J. Keller, et al., "In-silico modeling of atrial repolarization in normal and atrial fibrillation remodeled state," *Med Biol Eng Comput*, vol. 51, no. 10, pp. 1105–1119, 2013.

[159] C. C. Fink, B. Slepchenko, I. I. Moraru, et al., "An image-based model of calcium waves in differentiated neuroblastoma cells," *Biophys J*, vol. 79, no. 1, pp. 163–183, 2000.

[160] N. A. Trayanova and P. M. Boyle, *Modeling the heart and the circulatory system*. Cham: Springer International Publishing, 2015, ch. 1, pp. 1–27.

[161] M. Wallman, N. P. Smith, and B. Rodriguez, "A comparative study of graph-based, eikonal, and monodomain simulations for the estimation of cardiac activation times," *IEEE Trans Biomed Eng*, vol. 59, no. 6, pp. 1739–1748, 2012.

[162] E. Pernod, M. Sermesant, E. Konukoglu, et al., "Visual computing in biology and medicine: A multi-front eikonal model of cardiac electrophysiology for interactive simulation of radio-frequency ablation," *Comput Graph*, vol. 35, no. 2, pp. 431–440, 2011.

[163] L. Tung, "A bi-domain model for describing ischemic myocardial D-C potentials," PhD thesis, Dept. of Electrical Engineering and Computer Science, Massachusetts Institute of Technology, 1978.

[164] J. Keener and J. Sneyd, "Mathematical physiology: II: Systems physiology," New York, 2008.

[165] G. Seemann, *Modeling of electrophysiology and tension development in the human heart*, Karlsruhe Transactions on Biomedical Engineering, vol. 1. Karlsruhe: Universitätsverlag Karlsruhe, 2005.

[166] E. J. Vigmond, R. Weber dos Santos, A. J. Prassl, et al., "Solvers for the cardiac bidomain equations," *Prog Biophys Mol Biol*, vol. 96, no. 1-3, pp. 3–18, 2008.

[167] P. Pathmanathan, M. O. Bernabeu, R. Bordas, et al., "A numerical guide to the solution of the bidomain equations of cardiac electrophysiology," *Prog Biophys Mol Biol*, vol. 102, no. 2-3, pp. 136–155, 2010.

[168] E. M. Wülfers, "A comparison of mathematical models and numerical schemes for simulating body surface potential maps on realistic geometries," Master Thesis, Institute of Biomedical Engineering, Karlsruhe Institute of Technology (KIT), 2016.

[169] G. Seemann, F. B. Sachse, M. Karl, et al., "Framework for modular, flexible and efficient solving the cardiac bidomain equations using PETSc," *Prog Ind Math (ECMI 2008)*, vol. 15, pp. 363–369, 2010.

[170] S. A. Niederer, E. Kerfoot, A. P. Benson, et al., "Verification of cardiac tissue electrophysiology simulators using an N-version benchmark," *Philos Trans R Soc A Math Phys Eng Sci*, vol. 369, no. 1954, pp. 4331–4351, 2011.

[171] E. W. Dijkstra, "A note on two problems in connexion with graphs," *Numer Math*, vol. 1, no. 1, pp. 269–271, 1959.

[172] T. J. Misa, "An interview with Edsger W. Dijkstra," *Commun ACM*, vol. 53, no. 8, p. 41, 2010.

[173] P. Hart, N. Nilsson, and B. Raphael, "A formal basis for the heuristic determination of minimum cost paths," *IEEE Trans Syst Sci Cybern*, vol. 4, no. 2, pp. 100–107, 1968.

[174] E. Konukoglu, M. Sermesant, O. Clatz, et al., "A recursive anisotropic fast marching approach to reaction diffusion equation: Application to tumor growth modeling," *Inf Process Med imaging*, vol. 20, pp. 687–699, 2007.

[175] J. L. Qian and W. W. Symes, "Paraxial eikonal solvers for anisotropic quasi-p travel times," *J Comput Phys*, vol. 173, no. 1, pp. 256–278, 2001.

[176] M. Sermesant, E. Konukoglu, H. Delingette, et al., "An anisotropic multi-front fast marching method for real-time simulation of cardiac electrophysiology," in *Funct Imaging Model Hear*, Lecture Notes in Computer Science, F. Sachse and G. Seemann, Eds., vol. 4466. Berlin / Heidelberg: Springer, 2007, pp. 160–169.

[177] D. U. J. Keller, F. M. Weber, G. Seemann, et al., "Ranking the influence of tissue conductivities on forward-calculated ECGs," *IEEE Trans Biomed Eng*, vol. 57, no. 7, pp. 1568–1576, 2010.

[178] R. S. Oakes, T. J. Badger, E. G. Kholmovski, et al., "Detection and quantification of left atrial structural remodeling with delayed-enhancement magnetic resonance imaging in patients with atrial fibrillation," *Circulation*, vol. 119, no. 13, pp. 1758–1767, 2009.

[179] B. R. Knowles, D. Caulfield, M. Cooklin, et al., "3-D visualization of acute RF ablation lesions using MRI for the simultaneous determination of the patterns of necrosis and edema," *IEEE Trans Biomed Eng*, vol. 57, no. 6, pp. 1467–1475, 2010.

[180] R. Karim, A. Arujuna, A. Brazier, et al., "Automatic segmentation of left atrial scar from delayed-enhancement magnetic resonance imaging," in *Funct Imaging Model Hear*, Lecture Notes in Computer Science, D. N. Metaxas and L. Axel, Eds., vol. 6666. Berlin/Heidelberg: Springer, 2011, pp. 63–70.

[181] N. Akoum, M. Daccarett, C. McGann, et al., "Atrial fibrosis helps select the appropriate patient and strategy in catheter ablation of atrial fibrillation: A DE-MRI guided approach," *J Cardiovasc Electrophysiol*, vol. 22, no. 1, pp. 16–22, 2011.

[182] M. W. Krueger, K. S. Rhode, M. D. O'Neill, et al., "Patient-specific modeling of atrial fibrosis increases the accuracy of sinus rhythm simulations and may explain maintenance of atrial fibrillation," *J Electrocardiol*, vol. 47, no. 3, pp. 324–328, 2014.

[183] M. W. Krueger, G. Seemann, K. Rhode, et al., "Personalization of atrial anatomy and electrophysiology as a basis for clinical modeling of radio-frequency ablation of atrial fibrillation," *IEEE Trans Med Imaging*, vol. 32, no. 1, pp. 73–84, 2013.

[184] C. S. Henriquez, "Simulating the electrical behavior of cardiac tissue using the bidomain model," *Crit Rev Biomed Eng*, vol. 21, no. 1, pp. 1–77, 1993.

[185] A. SippensGroenewegen, H. A. Peeters, E. R. Jessurun, et al., "Body surface mapping during pacing at multiple sites in the human atrium: P-wave morphology of ectopic right atrial activation," *Circulation*, vol. 97, no. 4, pp. 369–380, 1998.

[186] K. S. Cole, "Dynamic electrical characteristics of the squid axon membrane," *Arch sci physiol*, vol. 3, no. 2, pp. 253–258, 1949.

[187] E. Neher and B. Sakmann, "Single-channel currents recorded from membrane of denervated frog muscle fibres," *Nature*, vol. 260, no. 5554, pp. 799–802, 1976.

[188] A. Loewe, M. Wilhelms, F. Fischer, et al., "Arrhythmic potency of human ether-à-go-go-related gene mutations L532P and N588K in a computational model of human atrial myocytes," *Europace*, vol. 16, no. 3, pp. 435–443, 2014.

[189] J. Dunlop, M. Bowlby, R. Peri, et al., "High-throughput electrophysiology: An emerging paradigm for ion-channel screening and physiology," *Nat Rev Drug Discov*, vol. 7, no. 4, pp. 358–368, 2008.

[190] T. F. Coleman and Y. Li, "An interior trust region approach for nonlinear minimization subject to bounds," *SIAM J Optim*, vol. 6, no. 2, pp. 418–445, 1996.

[191] B. B. C. B. Hui, S. Dokos, and N. H. Lovell, "Parameter identifiability of cardiac ionic models using a novel CellML least squares optimization tool," in *IEEE Eng Med Biol Soc EMBC*, 2007, pp. 5307–5310.

[192] A. Bueno-Orovio, E. M. Cherry, and F. H. Fenton, "Minimal model for human ventricular action potentials in tissue," *JournalAnnals ofTheoretical Biol*, vol. 253, no. 3, pp. 544–560, 2008.

[193] G. Seemann, S. Lurz, D. U. J. Keller, et al., "Adaption of mathematical ion channel models to measured data using the particle swarm optimization," in *IFMBE Proc*, vol. 22, 2008, pp. 2507–2510.

[194] F. Chen, A. Chu, X. Yang, et al., "Identification of the parameters of the beeler-reuter ionic equation with a partially perturbed particle swarm optimization," *IEEE Trans Biomed Eng*, vol. 59, no. 12, pp. 3412–3421, 2012.

[195] Z. Syed, E. Vigmond, S. Nattel, et al., "Atrial cell action potential parameter fitting using genetic algorithms," *Med Biol Eng Comput*, vol. 43, no. 5, pp. 561–571, 2005.

[196] D. Szekely, J. I. Vandenberg, S. Dokos, et al., "An improved curvilinear gradient method for parameter optimization in complex biological models," *Med Biol Eng Comput*, vol. 49, no. 3, pp. 289–296, 2011.

[197] C. T. Bot, A. R. Kherlopian, F. A. Ortega, et al., "Rapid genetic algorithm optimization of a mouse computational model: Benefits for anthropomorphization of neonatal mouse cardiomyocytes," *Front Physiol*, vol. 3, p. 421, 2012.

[198] S.-K. S. Fan, Y.-C. Liang, and E. Zahara, "A genetic algorithm and a particle swarm optimizer hybridized with Nelder-Mead simplex search," *Comput Ind Eng*, vol. 50, no. 4, pp. 401–425, 2006.

[199] C. Blum, "Hybrid metaheuristics," *Comput Oper Res*, vol. 37, no. 3, pp. 430–431, 2010.

[200] A. Loewe, M. Wilhelms, J. Schmid, et al., "Parameter estimation of ion current formulations requires hybrid optimization approach to be both accurate and reliable," *Front Bioeng Biotechnol*, vol. 3, p. 209, 2015.

[201] M. Wilhelms, J. Schmid, M. J. Krause, et al., "Calibration of human cardiac ion current models to patch clamp measurement data," in *Comput Cardiol*, vol. 39, 2012, pp. 229–232.

[202] A. Loewe, M. Wilhelms, F. Fischer, et al., "Impact of hERG mutations on simulated human atrial action potentials," in *Biomed Eng / Biomed Tech*, vol. 58, no. s1, 2013.

[203] A. Loewe, M. Wilhelms, J. Schmid, et al., "A hybrid optimization approach for the adaptation of cardiac ion current formulations to voltage and patch clamp data," in *Card Physiome Work*, Bar Harbor, 2013.

[204] J. Schmid, "Optimierte Parameteranpassung für Simulationen der menschlichen Vorhofelektrophysiologie," Diploma Thesis, Institute of Biomedical Engineering, Karlsruhe Institute of Technology (KIT), 2012.

[205] M. Wilhelms, *Multiscale modeling of cardiac electrophysiology: Adaptation to atrial and ventricular rhythm disorders and pharmacological treatment*, Karlsruhe Transactions on Biomedical Engineering, vol. 20. Karlsruhe: KIT Scientific Publishing, 2013.

[206] S. Rush and H. Larsen, "A practical algorithm for solving dynamic membrane equations," *IEEE Trans Biomed Eng*, vol. 25, no. 4, pp. 389–392, 1978.

[207] J. Kennedy and R. Eberhart, "Particle swarm optimization," in *Encycl Mach Learn*, vol. 4, 1995, pp. 1942–1948.

[208] R. Poli, J. Kennedy, and T. Blackwell, "Particle swarm optimization," *Swarm Intell*, vol. 1, no. 1, pp. 33–57, 2007.

[209] M. Clerc and J. Kennedy, "The particle swarm - explosion, stability, and convergence in a multidimensional complex space," *IEEE Trans Evol Comput*, vol. 6, no. 1, pp. 58–73, 2002.

[210] G. C. L. Bett, Q. Zhou, and R. L. Rasmusson, "Models of hERG gating," *Biophys J*, vol. 101, no. 3, pp. 631–642, 2011.

[211] E. A. Sobie, "Parameter sensitivity analysis in electrophysiological models using multivariable regression," *Biophys J*, vol. 96, no. 4, pp. 1264–1274, 2009.

[212] A. X. Sarkar and E. A. Sobie, "Regression analysis for constraining free parameters in electrophysiological models of cardiac cells," *PLoS Comput Biol*, vol. 6, no. 9, p. e1000914, 2010.

[213] K. Tøndel, S. A. Niederer, S. Land, et al., "Insight into model mechanisms through automatic parameter fitting: A new methodological framework for model development," *BMC Syst Biol*, vol. 8, p. 59, 2014.

[214] A. Sher, K. Wang, A. Wathen, et al., "A local sensitivity analysis method for developing biological models with identifiable parameters: Application to L-type calcium channel modelling," *IEEE Int Conf e-Science*, pp. 176–181, 2010.

[215] A. A. Sher, K. Wang, A. Wathen, et al., "A local sensitivity analysis method for developing biological models with identifiable parameters: Application to cardiac ionic channel modelling," *Futur Gener Comput Syst*, vol. 29, no. 2, pp. 591–598, feb 2013.

[216] M. Fink and D. Noble, "Markov models for ion channels: Versatility versus identifiability and speed," *Philos Trans A Math Phys Eng Sci*, vol. 367, no. 1896, pp. 2161–2179, 2009.

[217] A. Nygren, L. J. Leon, and W. R. Giles, "Simulations of the human atrial action potential," *Philos Trans R Soc A Math Phys Eng Sci*, vol. 359, no. 1783, pp. 1111–1125, 2001.

[218] M. M. Maleckar, J. L. Greenstein, W. R. Giles, et al., "K^+ current changes account for the rate dependence of the action potential in the human atrial myocyte," *Am J Physiol Heart Circ Physiol*, vol. 297, no. 4, pp. H1398–H1410, 2009.

[219] J. T. Koivumäki, T. Korhonen, and P. Tavi, "Impact of sarcoplasmic reticulum calcium release on calcium dynamics and action potential morphology in human atrial myocytes: A computational study," *PLoS Comput Biol*, vol. 7, no. 1, p. e1001067, 2011.

[220] E. Grandi, S. V. Pandit, N. Voigt, et al., "Human atrial action potential and Ca^{2+} model sinus rhythm and chronic atrial fibrillation," *Circ Res*, vol. 109, no. 9, pp. 1055–1066, 2011.

[221] K. H. W. J. ten Tusscher and a. V. Panfilov, "Alternans and spiral breakup in a human ventricular tissue model," *Am J Physiol Heart Circ Physiol*, vol. 291, no. 3, pp. H1088–H1100, 2006.

[222] T. O'Hara, L. Virág, A. Varró, et al., "Simulation of the undiseased human cardiac ventricular action potential: Model formulation and experimental validation," *PLoS Comput Biol*, vol. 7, no. 5, p. e1002061, 2011.

[223] M. Clerx, P. Collins, and P. G. Volders, "Applying novel identification protocols to markov models of I_{Na}," in *Comput Cardiol*, vol. 42, 2015, pp. 889–892.

[224] G. R. Mirams, K. Beattie, J. B. Louttit, et al., "Novel voltage protocols for determining hERG channel kinetics," *Biophys J*, vol. 108, no. 2, p. 121a, 2015.

[225] K. A. Beattie, T. de Boer, D. J. Gavaghan, et al., "Voltage protocol design for hERG channel model selection," *J Pharmacol Toxicol Methods*, vol. 75, p. 164, 2013.

[226] K. Tøndel, S. Land, S. A. Niederer, et al., "Quantifying inter-species differences in contractile function through biophysical modelling," *J Physiol*, vol. 593, no. 5, pp. 1083–1111, 2015.

[227] M. A. Khalef, "Comparison of statistic and optimization-based approaches for parameter estimation of ion current formulations," Bachelor Thesis, Institute of Biomedical Engineering, Karlsruhe Institute of Technology (KIT), 2015.

[228] H. Abdi, "Partial least squares regression and projection on latent structure regression (PLS regression)," *Wiley Interdiscip Rev Comput Stat*, vol. 2, no. 1, pp. 97–106, 2010.

[229] H. Martens and M. Martens, *Multivariate analysis of quality - an introduction*. Chichester: John Wiley & Sons Ltd, 2001.

[230] S. Wold, H. Martens, and H. Wold, *The multivariate calibration problem in chemistry solved by the PLS method*, Matrix pencils. Lecture Notes in Mathematics. Berlin/Heidelberg: Springer, 1983, vol. 973, pp. 286–293.

[231] K. Tøndel, U. G. Indahl, A. B. Gjuvsland, et al., "Multi-way metamodelling facilitates insight into the complex input-output maps of nonlinear dynamic models," *BMC Syst Biol*, vol. 6, no. 1, p. 88, 2012.

[232] K. Tøndel, U. G. Indahl, A. B. Gjuvsland, et al., "Hierarchical cluster-based partial least squares regression (HC-PLSR) is an efficient tool for metamodelling of nonlinear dynamic models," *BMC Syst Biol*, vol. 5, p. 90, 2011.

[233] J. C. Bezdek, "Pattern recognition with fuzzy objective function algorithms," *SIAM Rev*, vol. 25, no. 3, pp. 442–442, 1983.

[234] I. Berget, B. H. Mevik, and T. Næs, "New modifications and applications of fuzzy C-means methodology," *Comput Stat Data Anal*, vol. 52, no. 5, pp. 2403–2418, 2008.

[235] T. Næs, E. Kubberød, and H. Sivertsen, "Identifying and interpreting market segments using conjoint analysis," *Food Qual Prefer*, vol. 12, no. 2, pp. 133–143, 2001.

[236] T. Næs and T. Isaksson, "Splitting of calibration data by cluster-analysis," *J Chemom*, vol. 5, no. 1, pp. 49–65, 1991.

[237] A. M. D. McKay, R. J. Beckman, W. J. Conover, et al., "A comparison of three methods for selecting values of input variables in the analysis of output from a computer code," *Technometrics*, vol. 21, no. 2, pp. 239–245, 2016.

[238] D. Holtmann, *Grundlegende multivariate Modelle der sozialwissenschaftlichen Datenanalyse*. Potsdam: Universitätsverlag Potsdam, 2010.

[239] M. J. McPate, R. S. Duncan, J. T. Milnes, et al., "The N588K-hERG K^+ channel mutation in the 'short QT syndrome': Mechanism of gain-in-function determined at 37°C," *Biochem Biophys Res Commun*, vol. 334, no. 2, pp. 441–449, 2005.

[240] J. Eldstrom, Z. Wang, D. Werry, et al., "Microscopic mechanisms for long QT syndrome type 1 revealed by single-channel analysis of I_{Ks} with S3 domain mutations in KCNQ1," *Heart Rhythm*, vol. 12, no. 2, pp. 386–394, 2015.

[241] C. E. Woods and J. Olgin, "Atrial fibrillation therapy now and in the future: Drugs, biologicals, and ablation," *Circ Res*, vol. 114, no. 9, pp. 1532–1546, 2014.

[242] R. R. Tilz, A. Rillig, A. M. Thum, et al., "Catheter ablation of long-standing persistent atrial fibrillation: 5-year outcomes of the Hamburg sequential ablation strategy," *J Am Coll Cardiol*, vol. 60, no. 19, pp. 1921–1929, 2012.

[243] M. Takigawa, A. Takahashi, T. Kuwahara, et al., "Long-term follow-up after catheter ablation of paroxysmal atrial fibrillation the incidence of recurrence and progression of atrial fibrillation," *Circ Arrhythmia Electrophysiol*, vol. 7, no. 2, pp. 267–273, apr 2014.

[244] M. F. Sinner, P. T. Ellinor, T. Meitinger, et al., "Genome-wide association studies of atrial fibrillation: Past, present, and future," *Cardiovasc Res*, vol. 89, no. 4, pp. 701–709, 2011.

[245] R. Otway, J. I. Vandenberg, and D. Fatkin, "Atrial fibrillation - a new cardiac channelopathy," *Hear Lung Circ*, vol. 16, no. 5, pp. 356–360, 2007.

[246] N. R. Tucker and P. T. Ellinor, "Emerging directions in the genetics of atrial fibrillation," *Circ Res*, vol. 114, no. 9, pp. 1469–1482, 2014.

[247] M. F. Sinner, N. R. Tucker, K. L. Lunetta, et al., "Integrating genetic, transcriptional, and functional analyses to identify 5 novel genes for atrial fibrillation," *Circulation*, vol. 130, no. 15, pp. 1225–1235, 2014.

[248] D. Fatkin, R. Otway, and J. I. Vandenberg, "Genes and atrial fibrillation: a new look at an old problem," *Circulation*, vol. 116, no. 7, pp. 782–792, 2007.

[249] M. Courtemanche and A. T. Winfree, "Re-entract rotating waves in a Beeler-Reuter based model of two-dimensional cardiac electrical activity," *Int J Bifurc Chaos*, vol. 1, pp. 431–444, 1991.

[250] S. Nattel, "New ideas about atrial fibrillation 50 years on," *Nature*, vol. 415, no. 6868, pp. 219–226, 2002.

[251] K. Hong, D. R. Piper, A. Diaz-Valdecantos, et al., "De novo KCNQ1 mutation responsible for atrial fibrillation and short QT syndrome in utero," *Cardiovasc Res*, vol. 68, no. 3, pp. 433–440, 2005.

[252] D. Hassel, E. P. Scholz, N. Trano, et al., "Deficient zebrafish ether-à-go-go-related gene channel gating causes short-QT syndrome in zebrafish reggae mutants," *Circulation*, vol. 117, no. 7, pp. 866–875, 2008.

[253] T. Peitersen, M. Grunnet, A. P. Benson, et al., "Computational analysis of the effects of the hERG channel opener NS1643 in a human ventricular cell model," *Heart Rhythm*, vol. 5, no. 5, pp. 734–741, 2008.

[254] A. P. Benson, M. Al-Owais, and A. V. Holden, "Quantitative prediction of the arrhythmogenic effects of de novo hERG mutations in computational models of human ventricular tissues," *Eur Biophys J*, vol. 40, no. 5, pp. 627–639, 2011.

[255] C. E. Clancy and Y. Rudy, "Na^+ channel mutation that causes both Brugada and long-QT syndrome phenotypes: A simulation study of mechanism," *Circulation*, vol. 105, no. 10, pp. 1208–1213, 2002.

[256] A. P. Benson, M. Al-Owais, W. C. Tong, et al., "hERG effects on ventricular action potential duration and tissue vulnerability: A computational study," in *Funct Imaging Model Hear*, Lecture Notes in Computer Science, N. Ayache, H. Delingette, and M. Sermesant, Eds., vol. 5528. Berlin/Heidelberg: Springer, 2009, pp. 172–181.

[257] H. Zhang and J. C. Hancox, "In silico study of action potential and QT interval shortening due to loss of inactivation of the cardiac rapid delayed rectifier potassium current," *Biochem Biophys Res Commun*, vol. 322, no. 2, pp. 693–699, 2004.

[258] H. Itoh, M. Horie, M. Ito, et al., "Arrhythmogenesis in the short-QT syndrome associated with combined hERG channel gating defects: a simulation study," *Circ J*, vol. 70, no. 4, pp. 502–508, 2006.

[259] M. J. Mcpate, H. Zhang, I. Adeniran, et al., "Comparative effects of the short QT N588K mutation at 37°C on hERG K^+ channel current during ventricular, purkinje fibre and atrial action potentials: An action potential clamp study," *J Physiol Pharmacol*, vol. 60, no. 1, pp. 23–41, 2009.

[260] G. Seemann, P. Carrillo, D. L. Weiss, et al., "Investigating arrhythmogenic effects of the hERG mutation N588K in virtual human atria," in *Funct Imaging Model Hear*, Lecture Notes in Computer Science, N. Ayache, H. Delingette, and M. Sermesant, Eds., vol. 5528. Berlin / Heidelberg: Springer, 2009, pp. 144–153.

[261] P. Carrillo, G. Seemann, E. Scholz, et al., "Impact of the hERG channel mutation N588K on the electrical properties of the human atrium," in *IFMBE Proc*, vol. 22, no. 22, 2008, pp. 2583–2586.

[262] J. C. Hancox, S. Kharche, A. El Harchi, et al., "In silico investigation of a KCNQ1 mutation associated with familial atrial fibrillation," *J Electrocardiol*, vol. 47, no. 2, pp. 158–165, 2014.

[263] R. Imaniastuti, H. S. Lee, N. Kim, et al., "Computational prediction of proarrhythmogenic effect of the V241F KCNQ1 mutation in human atrium," *Prog Biophys Mol Biol*, vol. 116, no. 1, pp. 70–75, 2014.

[264] L. M. Hondeghem, L. Carlsson, and G. Duker, "Instability and triangulation of the action potential predict serious proarrhythmia, but action potential duration prolongation is antiarrhythmic," *Circulation*, vol. 103, no. 15, pp. 2004–2013, 2001.

[265] M. A. Bray, S. F. Lin, R. R. Aliev, et al., "Experimental and theoretical analysis of phase singularity dynamics in cardiac tissue," *J Cardiovasc Electrophysiol*, vol. 12, no. 6, pp. 716–722, 2001.

[266] R. H. Clayton, E. A. Zhuchkova, and A. V. Panfilov, "Phase singularities and filaments: Simplifying complexity in computational models of ventricular fibrillation," *Prog Biophys Mol Biol*, vol. 90, no. 1-3, pp. 378–398, 2006.

[267] L. J. Rantner, L. Wieser, M. C. Stühlinger, et al., "Detection of phase singularities in triangular meshes," *Methods Inf Med*, vol. 46, no. 6, pp. 646–654, 2007.

[268] R. Zou, J. Kneller, L. J. Leon, et al., "Development of a computer algorithm for the detection of phase singularities and initial application to analyze simulations of atrial fibrillation," *Chaos*, vol. 12, no. 3, pp. 764–778, 2002.

[269] M. A. Bray and J. P. Wikswo, "Use of topological charge to determine filament location and dynamics in a numerical model of scroll wave activity," *IEEE Trans Biomed Eng*, vol. 49, no. 10, pp. 1086–1093, 2002.

[270] T. Lankveld, C. B. de Vos, I. Limantoro, et al., "Systematic analysis of ECG predictors for sinus rhythm maintenance following electrical cardioversion for persistent atrial fibrillation," *Heart Rhythm*, 2016, epub ahead of print.

[271] J. Ng, A. H. Kadish, and J. J. Goldberger, "Technical considerations for dominant frequency analysis," *J Cardiovasc Electrophysiol*, vol. 18, no. 7, pp. 757–764, 2007.

[272] F. Atienza, J. Almendral, J. Jalife, et al., "Real-time dominant frequency mapping and ablation of dominant frequency sites in atrial fibrillation with left-to-right frequency

gradients predicts long-term maintenance of sinus rhythm," *Heart Rhythm*, vol. 6, no. 1, pp. 33–40, 2009.

[273] R. Mandapati, a. Skanes, J. Chen, et al., "Stable microreentrant sources as a mechanism of atrial fibrillation in the isolated sheep heart," *Circulation*, vol. 101, no. 2, pp. 194–199, 2000.

[274] A. C. Skanes, R. Mandapati, O. Berenfeld, et al., "Spatiotemporal periodicity during atrial fibrillation in the isolated sheep heart," *Circulation*, vol. 98, no. 12, pp. 1236–1248, 1998.

[275] R. Plonsey and R. C. Barr, *Bioelectricity: A quantitative approach*. Springer Science & Business Media, 2007.

[276] F. J. Harris, "On the use of windows for harmonic analysis with the discrete Fourier transform," *Proc IEEE*, vol. 66, no. 1, pp. 51–83, 1978.

[277] Y. Jiang, "Implementation of a stochastic regularization method to solve the inverse problem of electrocardiography," Master Thesis, Universität Karlsruhe (TH), 2005.

[278] C. K. Colenso, R. B. Sessions, Y. H. Zhang, et al., "Interactions between voltage sensor and pore domains in a hERG K^+ channel model from molecular simulations and the effects of a voltage sensor mutation," *J Chem Inf Model*, vol. 53, no. 6, pp. 1358–1370, 2013.

[279] N. Virag, O. Blanc, J. M. Vesin, et al., "Study of the mechanisms of arrhythmias in an anatomical computer model of human atria," in *Comput Cardiol*, vol. 26, 1999, pp. 113–116.

[280] P. Sanders, O. Berenfeld, M. Hocini, et al., "Spectral analysis identifies sites of high-frequency activity maintaining atrial fibrillation in humans," *Circulation*, vol. 112, no. 6, pp. 789–797, 2005.

[281] J. Ng and J. J. Goldberger, "Understanding and interpreting dominant frequency analysis of AF electrograms," *J Cardiovasc Electrophysiol*, vol. 18, no. 6, pp. 680–685, 2007.

[282] D. Noble, A. Varghese, P. Kohl, et al., "Improved guinea-pig ventricular cell model incorporating a diadic space, ikr and iks, and length- and tension-dependent processes," *Can J Cardiol*, vol. 14, no. 1, pp. 123–134, 1998.

[283] A. Nygren, C. Fiset, L. Firek, et al., "Mathematical model of an adult human atrial cell: The role of K^+ currents in repolarization," *Circ Res*, vol. 82, no. 1, pp. 63–81, 1998.

[284] R. Brugada, K. Hong, R. Dumaine, et al., "Sudden death associated with short-QT syndrome linked to mutations in hERG," *Circulation*, vol. 109, no. 1, pp. 30–35, 2004.

[285] J. I. Vandenberg, A. Varghese, Y. Lu, et al., "Temperature dependence of human ether-à-go-go-related gene k+ currents," *Am J Physiol Cell Physiol*, vol. 291, no. 1, pp. C165–C175, 2006.

[286] J. M. Cordeiro, R. Brugada, Y. S. Wu, et al., "Modulation of I_{Kr} inactivation by mutation N588K in KCNH2: A link to arrhythmogenesis in short QT syndrome," *Cardiovasc Res*, vol. 67, no. 3, pp. 498–509, 2005.

[287] Y. H. Zhang, C. K. Colenso, R. B. Sessions, et al., "The hERG K^+ channel S4 domain L532P mutation: Characterization at 37°C," *Biochim Biophys Acta - Biomembr*, vol. 1808, no. 10, pp. 2477–2487, 2011.

[288] M. A. Colman, O. V. Aslanidi, S. Kharche, et al., "Pro-arrhythmogenic effects of atrial fibrillation-induced electrical remodelling: Insights from the three-dimensional virtual human atria," *J Physiol*, vol. 591, no. 17, pp. 4249–4272, 2013.

[289] J. T. Koivumaki, G. Seemann, M. M. Maleckar, et al., "In silico screening of the key cellular remodeling targets in chronic atrial fibrillation," *PLoS Comput Biol*, vol. 10, no. 5, p. e1003620, 2014.

[290] E. Matene and V. Jacquemet, "Fully automated initiation of simulated episodes of atrial arrhythmias," *Europace*, vol. 14, no. S5, pp. v17–v24, 2012.

[291] G. Seemann, P. C. Bustamante, S. Ponto, et al., "Atrial fibrillation-based electrical remodeling in a computer model of the human atrium," in *Comput Cardiol*, vol. 37, 2010, pp. 417–420.

[292] L. Uldry, V. Jacquemet, N. Virag, et al., "Estimating the time scale and anatomical location of atrial fibrillation spontaneous termination in a biophysical model," *Med Biol Eng Comput*, vol. 50, no. 2, pp. 155–163, 2012.

[293] H. Zhang, C. J. Garratt, J. Zhu, et al., "Role of up-regulation of I_{K1} in action potential shortening associated with atrial fibrillation in humans," *Cardiovasc Res*, vol. 66, no. 3, pp. 493–502, 2005.

[294] A. Loewe, M. Wilhelms, O. Dössel, et al., "Influence of chronic atrial fibrillation induced remodeling in a computational electrophysiological model," *Biomed Tech / Biomed Eng*, vol. 59, no. S1, pp. S929–S932, 2014.

[295] D. Corradi, "Atrial fibrillation from the pathologist's perspective," *Cardiovasc Pathol*, vol. 23, no. 2, pp. 71–84, 2014.

[296] M. R. Franz, P. L. Karasik, C. Li, et al., "Electrical remodeling of the human atrium: Similar effects in patients with chronic atrial fibrillation and atrial flutter," *J Am Coll Cardiol*, vol. 30, no. 7, pp. 1785–1792, 1997.

[297] W. C. Yu, S. H. Lee, C. T. Tai, et al., "Reversal of atrial electrical remodeling following cardioversion of long-standing atrial fibrillation in man," *Cardiovasc Res*, vol. 42, no. 2, pp. 470–476, 1999.

[298] G. K. Feld, M. D. M. Mollerus, U. Birgersdotter-Green, et al., "Conduction velocity in the tricuspid valve-inferior vena cava isthmus is slower in patients with type I atrial flutter compared to those without a history of atrial flutter," *J Cardiovasc Electrophysiol*, vol. 8, no. 12, pp. 1338–1349, 1997.

[299] S. Nattel and M. Harada, "Atrial remodeling and atrial fibrillation: Recent advances and translational perspectives," *J Am Coll Cardiol*, vol. 63, no. 22, pp. 2335–2345, 2014.

[300] C. Sánchez, A. Bueno-Orovio, E. Wettwer, et al., "Inter-subject variability in human atrial action potential in sinus rhythm versus chronic atrial fibrillation," *PLoS One*, vol. 9, no. 8, p. e105897, 2014.

[301] M. R. Davies, K. Wang, G. R. Mirams, et al., "Recent developments in using mechanistic cardiac modelling for drug safety evaluation," *Drug Discov Today*, 2016, epub ahead of print.

[302] N. A. Trayanova, "Whole-heart modeling: Applications to cardiac electrophysiology and electromechanics," *Circ Res*, vol. 108, no. 1, pp. 113–128, 2011.

[303] E. P. Scholz, P. Carrillo-Bustamante, F. Fischer, et al., "Rotor termination is critically dependent on kinetic properties of I_{Kur} inhibitors in an in silico model of chronic atrial fibrillation," *PLoS One*, vol. 8, no. 12, p. e83179, 2013.

[304] J. C. Hancox, A. F. James, N. V. Marrion, et al., "Novel ion channel targets in atrial fibrillation," *Expert Opin Ther Targets*, 2016, epub ahead of print.

[305] S. Thomas, K. Wolstencroft, B. de Bono, et al., "A physiome interoperability roadmap for personalized drug development," *Interface Focus*, vol. 6, no. 2, p. 20150094, 2016.

[306] N. Zemzemi, M. O. Bernabeu, J. Saiz, et al., "Computational assessment of drug-induced effects on the electrocardiogram: From ion channel to body surface potentials," *Br J Pharmacol*, vol. 168, no. 3, pp. 718–733, 2013.

[307] M. Wilhelms, C. Rombach, E. P. Scholz, et al., "Impact of amiodarone and cisapride on simulated human ventricular electrophysiology and electrocardiograms," *Europace*, vol. 14, no. S5, pp. v90–v96, 2012.

[308] C. Obiol-Pardo, J. Gomis-Tena, F. Sanz, et al., "A multiscale simulation system for the prediction of drug-induced cardiotoxicity," *J Chem Inf Model*, vol. 51, no. 2, pp. 483–492, 2011.

[309] G. R. Mirams, M. R. Davies, S. J. Brough, et al., "Prediction of thorough QT study results using action potential simulations based on ion channel screens," *J Pharmacol Toxicol Methods*, vol. 70, no. 3, pp. 246–254, 2014.

[310] W. S. Redfern, L. Carlsson, A. S. Davis, et al., "Relationships between preclinical cardiac electrophysiology, clinical QT interval prolongation and torsade de pointes for a broad range of drugs: Evidence for a provisional safety margin in drug development," *Cardiovasc Res*, vol. 58, no. 1, pp. 32–45, 2003.

[311] S. Morotti, A. D. McCulloch, D. M. Bers, et al., "Atrial-selective targeting of arrhythmogenic phase-3 early afterdepolarizations in human myocytes," *J Mol Cell Cardiol*, 2015, epub ahead of print.

[312] K. Tsujimae, S. Suzuki, S. Murakami, et al., "Frequency-dependent effects of various ikr blockers on cardiac action potential duration in a human atrial model," *Am J Physiol Heart Circ Physiol*, vol. 293, no. 1, pp. H660–H669, 2007.

[313] K. Tsujimae, S. Murakami, and Y. Kurachi, "In silico study on the effects of ikur block kinetics on prolongation of human action potential after atrial fibrillation-induced electrical remodeling," *Am J Physiol Heart Circ Physiol*, vol. 294, no. 2, pp. H793–H800, 2008.

[314] M. Wilhelms, L. P. Holl, O. Dössel, et al., "Impact of antiarrhythmic drugs on a virtual model of atrial fibrillation," *Biomed Tech / Biomed Eng*, vol. 57, no. S1, 2012.

[315] O. V. Aslanidi, M. Al-Owais, A. P. Benson, et al., "Virtual tissue engineering of the human atrium: Modelling pharmacological actions on atrial arrhythmogenesis," *Eur J Pharm Sci*, vol. 46, no. 4, pp. 209–221, 2012.

[316] J. Heijman, A. Zaza, D. M. Johnson, et al., "Determinants of beat-to-beat variability of repolarization duration in the canine ventricular myocyte: A computational analysis," *PLoS Comput Biol*, vol. 9, no. 8, p. e1003202, 2013.

[317] C. Abrahamsson, C. Dota, B. Skallefell, et al., "DeltaT50 - a new method to assess temporal ventricular repolarization variability," *J Electrocardiol*, vol. 44, no. 4, pp. 477.e1–e9, 2011.

[318] B. N. Singh and E. M. V. Williams, "The effect of amiodarone, a new anti-anginal drug, on cardiac muscle," *Br J Pharmacol*, vol. 39, no. 4, pp. 657–667, 1970.

[319] Y. Lutz, "Specific antiarrhythmic therapy for familial atrial fibrillation in a numerical model of human atrial electrophysiology," Bachelor Thesis, Institute of Biomedical Engineering, Karlsruhe Institute of Technology (KIT), Karlsruhe, 2013.

[320] A. Hill, "The possible effects of the aggregation of the molecules of haemoglobin on its dissociation curves," *J Physiol*, vol. 40, no. 4, pp. 4–7, 1910.

[321] K. Kamiya, A. Nishiyama, K. Yasui, et al., "Short- and long-term effects of amiodarone on the two components of cardiac delayed rectifier K^+ current," *Circulation*, vol. 103, no. 9, pp. 1317–1324, 2001.

[322] D. P. Zankov, W. G. Ding, H. Matsuura, et al., "Open-state unblock characterizes acute inhibition of I_{Ks} potassium current by amiodarone in guinea pig ventricular myocytes," *J Cardiovasc Electrophysiol*, vol. 16, no. 3, pp. 314–322, 2005.

[323] N. Lalevée, S. Barrère-Lemaire, P. Gautier, et al., "Effects of amiodarone and dronedarone on voltage-dependent sodium current in human cardiomyocytes," *J Cardiovasc Electrophysiol*, vol. 14, no. 8, pp. 885–890, 2003.

[324] M. Nishimura, C. H. Follmer, and D. H. Singer, "Amiodarone blocks calcium current in single guinea pig ventricular myocytes," *J Pharmacol Exp Ther*, vol. 251, no. 2, pp. 650–659, 1989.

[325] Y. Watanabe, T. Iwamoto, I. Matsuoka, et al., "Effects of amiodarone on mutant Na^+/Ca^{2+} exchangers expressed in CCL 39 cells," *Eur J Pharmacol*, vol. 496, no. 1-3, pp. 49–54, 2004.

[326] D. F. Gray, A. S. Mihailidou, P. S. Hansen, et al., "Amiodarone inhibits the Na^+-K^+ pump in rabbit cardiac myocytes after acute and chronic treatment," *J Pharmacol Exp Ther*, vol. 284, no. 1, pp. 75–82, 1998.

[327] J. M. Ridley, J. T. Milnes, H. J. Witchel, et al., "High affinity hERG K^+ channel blockade by the antiarrhythmic agent dronedarone: Resistance to mutations of the S6 residues Y652 and F656," *Biochem Biophys Res Commun*, vol. 325, no. 3, pp. 883–891, 2004.

[328] P. Gautier, E. Guillemare, L. Djandjighian, et al., "In vivo and in vitro characterization of the novel antiarrhythmic agent SSR149744C," *J Cardiovasc Pharmacol*, vol. 44, no. 2, pp. 244–257, 2004.

[329] P. Gautier, E. Guillemare, A. Marion, et al., "Electrophysiologic characterization of dronedarone in guinea pig ventricular cells," *J Cardiovasc Pharmacol*, vol. 41, no. 2, pp. 191–202, 2003.

[330] P. J. Podrid, "Amiodarone: Reevaluation of an old drug," *Ann Intern Med*, vol. 122, no. 9, pp. 689–700, 1995.

[331] C. I. Haffajee, J. C. Love, A. T. Canada, et al., "Clinical pharmacokinetics and efficacy of amiodarone for refractory tachyarrhythmias," *Circulation*, vol. 67, no. 6, pp. 1347–1355, 1983.

[332] Sanofi-Aventis Canada Inc., "Product monograph multaq, dronedarone tablets," Laval, Quebec, 2011.

[333] S. M. Narayan, F. Bode, P. L. Karasik, et al., "Alternans of atrial action potential during atrial flutter as a percursor to atrial fibrillation," *Circulation*, vol. 106, pp. 1968–1973, 2002.

[334] Y. Gong, F. Xie, K. M. Stein, et al., "Mechanism underlying initiation of paroxysmal atrial flutter/atrial fibrillation by ectopic foci: A simulation study," *Circulation*, vol. 115, no. 16, pp. 2094–2102, 2007.

[335] K. Shinagawa, A. Shiroshita-Takeshita, G. Schram, et al., "Effects of antiarrhythmic drugs on fibrillation in the remodeled atrium: Insights into the mechanism of the superior efficacy of amiodarone," *Circulation*, vol. 107, no. 10, pp. 1440–1446, 2003.

[336] W. Sun, J. S. M. Sarma, and B. N. Singh, "Chronic and acute effects of dronedarone on the action potential of rabbit atrial muscle preparations: Comparison with amiodarone," *J Cardiovasc Pharmacol*, vol. 39, no. 5, pp. 677–684, 2002.

[337] J. Kramer, C. A. Obejero-Paz, G. Myatt, et al., "MICE models: Superior to the hERG model in predicting torsade de pointes," *Sci Rep*, vol. 3, p. 2100, 2013.

[338] M. R. Davies, H. B. Mistry, L. Hussein, et al., "An in silico canine cardiac midmyocardial action potential duration model as a tool for early drug safety assessment," *Am J Physiol Heart Circ Physiol*, vol. 302, no. 7, pp. H1466–H1480, 2012.

[339] G. R. Mirams, Y. Cui, A. Sher, et al., "Simulation of multiple ion channel block provides improved early prediction of compounds' clinical torsadogenic risk," *Cardiovasc Res*, vol. 91, no. 1, pp. 53–61, 2011.

[340] A. Caruso, N. Frances, C. Meille, et al., "Translational PK/PD modeling for cardiovascular safety assessment of drug candidates: Methods and examples in drug development," *J Pharmacol Toxicol Methods*, vol. 70, no. 1, pp. 73–85, 2014.

[341] H. B. Mistry, M. R. Davies, and G. Y. Di Veroli, "A new classifier-based strategy for in-silico ion-channel cardiac drug safety assessment," *Front Pharmacol*, vol. 24, no. 6, p. 59, 2015.

[342] J. J. Babcock, F. Du, K. Xu, et al., "Integrated analysis of drug-induced gene expression profiles predicts novel hERG inhibitors," *PLoS One*, vol. 8, no. 7, p. e69513, 2013.

[343] J. Kiehn, D. Thomas, C. a. Karle, et al., "Inhibitory effects of the class III antiarrhythmic drug amiodarone on cloned hERG potassium channels," *Naunyn Schmiedebergs Arch Pharmacol*, vol. 359, no. 3, pp. 212–219, 1999.

[344] L. Wu, S. Rajamani, J. C. Shryock, et al., "Augmentation of late sodium current unmasks the proarrhythmic effects of amiodarone," *Cardiovasc Res*, vol. 77, no. 3, pp. 481–488, 2008.

[345] Niwa R., Shimuzu A., Lu Z., et al., "Voltage-dependent effects of amiodarone on D540K hERG channels," *Environ Med*, no. vol. 47, pp. pp. 51–52, 2003.

[346] C. Lin, X. Ke, I. Cvetanovic, et al., "The effect of high extracellular potassium on I_{Kr} inhibition by anti-arrhythmic agents," *Cardiology*, vol. 108, no. 1, pp. 18–27, 2007.

[347] D. Stork, E. N. Timin, S. Berjukow, et al., "State dependent dissociation of hERG channel inhibitors," *Br J Pharmacol*, vol. 151, no. 8, pp. 1368–1376, 2007.

[348] L.-P. Lai, M.-J. Su, Y.-Z. Tseng, et al., "Sensitivity of the slow component of the delayed rectifier potassium current (I_{Ks}) to potassium channel blockers: Implications for clinical reverse use-dependent effects," *J Biomed Sci*, vol. 6, no. 4, pp. 251–259, 1999.

[349] W.-P. Yang, P. C. Levesque, W. A. Little, et al., "KvLQT1, a voltage-gated potassium channel responsible for human cardiac arrhythmias," *Proc Natl Acad Sci U S A*, vol. 94, no. 8, pp. 4017–4021, 1997.

[350] W. Guo, K. Kamiya, and J. Toyama, "Evidences of antagonism between amiodarone and triiodothyronine on the K^+ channel activities of cultured rat cardiomyocytes," *J Mol Cell Cardiol*, vol. 29, no. 2, pp. 617–627, 1997.

[351] R. S. Sheldon, R. J. Hill, N. J. Cannon, et al., "Amiodarone: Biochemical evidence for binding to a receptor for class I drugs associated with the rat cardiac sodium channel," *Circ Res*, vol. 65, no. 2, pp. 477–482, 1989.

[352] T. Suzuki, M. Morishima, S. Kato, et al., "Atrial selectivity in Na channel blockade by acute amiodarone," *Cardiovasc Res*, vol. 98, no. 1, pp. 136–144, 2013.

[353] C. H. Follmer, M. Aomine, J. Z. Yeh, et al., "Amiodarone-induced block of sodium current in isolated cardiac cells," *J Pharmacol Exp Ther*, vol. 243, no. 1, pp. 187–194, 1987.

[354] N. Yamashita, T. Kaku, T. Uchino, et al., "Short- and long-term amiodarone treatments regulate Cav3.2 low-voltage-activated T-type Ca^{2+} channel through distinct mechanisms," *Mol Pharmacol*, vol. 69, no. 5, pp. 1684–1691, 2006.

[355] A. Varro, L. Virag, and J. G. Papp, "Comparison of the chronic and acute effects of amiodarone on the calcium and potassium currents in rabbit isolated cardiac myocytes," *Br J Pharmacol*, vol. 117, no. 6, pp. 1181–1186, 1996.

[356] Y. Watanabe, Y. C. Hara, M. Tamagawa, et al., "Inhibitory effect of amiodarone on the muscarinic acetylcholine receptor-operated potassium current in guinea pig atrial cells," *J Pharmacol Exp Ther*, vol. 279, no. 2, pp. 617–624, 1996.

[357] D. Thomas, S. Kathofer, W. Zhang, et al., "Acute effects of dronedarone on both components of the cardiac delayed rectifier K^+ current, hERG and KvLQT1/minK potassium channels," *Br J Pharmacol*, vol. 140, no. 5, pp. 996–1002, 2003.

[358] A. Shimizu, R. Niwa, Z. Lu, et al., "Effects of dronedarone on hERG and KCNQ1/KCNE1 channels," *Environ Med Annu Rep Res Inst Environ Med Nagoya Univ*, vol. 47, pp. 48–50, 2003.

[359] J. T. Milnes, D. J. Madge, and J. W. Ford, "New pharmacological approaches to atrial fibrillation," *Drug Discov Today*, vol. 17, no. 13-14, pp. 654–659, 2012.

[360] E. Guillemare, A. Marion, D. Nisato, et al., "Inhibitory effects of dronedarone on muscarinic k+ current in guinea pig atrial cells," *J Cardiovasc Pharmacol*, vol. 36, no. 6, pp. 802–805, 2000.

[361] C. Altomare, A. Barbuti, C. Viscomi, et al., "Effects of dronedarone on acetylcholine-activated current in rabbit SAN cells," *Br J Pharmacol*, vol. 130, no. 6, pp. 1315–1320, 2000.

[362] G. R. Mirams, M. R. Davies, Y. Cui, et al., "Application of cardiac electrophysiology simulations to pro-arrhythmic safety testing," *Br J Pharmacol*, vol. 167, no. 5, pp. 932–945, 2012.

[363] R. C. Elkins, M. R. Davies, S. J. Brough, et al., "Variability in high-throughput ion-channel screening data and consequences for cardiac safety assessment," *J Pharmacol Toxicol Methods*, vol. 68, no. 1, pp. 112–122, 2013.

[364] O. J. Britton, A. Bueno-Orovio, K. Van Ammel, et al., "Experimentally calibrated population of models predicts and explains intersubject variability in cardiac cellular electrophysiology," *Proc Natl Acad Sci U S A*, vol. 110, no. 23, pp. E2098–E2105, 2013.

[365] R. H. Johnstone, E. T. Y. Chang, R. Bardenet, et al., "Uncertainty and variability in models of the cardiac action potential: Can we build trustworthy models?" *J Mol Cell Cardiol*, 2015, epub ahead of print.

[366] I. Kodama, K. Kamiya, and J. Toyama, "Cellular electropharmacology of amiodarone," *Cardiovasc Res*, vol. 35, no. 1, pp. 13–29, 1997.

[367] C. Patel, G. X. Yan, and P. R. Kowey, "Dronedarone," *Circulation*, vol. 120, pp. 636–644, 2009.

[368] D. U. J. Keller, A. Bohn, O. Dössel, et al., "In-silico evaluation of beta-adrenergic effects on the long-QT syndrome," in *Comput Cardiol*, vol. 37, 2010, pp. 825–828.

[369] T. Chiba, N. Kondo, and A. Takahara, "Influences of rapid pacing-induced electrical remodeling on pharmacological manipulation of the atrial refractoriness in rabbits," *J Pharmacol Sci*, 2016, epub ahead of print.

[370] C. Xie, S. Yang, D. Zhong, et al., "Simultaneous determination of dronedarone and its active metabolite debutyldronedarone in human plasma by liquid chromatography-tandem mass spectrometry: Application to a pharmacokinetic study," *J Chromatogr B Anal Technol Biomed Life Sci*, vol. 879, no. 28, pp. 3071–3075, 2011.

[371] M. E. Veronese, S. McLean, and R. Hendriks, "Plasma protein binding of amiodarone in a patient population: Measurement by erythrocyte partitioning and a novel glass-binding method," *Br J Clin Pharmacol*, vol. 26, no. 6, pp. 721–731, 1988.

[372] R. Latini, G. Tognoni, and R. E. Kates, "Clinical pharmacokinetics of amiodarone," *Clin Pharmacokinet*, vol. 9, no. 2, pp. 136–156, 1984.

[373] D. Roy, B. H. Rowe, I. G. Stiell, et al., "A randomized, controlled trial of RSD1235, a novel anti-arrhythmic agent, in the treatment of recent onset atrial fibrillation," *J Am Coll Cardiol*, vol. 44, no. 12, pp. 2355–2361, 2004.

[374] D. Roy, C. M. Pratt, C. Torp-Pedersen, et al., "Vernakalant hydrochloride for rapid conversion of atrial fibrillation: A phase 3, randomized, placebo-controlled trial," *Circulation*, vol. 117, no. 12, pp. 1518–1525, 2008.

[375] D. Fedida, P. M. R. Orth, J. Y. C. Chen, et al., "The mechanism of atrial antiarrhythmic action of RSD1235," *J Cardiovasc Electrophysiol*, vol. 16, no. 11, pp. 1227–1238, 2005.

[376] E. Wettwer, T. Christ, S. Endig, et al., "The new antiarrhythmic drug vernakalant: Ex vivo study of human atrial tissue from sinus rhythm and chronic atrial fibrillation," *Cardiovasc Res*, vol. 98, no. 1, pp. 145–154, 2013.

[377] P. Dorian, A. Pinter, I. Mangat, et al., "The effect of vernakalant (RSD1235), an investigational antiarrhythmic agent, on atrial electrophysiology in humans," *J Cardiovasc Pharmacol*, vol. 50, no. 1, pp. 35–40, 2007.

[378] A. Loewe, Y. Xu, E. P. Scholz, et al., "Understanding the cellular mode of action of vernakalant using a computational model: Answers and new questions," *Curr Dir Biomed Eng*, vol. 1, no. 1, pp. 418–422, 2015.

[379] J. Xu, A. R. Dehaghani, F. Gao, et al., "Noninvasive transmural electrophysiological imaging based on minimization of total-variation functional," *IEEE Trans Med Imaging*, vol. 33, no. 9, pp. 1860–1874, 2014.

[380] G. Frommeyer, C. Ellermann, M. Sterneberg, et al., "Comparison of the electrophysiologic effects of vernakalant and ranolazine in an experimental whole-heart model of atrial fibrillation," *Clin Res Cardiol*, vol. 105, p. P1704, 2016.

[381] A. Burashnikov, M. Pourrier, J. K. Gibson, et al., "Rate-dependent effects of vernakalant in the isolated non-remodeled canine left atria are primarily due to block of the sodium channel comparison with ranolazine and dl-sotalol," *Circ Arrhythmia Electrophysiol*, vol. 5, no. 2, pp. 400–408, 2012.

[382] J. D. Moreno, T. J. Lewis, and C. E. Clancy, "Parameterization for in-silico modeling of ion channel interactions with drugs," *PLoS One*, vol. 11, no. 3, p. e0150761, 2016.

[383] S. A. Lubitz, C. Ozcan, J. W. Magnani, et al., "Genetics of atrial fibrillation: Implications for future research directions and personalized medicine," *Circ Arrhythmia Electrophysiol*, vol. 3, no. 3, pp. 291–299, 2010.

[384] A. Loewe, Y. Lutz, M. Wilhelms, et al., "Optimization of pharmacotherapy for familial atrial fibrillation in a numerical model of human atrial electrophysiology," in *Comput Cardiol*, vol. 41, 2014, pp. 745–748.

[385] Y. Lutz, A. Loewe, M. Wilhelms, et al., "Specific antiarrhythmic therapy for familial atrial fibrillation in a numerical model of human atrial electrophysiology," in *Biomed Tech / Biomed Eng*, vol. 59, no. S1, 2014, pp. S933–S936.

[386] E. Jones, T. Oliphant, and P. Peterson, "Scipy: Open source scientific tools for Python. Version: 0.16.0," 2015.

[387] R. Ranjan, E. Kholmovski, J. Silvernagel, et al., "Late gadolinium enhanced MR images of acute ablation lesions significantly overestimates the chronic scar volume," *J Am Coll Cardiol*, vol. 63, no. 12s, 2014.

[388] A. Wachter, "Model-structure-independent, rule-based annotation of atrial fiber orientation and ablation patterns for an in silico assessment of their arrhythmogenic potential," Diploma Thesis, Institute of Biomedical Engineering, Karlsruhe Institute of Technology (KIT), 2015.

[389] A. Wachter, A. Loewe, M. W. Krueger, et al., "Mesh structure-independent modeling of patient-specific atrial fiber orientation," *Curr Dir Biomed Eng*, vol. 1, no. 1, pp. 409–412, 2015.

[390] S. Y. Ho, "Anatomy and myoarchitecture of the left ventricular wall in normal and in disease," *Eur J Echocardiogr*, vol. 10, no. 8, pp. iii3–iii7, 2009.

[391] S. Y. Ho, R. H. Anderson, and D. Sánchez-Quintana, "Atrial structure and fibres: Morphologic bases of atrial conduction," *Cardiovasc Res*, vol. 54, no. 2, pp. 325–336, 2002.

[392] J. A. Cabrera, S. Y. Ho, V. Climent, et al., "The architecture of the left lateral atrial wall: A particular anatomic region with implications for ablation of atrial fibrillation," *Eur Heart J*, vol. 29, no. 3, pp. 356–362, 2008.

[393] N. Toussaint, M. Sermesant, C. T. Stoeck, et al., "In vivo human 3D cardiac fibre architecture: Reconstruction using curvilinear interpolation of diffusion tensor images," in *Med Image Comput Comput Assist Interv*, vol. 13, no. Pt 1, 2010, pp. 418–425.

[394] F. O. Campos, T. Wiener, A. J. Prassl, et al., "A 2D-computer model of atrial tissue based on histographs describes the electro-anatomical impact of microstructure on endocardiac potentials and electric near-fields," in *IEEE Eng Med Biol Soc EMBC*, 2010, pp. 2541–2544.

[395] J. Zhao, M. L. Trew, I. J. Legrice, et al., "A tissue-specific model of reentry in the right atrial appendage," *J Cardiovasc Electrophysiol*, vol. 20, no. 6, pp. 675–684, 2009.

[396] D. A. Gerneke, G. B. Sands, R. Ganesaligam, et al., "Surface imaging microscopy using an ultramiller for large volume 3D reconstruction of wax- and resin-embedded tissues," *Microsc Res Tech*, vol. 70, no. 10, pp. 886–894, 2007.

[397] E. J. Vigmond, R. Ruckdeschel, and N. Trayanova, "Reentry in a morphologically realistic atrial model," *J Cardiovasc Electrophysiol*, vol. 12, no. 9, pp. 1046–1054, 2001.

[398] C. W. Zemlin, H. Herzel, S. Y. Ho, et al., "A realistic and efficient model of excitation propagation in the human atria," in *Comput Simul Exp Assess Card Electrophysiol*, N. Virag, O. Blanc, and L. Kappenberger, Eds. Futura, 2001, pp. 29–34.

[399] V. Jacquemet, N. Virag, Z. Ihara, et al., "Study of unipolar electrogram morphology in a computer model of atrial fibrillation," *J Cardiovasc Electrophysiol*, vol. 14, no. s10, pp. S172–S179, 2003.

[400] B. D. F. Hermosillo, "Semi-automatic enhancement of atrial models to include atrial architecture and patient specific data: For biophysical simulations," in *Comput Cardiol*, vol. 35, 2008, pp. 633–636.

[401] G. Plank, A. J. Prassl, J. I. Wang, et al., "Atrial fibrosis promotes the transistion of pulmonary vein ectopy into reentrant arrhathmias," in *Heart Rhythm*, vol. 5, no. S5, 2008, p. S162.

[402] M. W. Krueger, V. Schmidt, C. Tobón, et al., "Modeling atrial fiber orientation in patient-specific geometries: A semi-automatic rule-based approach," in *Funct Imaging Model Hear*, Lecture Notes in Computer Science, L. Axel and D. Metaxas, Eds., vol. 6666. Berlin / Heidelberg: Springer, 2011, pp. 223–232.

[403] R. A. B. Burton, G. Plank, J. E. Schneider, et al., "Three-dimensional models of individual cardiac histoanatomy: Tools and challenges," *Ann N Y Acad Sci*, vol. 1080, pp. 301–319, 2006.

[404] J. D. Bayer, R. C. Blake, G. Plank, et al., "A novel rule-based algorithm for assigning myocardial fiber orientation to computational heart models," *Ann Biomed Eng*, vol. 40, no. 10, pp. 2243–2254, 2012.

[405] F. Holmqvist, D. Husser, J. M. Tapanainen, et al., "Interatrial conduction can be accurately determined using standard 12-lead electrocardiography: Validation of P-wave morphology using electroanatomic mapping in man," *Heart Rhythm*, vol. 5, no. 3, pp. 413–418, 2008.

[406] T. R. Betts, P. R. Roberts, and J. M. Morgan, "High-density mapping of left atrial endocardial activation during sinus rhythm and coronary sinus pacing in patients with paroxysmal atrial fibrillation," *J Cardiovasc Electrophysiol*, vol. 15, no. 10, pp. 1111–1117, 2004.

[407] G. Hindricks and H. Kottkamp, "Simultaneous noncontact mapping of left atrium in patients with paroxysmal atrial fibrillation," *Circulation*, vol. 104, no. 3, pp. 297–303, 2001.

[408] V. Markides, R. J. Schilling, S. Y. Ho, et al., "Characterization of left atrial activation in the intact human heart," *Circulation*, vol. 107, no. 5, pp. 733–739, 2003.

[409] W. J. Schroeder, B. Lorensen, and K. Martin, *The visualization toolkit*. Kitware, 2004.

[410] H. Si and K. Gärtner, "Meshing piecewise linear complexes by constrained delaunay tetrahedralizations," in *Int Meshing Roundtable*, B. W. Hanks, Ed. Berlin/Heidelberg: Springer, 2005, pp. 147–163.

[411] M. Reumann, J. Bohnert, G. Seemann, et al., "Preventive ablation strategies in a biophysical model of atrial fibrillation based on realistic anatomical data," *IEEE Trans Biomed Eng*, vol. 55, no. 2, pp. 399–406, 2008.

[412] I. Deisenhofer, M. A. E. Schneider, M. Böhlen-Knauf, et al., "Circumferential mapping and electric isolation of pulmonary veins in patients with atrial fibrillation," *Am J Cardiol*, vol. 91, no. 2, pp. 159–163, 2003.

[413] F. Sachse, R. Frech, C. Werner, et al., "A model based approach to assignment of myocardial fibre orientation," in *Comput Cardiol*, vol. 26, 1999, pp. 145–148.

[414] C. D. Werner, O. Dössel, and F. B. Sachse, "Electrical excitation propagation in the human heart," *Int J Bioelectromagn*, vol. 2, no. 2, 2000.

[415] J. Zhao, T. D. Butters, H. Zhang, et al., "An image-based model of atrial muscular architecture effects of structural anisotropy on electrical activation," *Circ Arrhythmia Electrophysiol*, vol. 5, no. 2, pp. 361–370, 2012.

[416] A. Frangi, W. J. Niessen, K. L. Vincken, et al., "Multiscale vessel enhancement filtering," in *Med Image Comput Comput Interv*, Lecture Notes in Computer Science, W. Wells, A. Colchester, and S. Delp, Eds., vol. 1496. Berlin/Heidelberg: Springer, 1998, pp. 130–137.

[417] T. J. Bunch, H. T. May, T. L. Bair, et al., "The impact of age on 5-year outcomes after atrial fibrillation catheter ablation," *J Cardiovasc Electrophysiol*, vol. 27, no. 2, pp. 141–146, 2016.

[418] L. Dong, Z. Bie, L. Sun, et al., "Long-term clinical outcome and risk of catheter ablation in elderly with non-paroxysmal atrial fibrillation," *Int J Clin Exp Med*, vol. 8, no. 9, pp. 16 050–16 056, 2015.

[419] E. Gucuk Ipek, J. E. Marine, M. Habibi, et al., "Association of left atrial function with incident atypical atrial flutter after atrial fibrillation ablation," *Heart Rhythm*, vol. 13, no. 2, pp. 391–398, 2015.

[420] J. J. Liang, M. A. Elafros, W. W. Chik, et al., "Early recurrence of atrial arrhythmias following pulmonary vein antral isolation: Timing and frequency of early recurrences predicts long-term ablation success," *Heart Rhythm*, vol. 12, no. 12, pp. 2461–2468, 2015.

[421] A. L. Waldo and G. K. Feld, "Inter-relationships of atrial fibrillation and atrial flutter. mechanisms and clinical implications," *J Am Coll Cardiol*, vol. 51, no. 8, pp. 779–786, 2008.

[422] I. Deisenhofer, H. Estner, B. Zrenner, et al., "Left atrial tachycardia after circumferential pulmonary vein ablation for atrial fibrillation: Incidence, electrophysiological characteristics, and results of radiofrequency ablation," *Europace*, vol. 8, no. 8, pp. 573–582, 2006.

[423] P. Jaïs, P. Sanders, L. F. Hsu, et al., "Flutter localized to the anterior left atrium after catheter ablation of atrial fibrillation," *J Cardiovasc Electrophysiol*, vol. 17, no. 3, pp. 279–285, 2006.

[424] C. E. Mesas, C. Pappone, C. C. E. Lang, et al., "Left atrial tachycardia after circumferential pulmonary vein ablation for atrial fibrillation: Electroanatomic characterization and treatment," *J Am Coll Cardiol*, vol. 44, no. 5, pp. 1071–1079, 2004.

[425] S. Castrejón-Castrejón, M. Ortega, A. Pérez-Silva, et al., "Organized atrial tachycardias after atrial fibrillation ablation," *Cardiol Res Pract*, vol. 2011, p. 957538, 2011.

[426] A. Garny, D. Noble, and P. Kohl, "Dimensionality in cardiac modelling," *Prog Biophys Mol Biol*, vol. 87, no. 1 SPEC. ISS., pp. 47–66, 2005.

[427] J. P. Keener, "An eikonal-curvature equation for action potential propagation in myocardium," *J Math Biol*, vol. 29, no. 7, pp. 629–651, 1991.

[428] P. C. Franzone and L. Guerri, "Spreading of excitation in 3-D models of the anisotropic cardiac tissue. I. validation of the eikonal model," *Math Biosci*, vol. 113, no. 2, pp. 145–209, 1993.

[429] P. M. van Dam and A. van Oosterom, "Atrial excitation assuming uniform propagation," *J Cardiovasc Electrophysiol*, vol. 14, no. S10, pp. S166–S171, 2003.

[430] J. A. Bærentzen, "On the implementation of fast marching methods for 3D lattices," Lyngby, Denmark, Tech. Rep., 2001.

[431] M. Sermesant, Y. Coudière, V. Moreau-Viléger, et al., "A fast-marching approach to cardiac electrophysiology simulation for XMR interventional imaging," in *Med Image Comput Comput Interv*, Lecture Notes in Computer Science, vol. 3750, no. Pt 2. Berlin / Heidelberg: Springer, 2005, pp. 607–615.

[432] J. A. Sethian, *Level set methods and fast marching methods*, Cambridge Monographs on Applied and Computational Mathematics. Cambridge: Cambridge University Press, 1999.

[433] J. A. Sethian, "A fast marching level set method for monotonically advancing fronts," *Proc Natl Acad Sci U S A*, vol. 93, no. 4, pp. 1591–1595, 1996.

[434] J. A. Sethian and A. Vladimirsky, "Fast methods for the eikonal and related Hamilton-Jacobi equations on unstructured meshes," *Proc Natl Acad Sci U S A*, vol. 97, no. 11, pp. 5699–5703, 2000.

[435] J. A. Sethian and A. Vladimirsky, "Ordered upwind methods for static Hamilton-Jacobi equations," *Proc Natl Acad Sci*, vol. 98, no. 20, pp. 11 069–11 074, 2001.

[436] L. Dang, N. Virag, Z. Ihara, et al., "Evaluation of ablation patterns using a biophysical model of atrial fibrillation," *Ann Biomed Eng*, vol. 33, no. 4, pp. 465–474, 2005.

[437] M. Hwang, S. S. Kwon, J. Wi, et al., "Virtual ablation for atrial fibrillation in personalized in-silico three-dimensional left atrial modeling: Comparison with clinical catheter ablation," *Prog Biophys Mol Biol*, vol. 116, no. 1, pp. 40–47, 2014.

[438] K. S. McDowell, S. Zahid, F. Vadakkumpadan, et al., "Virtual electrophysiological study of atrial fibrillation in fibrotic remodeling," *PLoS One*, vol. 10, no. 2, p. e0117110, 2015.

[439] J. D. Bayer, C. Roney, A. Pashaei, et al., "Novel radiofrequency ablation strategies for terminating atrial fibrillation in the left atrium: A simulation study," *Front Physiol*, vol. 7, p. 108, 2016.

[440] S. Zahid, K. N. Whyte, E. L. Schwarz, et al., "Feasibility of using patient-specific models and the "minimum cut" algorithm to predict optimal ablation targets for left atrial flutter," *Heart Rhythm*, 2016, epub ahead of print.

[441] J. Zhao, S. R. Kharche, B. J. Hansen, et al., "Optimization of catheter ablation of atrial fibrillation: Insights gained from clinically-derived computer models," *Int J Mol Sci*, vol. 16, no. 5, pp. 10 834–10 854, 2015.

[442] G. T. Lines, M. C. MacLachlan, S. Linge, et al., "Synchronizing computer simulations with measurement data for a case of atrial flutter," *Ann Biomed Eng*, vol. 37, no. 7, pp. 1287–1293, 2009.

[443] E. Poremba, "Implementation of a fast simulation C++ framework for the computation of vulnerability to artial arrhythmias using the fast marching algorithm," Bachelor Thesis, Institute of Biomedical Engineering, Karlsruhe Institute of Technology (KIT), 2013.

[444] S. Bischoff and L. P. Kobbelt, "Parameterizaiton-free active contour models with topology control," *Vis Comput*, vol. 20, no. 4, pp. 217–228, 2004.

[445] S. Bischoff, T. Weyand, and L. Kobbelt, "Snakes on triangle meshes," in *Bild für die Medizin*, Informatik aktuell, H.-P. Meinzer, H. Handels, A. Horsch, et al., Eds. Berlin/Heidelberg: Springer, 2005, pp. 208–212.

[446] Y. Lee and S. Lee, "Geometric snakes for triangular meshes," in *Comput Graph Forum*, vol. 21, no. 3. Wiley Online Library, 2002, pp. 229–238.

[447] Y. Lee, S. Lee, A. Shamir, et al., "Intelligent mesh scissoring using 3D snakes," in *Pacific Conf Comput Graph Appl*, 2004, pp. 279–287.

[448] F. Hetroy and D. Attali, "From a closed piecewise geodesic to a constriction on a closed triangulated surface," in *Pacific Conf Comput Graph Appl*, 2003, pp. 394–398.

[449] V. Jacquemet, "An eikonal approach for the initiation of reentrant cardiac propagation in reactiondiffusion models," *IEEE Trans Biomed Eng*, vol. 57, no. 9, pp. 2090–2098, 2010.

[450] V. Jacquemet, "An eikonal-diffusion solver and its application to the interpolation and the simulation of reentrant cardiac activations," *Comput Methods Programs Biomed*, vol. 108, no. 2, pp. 548–558, 2012.

[451] K. A. Tomlinson, P. J. Hunter, and A. J. Pullan, "A finite element method for an eikonal equation model of myocardial excitation wavefront propagation," *SIAM J Appl Math*, vol. 63, no. 1, pp. 324–350, 2002.

[452] P. Colli Franzone, L. Guerri, and S. Rovida, "Wavefront propagation in an activation model of the anisotropic cardiac tissue: Asymptotic analysis and numerical simulations," *J Math Biol*, vol. 28, no. 2, pp. 121–176, 1990.

[453] T. F. Oostendorp, A. van Oosterom, and G. Huiskamp, "Interpolation on a triangulated 3D surface," *J Comput Phys*, vol. 80, no. 2, pp. 331–343, 1989.

[454] T. Alkhalifah, "Traveltime computation with the linearized eikonal equation for anisotropic media," *Geophys Prospect*, vol. 50, no. 4, pp. 373–382, 2002.

[455] F. M. Weber, C. Schilling, G. Seemann, et al., "Wave-direction and conduction-velocity analysis from intracardiac electrograms - a single-shot technique," *IEEE Trans Biomed Eng*, vol. 57, no. 10, pp. 2394–2401, 2010.

[456] F. M. Weber, A. Luik, C. Schilling, et al., "Conduction velocity restitution of the human atriuman - an efficient measurement protocol for clinical electrophysiological studies," *IEEE Trans Biomed Eng*, vol. 58, no. 9, pp. 2648–2655, 2011.

[457] D. G. Latcu and N. Saoudi, "How fast does the electrical impulse travel within the myocardium? The need for a new clinical electrophysiology tool: The conduction velocity mapping," pp. 395–397, 2014.

[458] C. D. Cantwell, C. H. Roney, F. S. Ng, et al., "Techniques for automated local activation time annotation and conduction velocity estimation in cardiac mapping," *Comput Biol Med*, vol. 65, pp. 229–242, 2015.

[459] M. Wallman, N. Smith, and B. Rodriguez, "Estimation of activation times in cardiac tissue using graph based methods," in *Funct Imaging Model Hear*. Springer, 2011, pp. 71–79.

[460] P. M. van Dam, T. F. Oostendorp, and A. van Oosterom, "Application of the fastest route algorithm in the interactive simulation of the effect of local ischemia on the ECG," *Med Biol Eng Comput*, vol. 47, no. 1, pp. 11–20, 2009.

[461] C. D. Werner, *Simulation der elektrischen Erregungsausbreitung in anatomischen Herzmodellen mit adaptiven zellulären Automaten*. Berlin: TENEA Verlag für Medien, 2001.

[462] N. Child, M. J. Bishop, B. Hanson, et al., "An activation-repolarization time metric to predict localized regions of high susceptibility to reentry," *Heart Rhythm*, vol. 12, no. 7, pp. 1644–1653, 2015.

[463] Y. R. Hill, N. Child, B. Hanson, et al., "Investigating a novel activation-repolarisation time metric to predict localised vulnerability to reentry using computational modelling," *PLoS One*, vol. 11, no. 3, p. e0149342, 2016.

[464] M. Wallman, A. Bueno-Orovio, and B. Rodriguez, "Computational probabilistic quantification of pro-arrhythmic risk from scar and left-to-right heterogeneity in the human ventricles," in *Comput Cardiol*, 2013, pp. 711–714.

[465] J. Trächtler, "Analysis of electrogram morphology and parameterization of a simulation environment for clinical cases of atrial flutter," Bachelor Thesis, Institute of Biomedical Engineering, Karlsruhe Institute of Technology (KIT), 2014.

[466] J. Trächtler, T. G. Oesterlein, A. Loewe, et al., "Virtualizing clinical cases of atrial flutter in a fast marching simulation including conduction velocity and ablation scars," *Curr Dir Biomed Eng*, vol. 1, no. 1, pp. 405–408, 2015.

[467] V. Jacquemet, "The inverse problem of phase singularity distribution: An eikonal approach," in *Comput Cardiol*, vol. 37, 2010, pp. 863–866.

[468] A. Herlin and V. Jacquemet, "Eikonal-based initiation of fibrillatory activity in thin-walled cardiac propagation models," *Chaos*, vol. 21, no. 4, pp. 431–436, 2011.

[469] T. Krogh-Madsen and D. J. Christini, "Nonlinear dynamics in cardiology," *Annu Rev Biomed Eng*, vol. 14, no. 1, pp. 179–203, 2012.

[470] V. Jacquemet, N. Virag, and L. Kappenberger, "Wavelength and vulnerability to atrial fibrillation: Insights from a computer model of human atria," *Europace*, vol. 7, no. S2, pp. 83–92, 2005.

[471] E. Konukoglu, J. Relan, U. Cilingir, et al., "Efficient probabilistic model personalization integrating uncertainty on data and parameters: Application to eikonal-diffusion models in cardiac electrophysiology," *Prog Biophys Mol Biol*, vol. 107, no. 1, pp. 134–146, 2011.

[472] F. E. Marchlinski, "Atrial fibrillation catheter ablation," *J Am Coll Cardiol*, vol. 51, no. 10, pp. 1011–1013, 2008.

[473] M. Mansour, "Learning while burning: Further evidence for drivers and fibrillatory conduction as a mechanism for atrial fibrillation," *J Cardiovasc Electrophysiol*, vol. 15, no. 5, pp. 522–523, 2004.

[474] B. S. Lipman and E. Massie, *Clinical scalar electrocardiography*, 5th ed. Chicago: Year Book Medical Publishers, 1965.

[475] J. J. Morris, E. H. Estes, R. E. Whalen, et al., "P-wave analysis in valvular heart disease," *Circulation*, vol. 29, no. 2, pp. 242–252, 1964.

[476] J. W. Magnani, "Risk assessment for atrial fibrillation: Enter the P-wave," *Heart Rhythm*, vol. 12, no. 9, pp. 1896–1897, 2015.

[477] G. Ndrepepa, B. Zrenner, I. Deisenhofer, et al., "Relationship between surface electrocardiogram characteristics and endocardial activation sequence in patients with typical atrial flutter," *Z Kardiol*, vol. 89, no. 6, pp. 527–537, 2000.

[478] O. Ozdemir, "P-wave durations as a predictor for atrial fibrillation development in patients with hypertrophic cardiomyopathy," *Int J Cardiol*, vol. 94, no. 2-3, pp. 163–166, 2004.

[479] E. W. Hancock, B. J. Deal, D. M. Mirvis, et al., "AHA/ACCF/HRS recommendations for the standardization and interpretation of the electrocardiogram. Part V: Electrocardiogram changes associated with cardiac chamber hypertrophy," *J Am Coll Cardiol*, vol. 53, no. 11, pp. 992–1002, 2009.

[480] V. Ariyarajah, K. Mercado, S. Apiyasawat, et al., "Correlation of left atrial size with P-wave duration in interatrial block," *Chest*, vol. 128, no. 4, pp. 2615–2618, 2005.

[481] R. Chirife, G. S. Feitosa, and W. S. Frankl, "Electrocardiographic detection of left atrial enlargement. Correlation of P wave with left atrial dimension by echocardiography," *Br Heart J*, vol. 37, no. 12, pp. 1281–1285, 1975.

[482] C. B. Hopkins and O. Barrett, "Electrocardiographic diagnosis of left atrial enlargement. Role of the P terminal force in lead v_1," *J Electrocardiol*, vol. 22, no. 4, pp. 359–363, 1989.

[483] A. Michelucci, G. Bagliani, A. Colella, et al., "P wave assessment: State of the art update," *Card Electrophysiol Rev*, vol. 6, no. 3, pp. 215–220, 2002.

[484] A. van Oosterom and V. Jacquemet, "Genesis of the P wave: Atrial signals as generated by the equivalent double layer source model," *Europace*, vol. 7, no. S2, pp. 21–29, 2005.

[485] M. Potse, B. Dubé, and A. Vinet, "Cardiac anisotropy in boundary-element models for the electrocardiogram," *Med Biol Eng Comput*, vol. 47, no. 7, pp. 719–729, 2009.

[486] W. Lu, D. Wei, X. Zhu, et al., "A computer model based on real anatomy for electrophysiology study," *Adv Eng Softw*, vol. 42, no. 7, pp. 463–476, 2011.

[487] P. M. van Dam and A. van Oosterom, "Volume conductor effects involved in the genesis of the P wave," *Europace*, vol. 7, no. S2, pp. 30–38, 2005.

[488] M. A. Colman, D. Giacopelli, P. Langley, et al., "Elucidating the body surface P-wave using a detailed computer model of atrial activation," in *Comput Cardiol*, vol. 39, 2012, pp. 129–132.

[489] M. A. Colman, O. V. Aslanidi, J. Stott, et al., "Correlation between P-wave morphology and origin of atrial focal tachycardia - insights from realistic models of the human atria and torso," *IEEE Trans Biomed Eng*, vol. 58, no. 10, pp. 2952–2955, 2011.

[490] M. W. Krueger, S. Severi, K. Rhode, et al., "Alterations of atrial electrophysiology related to hemodialysis session: Insights from a multiscale computer model," *J Electrocardiol*, vol. 44, no. 2, pp. 176–183, 2011.

[491] O. V. Aslanidi, M. A. Colman, J. Stott, et al., "3D virtual human atria: A computational platform for studying clinical atrial fibrillation," *Prog Biophys Mol Biol*, vol. 107, no. 1, pp. 156–168, 2011.

[492] V. Jacquemet, A. van Oosterom, J. M. Vesin, et al., "Analysis of electrocardiograms during atrial fibrillation. A biophysical model approach," *IEEE Eng Med Biol Mag*, vol. 25, no. 6, pp. 79–88, 2006.

[493] A. van Oosterom, Z. Ihara, V. Jacquemet, et al., "Vectorcardiographic lead systems for the characterization of atrial fibrillation," *J Electrocardiol*, vol. 40, no. 4, pp. 343.e1–e11, 2007.

[494] Z. Ihara, A. van Oosterom, V. Jacquemet, et al., "Adaptation of the standard 12-lead electrocardiogram system dedicated to the analysis of atrial fibrillation," *J Electrocardiol*, vol. 40, no. 1, pp. 68.e1–e8, 2007.

[495] V. Jacquemet, "Modeling left and right atrial contributions to the ECG: A dipole-current source approach," *Comput Biol Med*, vol. 65, pp. 192–199, 2015.

[496] A. Ferrer, R. Sebastián, D. Sánchez-Quintana, et al., "Detailed anatomical and electrophysiological models of human atria and torso for the simulation of atrial activation," *PLoS One*, vol. 10, no. 11, p. e0141573, 2015.

[497] A. Loewe, M. W. Krueger, P. G. Platonov, et al., "Left and right atrial contribution to the P-wave in realistic computational models," in *Funct Imaging Model Hear*, Lecture Notes

in Computer Science, H. van Assen, P. Bovendeerd, and T. Delhaas, Eds., vol. 9126. Berlin / Heidelberg: Springer, 2015, pp. 439–447.

[498] A. Loewe, M. W. Krueger, F. Holmqvist, et al., "P-wave terminal force is affected by site of earliest right atrial activation and its proximity to inter-atrial connections," *Europace*, vol. under review, 2016.

[499] A. Loewe, M. W. Krueger, F. Holmqvist, et al., "P-wave terminal force is affected by site of earliest right atrial activation and its proximity to inter-atrial connections," in *International Conference on Electrocardiology*, 2016, accepted for presentation in June 2016.

[500] The CGAL Project, *CGAL user and reference manual*, 4.7 ed., 2015.

[501] S. Gabriel, C. Gabriel, and L. R. W, "The dielectric properties of biological tissues: II. Measurements in the frequency range 10 Hz to 20 GHz," *Phys Med Biol*, vol. 41, no. 11, pp. 2251–2269, 1996.

[502] R. Lemery, D. Birnie, A. S. L. Tang, et al., "Normal atrial activation and voltage during sinus rhythm in the human heart: An endocardial and epicardial mapping study in patients with a history of atrial fibrillation," *J Cardiovasc Electrophysiol*, vol. 18, no. 4, pp. 402–408, 2007.

[503] A. K. Agarwal, "Spatial-temporal analysis of multi-channel electrocardiogram with special focus on T-wave," Master Thesis, Institute of Biomedical Engineering, Universität Karlsruhe (TH), Karlsruhe, 2008.

[504] M. E. Josephson, J. A. Kastor, and J. Morganroth, "Electrocardiographic left atrial enlargement. Electrophysiologic, echocardiographic and hemodynamic correlates," *Am J Cardiol*, vol. 39, no. 7, pp. 967–971, 1977.

[505] Q. A. Truong, E. M. Charipar, L. M. Ptaszek, et al., "Usefulness of electrocardiographic parameters as compared with computed tomography measures of left atrial volume enlargement: From the ROMICAT trial," *J Electrocardiol*, vol. 44, no. 2, pp. 257–264, 2011.

[506] M. S. Hazen, T. H. Marwick, and D. A. Underwood, "Diagnostic accuracy of the resting electrocardiogram in detection and estimation of left atrial enlargement: An echocardiographic correlation in 551 patients," *Am Heart J*, vol. 122, no. 3, pp. 823–828, 1991.

[507] K. Forfang and J. Erikssen, "Significance of P wave terminal force in presumably healthy middle-aged men," *Am Heart J*, vol. 96, no. 6, pp. 739–743, dec 1978.

[508] R. Petersson, H. M. Berge, G. F. Gjerdalen, et al., "P-wave morphology is unaffected by atrial size: A study in healthy athletes," *Ann Noninvasive Electrocardiol*, vol. 19, no. 4, pp. 366–373, 2014.

[509] J. W. Magnani, M. A. Williamson, P. T. Ellinor, et al., "P wave indices current status and future directions in epidemiology, clinical, and research applications," *Circ Arrhythmia Electrophysiol*, vol. 2, no. 1, pp. 72–79, 2009.

[510] G. S. Wagner and D. G. Strauss, *Marriott's practical electrocardiography*, 12th ed. Philadelphia: Lippincott Williams & Wilkins, 2014.

[511] N. M. G. Debbas, S. H. D. Jackson, D. De Jonghe, et al., "Human atrial repolarization: Effects of sinus rate, pacing and drugs on the surface electrocardiogram," *J Am Coll Cardiol*, vol. 33, no. 2, pp. 358–365, 1999.

[512] Z. Ihara, A. van Oosterom, and R. Hoekema, "Atrial repolarization as observable during the PQ interval," *J Electrocardiol*, vol. 39, no. 3, pp. 290–297, 2006.

[513] A. van Oosterom, E. Macchi, T. F. Oostendorp, et al., "Model-based inferences for clinical applications of the ECG," *J Electrocardiol*, vol. 40, no. 1S, pp. S17–S18, 2007.

[514] V. Jacquemet, M. Lemay, A. van Oosterom, et al., "The equivalent dipole used to characterize atrial fibrillation," in *Comput Cardiol*, vol. 33, 2006, pp. 149–152.

[515] U. C. Nguyên, M. Potse, F. Regoli, et al., "An in-silico analysis of the effect of heart position and orientation on the ECG morphology and vectorcardiogram parameters in patients with heart failure and intraventricular conduction defects," *J Electrocardiol*, vol. 48, no. 4, pp. 617–625, 2015.

[516] H. Ashikaga, H. Arevalo, F. Vadakkumpadan, et al., "Feasibility of image-based simulation to estimate ablation target in human ventricular arrhythmia," *Heart Rhythm*, vol. 10, no. 8, pp. 1109–1116, 2013.

[517] D. Deng, H. Arevalo, F. Pashakhanloo, et al., "Accuracy of prediction of infarct-related arrhythmic circuits from image-based models reconstructed from low and high resolution MRI," *Front Physiol*, vol. 6, p. 282, 2015.

[518] S. Zahid, P. M. Boyle, P. Malamas, et al., "Reentrant sources in persistent AF are located in regions with specific spatial patterns of fibrosis," *Circulation*, vol. 130, no. S2, p. A13235, 2014.

[519] F. M. Weber, D. U. J. Keller, S. Bauer, et al., "Predicting tissue conductivity influences on body surface potentials - an efficient approach based on principal component analysis," *IEEE Trans Biomed Eng*, vol. 58, no. 2, pp. 265–273, 2011.

[520] A. Bayés De Luna, P. Platonov, F. G. Cosio, et al., "Interatrial blocks. A separate entity from left atrial enlargement: A consensus report," *J Electrocardiol*, vol. 45, no. 5, pp. 445–451, 2012.

[521] G. S. Wagner, P. Macfarlane, H. Wellens, et al., "AHA/ACCF/HRS recommendations for the standardization and interpretation of the electrocardiogram. Part VI: Acute ischemia/infarction," *J Am Coll Cardiol*, vol. 53, no. 11, pp. 1003–1011, 2009.

[522] M. Yokoyama, A. Sakamoto, S. Konno, et al., "P wave changes on exercise in patients with isolated mitral stenosis," *Am Heart J*, vol. 87, no. 1, pp. 15–20, 1974.

[523] S. B. Jones, D. E. Euler, E. Hardie, et al., "Comparison of SA nodal and subsidiary atrial pacemaker function and location in the dog," *Am J Physiol*, vol. 234, no. 4, pp. H471–H476, 1978.

[524] J. P. Boineau, R. B. Schuessler, W. R. Roeske, et al., "Quantitative relation between sites of atrial impulse origin and cycle length," *Am J Physiol*, vol. 245, no. 5 Pt 1, pp. H781–H789, 1983.

[525] M. Yokota, S. Noda, M. Koide, et al., "Analysis of the exercise-induced orthogonal P wave changes in normal subjects and patients with coronary artery disease," *Jpn Heart J*, vol. 27, no. 4, pp. 443–460, 1986.

[526] J. M. Tapanainen, R. Jurkko, F. Holmqvist, et al., "Interatrial right-to-left conduction in patients with paroxysmal atrial fibrillation," *J Interv Card Electrophysiol*, vol. 25, no. 2, pp. 117–122, 2009.

[527] Y. Huo, L. Mitrofanova, V. Orshanskaya, et al., "P-wave characteristics and histological atrial abnormality," *J Electrocardiol*, vol. 47, no. 3, pp. 275–280, 2014.

[528] J. B. Nielsen, J. T. Kühl, A. Pietersen, et al., "P-wave duration and the risk of atrial fibrillation: Results from the Copenhagen ECG study," *Heart Rhythm*, vol. 12, no. 9, pp. 1887–1895, 2015.

[529] F. Holmqvist, P. G. Platonov, S. McNitt, et al., "Abnormal P-wave morphology is a predictor of atrial fibrillation development and cardiac death in MADIT II patients," *Ann Noninvasive Electrocardiol*, vol. 15, no. 1, pp. 63–72, 2010.

[530] F. Holmqvist, P. G. Platonov, J. Carlson, et al., "Altered interatrial conduction detected in MADIT II patients bound to develop atrial fibrillation," *Ann Noninvasive Electrocardiol*, vol. 14, no. 3, pp. 268–275, 2009.

[531] C. W. Tsao, M. E. Josephson, T. H. Hauser, et al., "Accuracy of electrocardiographic criteria for atrial enlargement: Validation with cardiovascular magnetic resonance," *J Cardiovasc Magn Reson*, vol. 10, p. 7, 2008.

[532] T. Tsang, M. Barnes, B. Gersh, et al., "Risks for atrial fibrillation and congestive heart failure in patients >=65 years of age with abnormal left ventricular diastolic relaxation," *Am J Cardiol*, vol. 93, no. 1, pp. 54–58, 2004.

[533] B. B. Altunkeser, K. Ozdemir, H. Gok, et al., "Can P wave parameters obtained from 12-lead surface electrocardiogram be a predictor for atrial fibrillation in patients who have structural heart disease?" *Angiology*, vol. 54, no. 4, pp. 475–479, 2003.

[534] E. Gerdts, L. Oikarinen, V. Palmieri, et al., "Correlates of left atrial size in hypertensive patients with left ventricular hypertrophy: The losartan intervention for endpoint reduction in hypertension (LIFE) study," *Hypertension*, vol. 39, no. 3, pp. 739–743, 2002.

[535] T. S. Tsang, M. E. Barnes, K. R. Bailey, et al., "Left atrial volume: important risk marker of incident atrial fibrillation in 1655 older men and women," *Mayo Clin Proc*, vol. 76, no. 5, pp. 467–75, 2001.

[536] M. E. Barnes, Y. Miyasaka, J. B. Seward, et al., "Left atrial volume in the prediction of first ischemic stroke in an elderly cohort without atrial fibrillation," *Mayo Clin Proc*, vol. 79, no. 8, pp. 1008–1014, 2004.

[537] T. S. M. Tsang, M. E. Barnes, B. J. Gersh, et al., "Left atrial volume as a morphophysiologic expression of left ventricular diastolic dysfunction and relation to cardiovascular risk burden," *Am J Cardiol*, vol. 90, no. 12, pp. 1284–1289, 2002.

[538] M. G. Modena, N. Muia, F. A. Sgura, et al., "Left atrial size is the major predictor of cardiac death and overall clinical outcome in patients with dilated cardiomyopathy: A long-term follow-up study," *Clin Cardiol*, vol. 20, no. 6, pp. 553–560, 1997.

[539] T. S. M. Tsang, W. P. Abhayaratna, M. E. Barnes, et al., "Prediction of cardiovascular outcomes with left atrial size," *J Am Coll Cardiol*, vol. 47, no. 5, pp. 1018–1023, 2006.

[540] A. Verma, N. S. Anavekar, A. Meris, et al., "The relationship between renal function and cardiac structure, function, and prognosis after myocardial infarction. The VALIANT echo study," *J Am Coll Cardiol*, vol. 50, no. 13, pp. 1238–1245, 2007.

[541] T. S. M. Tsang, M. E. Barnes, B. J. Gersh, et al., "Prediction of risk for first age-related cardiovascular events in an elderly population: The incremental value of echocardiography," *J Am Coll Cardiol*, vol. 2007, no. 7, pp. 1199–1205, 2003.

[542] R. Macruz, J. K. Perloff, and R. B. Case, "A method for the electrocardiographic recognition of atrial enlargement," *Circulation*, vol. 17, no. 5, pp. 882–889, 1958.

[543] J. P. Birkbeck, D. B. Wilson, M. A. Hall, et al., "P-wave morphology correlation with left atrial volumes assessed by 2-dimensional echocardiography," *J Electrocardiol*, vol. 39, no. 2, pp. 225–229, 2006.

[544] K. Munuswamy, M. A. Alpert, R. H. Martin, et al., "Sensitivity and specificity of commonly used electrocardiographic criteria for left atrial enlargement determined by M-mode echocardiography," *Am J Cardiol*, vol. 53, no. 6, pp. 829–832, 1984.

[545] M. A. Alpert and K. Munuswamy, "Electrocardiographic diagnosis of left atrial enlargement," *Postgrad Med*, vol. 20, no. 3, pp. 231–232, 1968.

[546] A. M. Perosio, L. D. Suarez, A. Torino, et al., "Reassessment of electrovectorcardiographic signs of left atrial enlargement," *Clin Cardiol*, vol. 5, no. 12, pp. 640–646, 1982.

[547] C. Zeng, T. Wei, R. Zhao, et al., "Electrocardiographic diagnosis of left atrial enlargement in patients with mitral stenosis: The value of the P-wave area," *Acta Cardiol*, vol. 58, no. 2, pp. 139–141, 2003.

[548] P. G. Platonov, "Atrial conduction and atrial fibrillation: What can we learn from surface ECG?" *Cardiol J*, vol. 15, no. 5, pp. 402–407, 2008.

[549] R. Andlauer, "Investigation of the effect of left atrial anatomy alterations on P-wave morphology in a computational model," Bachelor Thesis, Institute of Biomedical Engineering, Karlsruhe Institute of Technology (KIT), 2016.

[550] A. Loewe, R. Andlauer, P. G. Platonov, et al., "Left atrial hypertrophy increases P-wave terminal force through amplitude but not duration," in *Comput Cardiol*, 2016, under review for presentation in September.

[551] R. Andlauer, A. Loewe, P. G. Platonov, et al., "Effect of left atrial hypertrophy on P-wave morphology in a computational model," in *Biomed Tech*, 2016, under review for presentation in October.

[552] T. Fritz, C. Wieners, G. Seemann, et al., "Simulation of the contraction of the ventricles in a human heart model including atria and pericardium: Finite element analysis of a frictionless contact problem," *Biomech Model Mechanobiol*, vol. 13, no. 3, pp. 627–641, 2014.

[553] Blender Online Community, *Blender - a 3D modelling and rendering package*, Blender Foundation, Blender Institute, Amsterdam, 2015.

[554] C. Geuzaine and J.-F. Remacle, "Gmsh: A 3-D finite element mesh generator with built-in pre-and post-processing facilities," *International Journal for Numerical Methods in Engineering*, vol. 79, no. 11, pp. 1309–1331, 2009.

[555] G. R. Mirams, P. Pathmanathan, R. A. Gray, et al., "White paper: Uncertainty and variability in computational and mathematical models of cardiac physiology," *J Physiol*, 2016, epub ahead of print.

List of Publications and Supervised Theses

Journal Articles

- **Axel Loewe**, Mathias Wilhelms, Fathima Fischer, Eberhard P Scholz, Olaf Dössel, Gunnar Seemann, *Arrhythmic Potency of Human Ether-à-Go-Go-Related Gene Mutations L532P and N588K in a Computational Model of Human Atrial Myocytes*, Europace 2014;16:435–443
- **Axel Loewe**, Yannick Lutz, Matthias Wilhelms, Daniel Sinnecker, Petra Barthel, Eberhard P Scholz, Olaf Dössel, Georg Schmidt, Gunnar Seemann, *In-silico Assessment of the Dynamic Effects of Amiodarone and Dronedarone on Human Atrial Patho-Electrophysiology*, Europace 2014;16:iv30–38
- **Axel Loewe**, Walther HW Schulze, Yuan Jiang, Mathias Wilhelms, Armin Luik, Olaf Dössel, Gunnar Seemann, *ECG-based Detection of Myocardial Ischemia in a Computational Model: Impact of Additional Electrodes, Optimal Placement and a New Feature of ST Deviation*, Biomed Research International, 2015, ID 530352
- **Axel Loewe**, Mathias Wilhelms, Jochen Schmid, Mathias J Krause, Fathima Fischer, Dierk Thomas, Eberhard P Scholz, Olaf Dössel, Gunnar Seemann, *Parameter Estimation of Ion Current Formulations Requires Hybrid Optimization Approach to be Both Accurate and Reliable*, Frontiers in Bioengineering and Biotechnology, 2015;3:209

- **Axel Loewe**, Martin W. Krueger, Fredrik Holmqvist, Olaf Dössel, Gunnar Seemann, Pyotr G. Platonov, *P-Wave Terminal Force is Affected by Site of Earliest Right Atrial Activation*, Europace, under review
- Olaf Dössel, Gustavo Lenis, **Axel Loewe**, Markus Rottmann, Gunnar Seemann, Tobias Oesterlein, *Model Assisted Biosignal Analysis of Atrial Electrograms*, technisches messen, 2016;83:102–111
- Stefan Pollnow, Robert Arnold, Matthias Werber, **Axel Loewe**, Olaf Dössel, Gunnar Seemann, *Hyperthermia Dependence of Cardiac Conduction Velocity in Rat Myocardium: Optical Mapping, Cardiac Near Field Measurements and In-Silico Modelling*, Biomedical Engineering / Biomedizinische Technik, under review
- Tobias Oesterlein, Daniel Frisch, **Axel Loewe**, Gunnar Seemann, Claus Schmitt, Olaf Dössel, Armin Luik, *Basket-Type Catheters: Diagnostic Pitfalls Caused by Deformation and Limited Coverage*, Journal of Cardiovascular Electrophysiology, in preparation

Refereed Conference Articles

- **Axel Loewe**, Walther HW Schulze, Yuan Jiang, Mathias Wilhelms, Olaf Dössel, *Determination of Optimal Electrode Positions of a Wearable ECG Monitoring System for Detection of Myocardial Ischemia: A Simulation Study*, Computing in Cardiology, 2011;38:741–744
- **Axel Loewe**, Mathias Wilhelms, Fathima Fischer, Eberhard P Scholz, Olaf Dössel, Gunnar Seemann, *Impact of hERG Mutations on Simulated Human Atrial Action Potentials*, Biomedical Engineering / Biomedizinische Technik 2013;58:SI–1N
- **Axel Loewe**, Mathias Wilhelms, Eberhard P Scholz, Olaf Dössel, Gunnar Seemann, *Influence of Chronic Atrial Fibrillation Induced Remodeling in a Computational Electrophysiological Model*, Biomedical Engineering / Biomedizinische Technik 2014;59:S929–932
- **Axel Loewe**, Yannick Lutz, Mathias Wilhelms, Eberhard P Scholz, Olaf Dössel, Gunnar Seemann, *Optimization of Pharmacotherapy for Familial Atrial Fibrillation in a Numerical Model of Human Atrial Electrophysiology*, Computing in Cardiology 2014;41:745–748

- **Axel Loewe**, Martin W Krueger, Pyotr G Platonov, Fredrik Holmqvist, Olaf Dössel, Gunnar Seemann, *Left and Right Atrial Contribution to the P-Wave in Realistic Computational Models*, Functional Imaging and Modeling of the Heart, Lecture Notes in Computer Science, 2015;9126:439-47
- **Axel Loewe**, Yan Xu, Eberhard P Scholz, Olaf Dössel, Gunnar Seemann, *Understanding the Cellular Mode of Action of Vernakalant Using a Computational Model: Answers and New Questions*, Current Directions in Biomedical Engineering, 2015;1:418–422
- Walther HW Schulze, Francesc E Henar, Danila Potyagaylo, **Axel Loewe**, Matti Stenroos, Olaf Dössel, *Kalman Filter with Augmented Measurement Model: an ECG Imaging Simulation Study*, Functional Imaging and Modeling of the Heart, Lecture Notes in Computer Science, 2013;7945:200–207
- Yannick Lutz, **Axel Loewe**, Mathias Wilhelms, Olaf Dössel, Gunnar Seemann, *Specific Antiarrhythmic Therapy for Familial Atrial Fibrillation in a Numerical Model of Human Atrial Electrophysiology*, Biomedical Engineering / Biomedizinische Technik 2014;59:S933–936
- Markus Rottmann, Laura A Unger, Wenzel Kaltenbacher, **Axel Loewe**, Martin W Krueger, Gunnar Seemann, Thomas Arentz, Amir Jadidi, Olaf Dössel, *Methods for Analyzing Signal Characteristics of Stable and Unstable Rotors in a Realistic Heart Model*, Computing in Cardiology, 2015;42:485–488
- Andreas Wachter, **Axel Loewe**, Martin W Krueger, Olaf Dössel, Gunnar Seemann, *Mesh Structure-independent Modeling of Patient-specific Atrial Fiber Orientation*, Current Directions in Biomedical Engineering, 2015;1:409–412
- Nicolas Pilia, Gustavo Lenis, **Axel Loewe**, Walther HW Schulze, Olaf Dössel, *The Impact of Baseline Wander Removal Techniques on the ST Segment in Simulated Ischemic 12-Lead ECGs*, Current Directions in Biomedical Engineering, 2015;1:96–99
- Julia Trächtler, Tobias Oesterlein, **Axel Loewe**, Emanuel Poremba, Armin Luik, Claus Schmitt, Olaf Dössel, *Virtualizing Clinical Cases of Atrial Flutter in a Fast Marching Simulation Including Conduction Velocity and Ablation Scars*, Current Directions in Biomedical Engineering, 2015;1:405–408
- **Axel Loewe**, Robin Andlauer, Pyotr G Platonov, Olaf Dössel, Gunnar Seemann, *Left Atrial Hypertrophy Increases P-Wave Terminal Force Through*

Amplitude but not Duration, Computing in Cardiology, under review for presentation in September 2016
- Bhawna Verma, **Axel Loewe**, Armin Luik, Claus Schmitt, Olaf Dössel, *Regional Conduction Velocity Calculation Based on Local Activation Times: A Simulation Study on Clinical Geometries*, Computing in Cardiology, under review for presentation in September 2016
- Robin Andlauer, **Axel Loewe**, Pyotr G Platonov, Olaf Dössel, Gunnar Seemann, *Effect of Left Atrial Hypertrophy on P-Wave Morphology in a Computational Model*, Meeting of the Swiss, Austrian, and German Societies of Biomedical Engineering, under review for presentation in October 2016

Refereed Conference Abstracts

- **Axel Loewe**, Martin W Krueger, Fredrik Holmqvist, Olaf Dössel, Gunnar Seemann, Pyotr G Platonov, *P-Wave Morphology is Affected by Site of Earliest Right Atrial Activation Independent from Atrial Size in Silico*, International Congress on Electrocardiology 2016, accepted for presentation in June 2016
- **Axel Loewe**, Martin W Krueger, Fredrik Holmqvist, Olaf Dössel, Gunnar Seemann, Pyotr G Platonov, *P-Wave Morphology is Affected by the Site of Earliest Right Atrial Activation and its Proximity to Inter-Atrial Connections Independent from Atrial Size*, Meeting of the Swiss, Austrian, and German Societies of Biomedical Engineering, under review for presentation in October 2016
- Jun Liu, **Axel Loewe**, Michael Zenge, Alban Lefebvre, Edgar Mueller, Mariappan S Nadar, *Elora: Enforcing Low Rank for Parallel MR Reconstruction*, Proceedings of the 21st Annual Meeting of the International Society of Magnetic Resonance in Medicine (ISMRM) 2013, Abstract 3302, p. 2652
- Danila Potyagaylo, **Axel Loewe**, Olaf Dössel, *ECG Imaging of Ectopic Atrial Excitation: Evaluation in a Realistic Simulation Setup*, Computing in Cardiology, under review for presentation in September 2016

Conference Presentations

- **Axel Loewe**, Mathias Wilhelms, Jochen Schmid, Mathias J Krause, Fathima Fischer, Eberhard P Scholz, Olaf Dössel, Gunnar Seemann, *A Hybrid Optimization Approach for the Adaptation of Cardiac Ion Current Formulations to Voltage and Patch Clamp Data*, Cardiac Physiome Project Workshop (poster), Bar Harbor, ME, USA, 2013
- **Axel Loewe**, Emanuel Poremba, Martin W Krueger, Olaf Dössel, Gunnar Seemann, *Fast Marching Simulation of Atrial Excitation: Towards Personalized Ablation Planning*, TRM Forum (poster), Lugano, Switzerland, 2013
- **Axel Loewe**, Yannick Lutz, Matthias Wilhelms, Daniel Sinnecker, Petra Barthel, Eberhard P Scholz, Olaf Dössel, Georg Schmidt, Gunnar Seemann, *In-silico Assessment of the Dynamic Effects of Amiodarone and Dronedarone on Human Atrial Patho-Electrophysiology*, Cardiac Physiome Project Workshop (talk), Auckland, New Zealand, 2015
- **Axel Loewe**, Yannick Lutz, Matthias Wilhelms, Daniel Sinnecker, Petra Barthel, Eberhard P Scholz, Olaf Dössel, Georg Schmidt, Gunnar Seemann, *In-silico Assessment of the Dynamic Effects of Amiodarone and Dronedarone on Human Atrial Patho-Electrophysiology*, Atrial Signals (poster), Karlsruhe, Germany, 2015
- **Axel Loewe**, Martin W Krueger, Fredrik Holmqvist, Olaf Dössel, Gunnar Seemann, Pyotr G Platonov, *P-wave Morphology is Affected by Site of Earliest Right Atrial Activation: a Simulation Study*, TRM Forum (poster), Lugano, Switzerland, 2015
- Gunnar Seemann, **Axel Loewe**, Yannick Lutz, Mathias Wilhelms, Olaf Dössel, *Simulating the Effects of Drugs and Genetic Defects on Atrial Electrophysiology*, TRM Forum (talk), Lugano, Switzerland, 2013
- Markus Rottmann, Laura A Unger, Wenzel Kaltenbacher, **Axel Loewe**, Martin W Krueger, Gunnar Seemann, Thomas Arentz, Amir Jadidi, Olaf Dössel, *Methods for Analyzing Signal Characteristics of Stable and Unstable Rotors in a Realistic Heart Model*, Atrial Signals (poster), Karlsruhe, Germany, 2015

Invited Talks

- *Modeling Human Atrial Patho-Electrophysiology: Genetic Defects and Pharmacological Agents*, Simula Cardiac Modeling Workshop, Oslo, Norway, 06 Nov 2014
- *In-silico Assessment of the Dynamic Effects of Amiodarone and Dronedarone on Human Atrial Patho-Electrophysiology*, Workshop "Emerging Mathematical Topics in Biology and Life Sciences", Research Core Area "Modeling and Simulation", Karl-Franzens-Universität Graz, Austria, 07 May 2015

Other Talks

- *Multi-Scale in Silico Modeling of Human Atrial Electrophysiology*, Computational Cardiology Lab (Prof. Natalia Trayanova), Institute for Computational Medicine, Johns Hopkins University, Baltimore, MD, USA, 03 Sep 2014 via Contact scholarship of Karlsruhe House of Young Scientists (KHYS)

Patents

- Alban Lefebvre, **Axel Loewe**, Mariappan S Nadar, Jun Liu, *Zero Communication Block Partitioning*, US Patent App. 2014/0037228 A1 (2012P18991 US01, 13/950,535, 2012P18991 US, 61/679,132)
- Jun Liu, Zhili Yang, Mariappan S Nadar, Nirmal Janardhanan, Qiu Wang, **Axel Loewe**, *Multi-stage Magnetic Resonance Reconstruction for Parallel Imaging Applications*, US Patent App. 2014/0133724 A1 (2012P26350 US01, 14/054,003, 2012P26350 US, 61/724,470)

Reports and Theses

- **Axel Loewe**, *Comparison of Cardiac Simulation Tools Regarding the Modeling of Acute Ischemia*, Bachelor Thesis, Institute of Biomedical Engineering, Karlsruhe Institute of Technology (KIT), 2010

- **Axel Loewe**, *Arrhythmic Potency of Human Electrophysiological Models Adapted to Chronic and Familial Atrial Fibrillation*, Master Thesis, Institute of Biomedical Engineering, Karlsruhe Institute of Technology (KIT), 2013
- Milena Hugenschmidt, Stefan Pollnow, **Axel Loewe**, *Bildrekonstruktionsalgorithmen für die Computertomographie in Matlab*, Hands on module for the class "Bildgebende Verfahren in der Medizin", Institute of Biomedical Engineering, Karlsruhe Institute of Technology (KIT), 2015

Supervised Student Theses

- Emanuel Poremba, *Implementation of a Fast Simulation C++ Framework for the Computation of Vulnerability to Atrial Arrhythmias Using the Fast Marching Algorithm*, Bachelor Thesis, Institute of Biomedical Engineering, Karlsruhe Institute of Technology (KIT), 2013
- Yannick Lutz, *Specific Antiarrhythmic Therapy for Familial Atrial Fibrillation in a Numerical Model of Human Atrial Electrophysiology*, Bachelor Thesis, Institute of Biomedical Engineering, Karlsruhe Institute of Technology (KIT), 2013
- Yan Xu, *In-silico Characterization of the Atrial Mode of Action of Ajmaline and Vernakalant and their Effect on Spiral Waves*, Bachelor Thesis, Institute of Biomedical Engineering, Karlsruhe Institute of Technology (KIT), 2014
- Andreas Wachter, *In-silico Assessment of Arrhythmogenic Potential of Atrial Ablation Patterns: A Sensitivity Analysis*, Diploma Thesis, Institute of Biomedical Engineering, Karlsruhe Institute of Technology (KIT), 2015
- Amine Khalef, *Comparison of Statistic and Optimization-based Approaches for Parameter Estimation of Ion Current Formulations*, Bachelor Thesis, Institute of Biomedical Engineering, Karlsruhe Institute of Technology (KIT), 2015
- Robin Andlauer, *Investigation of the Effect of Left Atrial Anatomy Alterations on P-Wave Morphology in a Computational Model*, Bachelor Thesis, Institute of Biomedical Engineering, Karlsruhe Institute of Technology (KIT), 2015
- Huy Nguyen Cong, *Estimation of Local Cardiac Conduction Velocity Based on Intra-cardiac Recordings*, Bachelor Thesis, Institute of Biomedical Engineering, Karlsruhe Institute of Technology (KIT), ongoing

- Nicolas Pilia, *Characterization and Reconstruction of Ionic Concentrations in the Human Ventricles Analyzing the Action Potential and the Surface ECG*, Master Thesis, Institute of Biomedical Engineering, Karlsruhe Institute of Technology (KIT), ongoing

Awards & Grants

- 1st price in student competition, 48th DGBMT Annual Conference, 2014, Yannick Lutz, **Axel Loewe**, Mathias Wilhelms, Olaf Dössel, Gunnar Seemann, *Specific Antiarrhythmic Therapy for Familial Atrial Fibrillation in a Numerical Model of Human Atrial Electrophysiology*
- Best graduate student poster, Cardiac Physiome Workshop, 2013, **Axel Loewe**, Mathias Wilhelms, Jochen Schmid, Mathias J Krause, Fathima Fischer, Eberhard P Scholz, Olaf Dössel, Gunnar Seemann, *A Hybrid Optimization Approach for the Adaptation of Cardiac Ion Current Formulations*
- 2nd price in student competition, 47th DGBMT Annual Conference, 2013, **Axel Loewe**, Mathias Wilhelms, Fathima Fischer, Eberhard P Scholz, Olaf Dössel, Gunnar Seemann, *Impact of hERG Mutations on Simulated Human Atrial Action Potentials*
- Best poster awards, Computing in Cardiology, 2011, **Axel Loewe**, Walther HW Schulze, Yuan Jiang, Mathias Wilhelms, Olaf Dössel, *Determination of Optimal Electrode Positions of a Wearable ECG Monitoring System for Detection of Myocardial Ischemia: A Simulation Study*
- Congress Scholarship, German Academic Exchange Service (DAAD), Cardiac Physiome Workshop, Seoul, South Korea, 2016
- Contact Scholarship, Karlsruhe House of Young Scientists (KHYS), 2014
- Student Scholarship, e-fellows.net, 2006 – 2016

Karlsruhe Transactions on Biomedical Engineering (ISSN 1864-5933)

Karlsruhe Institute of Technology / Institute of Biomedical Engineering (Ed.)

Die Bände sind unter www.ksp.kit.edu als PDF frei verfügbar oder als Druckausgabe bestellbar.

Band 2 Matthias Reumann
Computer assisted optimisation on non-pharmacological treatment of congestive heart failure and supraventricular arrhythmia. 2007
ISBN 978-3-86644-122-4

Band 3 Antoun Khawaja
Automatic ECG analysis using principal component analysis and wavelet transformation. 2007
ISBN 978-3-86644-132-3

Band 4 Dmytro Farina
Forward and inverse problems of electrocardiography: clinical investigations. 2008
ISBN 978-3-86644-219-1

Band 5 Jörn Thiele
Optische und mechanische Messungen von elektrophysiologischen Vorgängen im Myokardgewebe. 2008
ISBN 978-3-86644-240-5

Band 6 Raz Miri
Computer assisted optimization of cardiac resynchronization therapy. 2009
ISBN 978-3-86644-360-0

Band 7 Frank Kreuder
2D-3D-Registrierung mit Parameterentkopplung für die Patientenlagerung in der Strahlentherapie. 2009
ISBN 978-3-86644-376-1

Band 8 Daniel Unholtz
Optische Oberflächensignalmessung mit Mikrolinsen-Detektoren für die Kleintierbildgebung. 2009
ISBN 978-3-86644-423-2

Band 9 Yuan Jiang
Solving the inverse problem of electrocardiography in a realistic environment. 2010
ISBN 978-3-86644-486-7

Karlsruhe Transactions on Biomedical Engineering (ISSN 1864-5933)

Band 10 Sebastian Seitz
Magnetic Resonance Imaging on Patients with Implanted Cardiac Pacemakers. 2011
ISBN 978-3-86644-610-6

Band 11 Tobias Voigt
Quantitative MR Imaging of the Electric Properties and Local SAR based on Improved RF Transmit Field Mapping. 2011
ISBN 978-3-86644-598-7

Band 12 Frank Michael Weber
Personalizing Simulations of the Human Atria: Intracardiac Measurements, Tissue Conductivities, and Cellular Electrophysiology. 2011
ISBN 978-3-86644-646-5

Band 13 David Urs Josef Keller
Multiscale Modeling of the Ventricles: from Cellular Electrophysio-logy to Body Surface Electrocardiograms. 2011
ISBN 978-3-86644-714-1

Band 14 Oussama Jarrousse
Modified Mass-Spring System for Physically Based Deformation Modeling. 2012
ISBN 978-3-86644-742-4

Band 15 Julia Bohnert
Effects of Time-Varying Magnetic Fields in the Frequency Range 1 kHz to 100 kHz upon the Human Body: Numerical Studies and Stimulation Experiment. 2012
ISBN 978-3-86644-782-0

Band 16 Hanno Homann
SAR Prediction and SAR Management for Parallel Transmit MRI. 2012
ISBN 978-3-86644-800-1

Band 17 Christopher Schilling
Analysis of Atrial Electrograms. 2012
ISBN 978-3-86644-894-0

Band 18 Tobias Baas
ECG Based Analysis of the Ventricular Repolarisation in the Human Heart. 2012
ISBN 978-3-86644-882-7

Karlsruhe Transactions on Biomedical Engineering (ISSN 1864-5933)

Band 19 Martin Wolfgang Krüger
Personalized Multi-Scale Modeling of the Atria: Heterogeneities, Fiber Architecture, Hemodialysis and Ablation Therapy. 2012
ISBN 978-3-86644-948-0

Band 20 Mathias Wilhelms
Multiscale Modeling of Cardiac Electrophysiology: Adaptation to Atrial and Ventricular Rhythm Disorders and Pharmacological Treatment. 2013
ISBN 978-3-7315-0045-2

Band 21 Matthias Keller
Formation of Intracardiac Electrograms under Physiological and Pathological Conditions. 2014
ISBN 978-3-7315-0228-9

Band 22 Walther H. W. Schulze
ECG Imaging of Ventricular Activity in Clinical Applications. 2015
ISBN 978-3-7315-0374-3

Band 23 Axel Loewe
Modeling Human Atrial Patho-Electrophysiology from Ion Channels to ECG. Substrates, Pharmacology, Vulnerability, and P-Waves. 2016
ISBN 978-3-7315-0528-0